Female Reproductive Aging

STUDIES IN PROFERTILITY SERIES

VOLUME 9

Female Reproductive Aging

The Proceedings of the 10th Reinier de Graaf Symposium, Zeist, The Netherlands, 9–11 September 1999

EDITED BY E. R. TE VELDE, P. L. PEARSON AND F. J. BROEKMANS

The publication of this book has been made possible by an educational grant from NV Organon

The Parthenon Publishing Group

International Publishers in Medicine, Science & Technology

NEW YORK LONDON

Published in the USA by
The Parthenon Publishing Group Inc.
One Blue Hill Plaza
PO Box 1564, Pearl River,
New York 10965, USA

Published in the UK by
The Parthenon Publishing Group Limited
Casterton Hall, Carnforth,
Lancs, LA6 2LA, UK

Library of Congress Cataloging-in-Publication Data

Reinier de Graaf Symposium (10th: 1999: Zeist, Netherlands)
Female reproductive aging: the proceedings of the 10th Reinier de Graaf Symposium. Zeist, the Netherlands, 9–11 September 1999 / edited by E.R. te Velde, P. Pearson, and F.J. Broekmans.
p.; cm.—(Studies in profertility series; v. 9)
Includes bibliographical references and index.
ISBN 1-85070-676-X
1. Ovaries—Aging—Congresses. 2. Infertility, Female—Congresses. I. Velde, E.R. te. II. Pearson, P.L. III. Broekmans, F.J. IV. Title. V. Series.
[DNLM: 1. Ovary–physiology—Congresses. 2. Aging–physiology–Congresses. 3. Fertility–physiology–Congresses. 4. Infertility, Female–therapy–Congresses. 5. Menopause—physiology —Congresses. 6. Oocytes—physiology—Congresses. WP 540 R367f 2000]
QP261.R38 1999
612. 6'2—dc21

00-025520

British Library Cataloguing in Publication Data

Female reproductive aging: the proceedings of the 10th Reinier de Graaf Symposium, Zeist, the Netherlands, 9–11 September 1999.— (Studies in profertility series; v. 9)
1. Fertility, Human 2. Human reproduction – Age factors – Congresses 3. Generative organs, Female – Congresses I. Velde, E.R. te II. Pearson, P. III. Broekmans, F.J. IV. Reinier de Graaf Symposium (10th: 1999: Zeist, Netherlands)
612.6′2
ISBN 185070676X

First published 2000

Composition by SIVA Math Setters, Chennai, India
Printed and bound by Butler and Tanner Ltd., Frome and London, UK

Contents

List of principal contributors

F.J. Broekmans
Department of Reproductive Medicine
Division of Obstetrics and Gynecology
University Medical Centre Utrecht
PO Box 85500
3508 GA Utrecht
The Netherlands

J.M. Cummins
Division of Veterinary and Biomedical Sciences
Murdoch University
PO Box S1400
Perth
Western Australia 6849

U. Eichenlaub-Ritter
Fakultat Biologie
Gentechnologie/Mikrobiologie
University of Bielefeld
Postfach 100131
D-33501 Bielefeld
Germany

M.J. Faddy
Department of Mathematics and Statistics
University of Canterbury
Private Bag 4800
Christchurch
New Zealand

B.C.J.M. Fauser
Department of Obstetrics and Gynecology
Erasmus University Medical Centre Rotterdam
Dr. Molewaterplein 40
3015 GD Rotterdam
The Netherlands

R.G. Gosden
Division of Obstetrics and Gynecology
McGill University
Royal Victoria Hospital, Women's Pavilion (F3. 38)
687 Pine Avenue West
Montreal QC H3A IAI
Canada

K. Hawkes
Department of Anthropology
University of Utah
270 S 1400 E, Room 102
Salt Lake City
UT 84112–0060
USA

D.J. Holman
Department of Anthropology
Box 353100
University of Washington
Seattle, WA 98195
USA

A.J.W. Hsueh
Department of Obstetrics and Gynecology
Division of Reproductive Biology
Stanford University School of Medicine
300 Pasteur Drive, Room A344
Stanford, CA 94305–5317
USA

P.A. Hunt
Department of Genetics and Center for Human Genetics
Case Western Reserve University
Cleveland, OH 44106–4955
USA

T.B.L. Kirkwood
Department of Gerontology
University of Newcastle upon Tyne
Institute for the Health of the Elderly
Wolfson Research Centre
Newcastle General Hospital
Westgate Road
Newcastle upon Tyne
NE4 6BE
UK

C.B. Lambalk
University Hospital
Free University Amsterdam
PO Box 7057
1007 MB Amsterdam
The Netherlands

N.S. Macklon
Department of Obstetrics and Gynecology
University Hospital Rotterdam
Dr. Molewaterplein 40
3015 GD Rotterdam
The Netherlands

P.L. Pearson
Department of Medical Genetics
University Medical Centre Utrecht
Wilhelmina Children's Hospital
3584 EA Utrecht
The Netherlands

A. Pellicer
Instituto Valenciano de Infertilidad
Guardia Civil 23
46020 Valencia
Spain

R.V. Short
Department of Obstetrics and Gynecology
Royal Woman's Hospital
University of Melbourne
132 Grattan Street
Carlton
Victoria 3053
Australia

C. Simón
Instituto Valenciano de Infertilidad
Guardia Civil 23
46020 Valencia
Spain

M.R. Soules
Department of Obstetrics and Gynecology
Division of Reproductive Endocrinology
University of Washington School of Medicine
Box 354793
4225 Roosevelt Way NE, Suite 305
Seattle, WA 98105
USA

E.H. Stephen
Department of Demography
Georgetown University
PO Box 571214
Washington, DC 20057–1214
USA

E.R. te Velde
Department of Reproductive Medicine
Division of Obstetrics and Gynecology
University Medical Centre Utrecht
PO Box 85500
3508 GA Utrecht
The Netherlands

A.P.N. Themmen
Department of Endocrinology and Reproduction
Erasmus University Rotterdam
PO Box 1738
3000 DR Rotterdam
The Netherlands

Y.M. van Kasteren
Medical Center Alkmaar
PO Box 501
1800 AM Alkmaar
The Netherlands

Preface: Reinier de Graaf and his symposium

E.R. te Velde

Reinier de Graaf, born in 1641, lived a short, but intense and extremely fruitful life. He was born in Schoonhoven, in the Netherlands, to Roman Catholic parents and always remained faithful to his religion. In a predominantly Calvinistic country, this circumstance is likely to have negatively influenced his career which may have been the reason why he did not succeed Professor Sylvius, his valued and trusted mentor, in Leiden.

In 1658 he started his medical study in Leuven, Belgium. He continued his studies in the cities of Utrecht and Leiden, after which he spent some exciting and adventurous years in France. In 1666, he settled in the city of Delft and started to practice as a medical doctor. It was in Delft that he published his famous treatises on the male and female reproductive organs. In 1672 he married Maria van Dijck from Gouda; however, only 1 year later, in 1673, he died, probably of an infectious disease which may have been the plague.

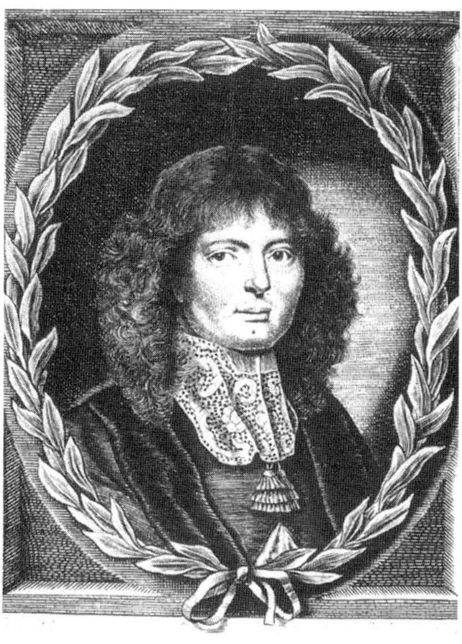

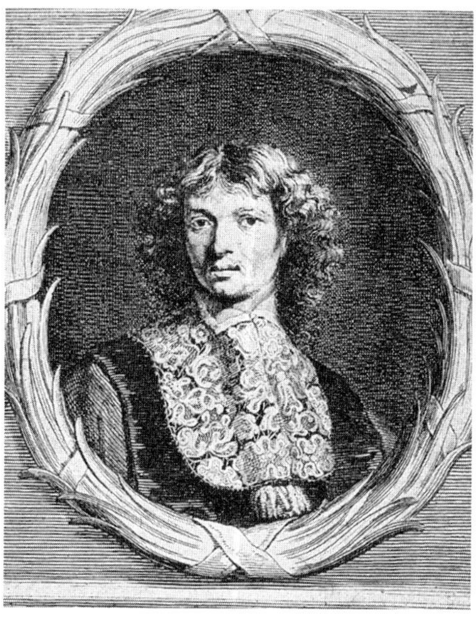

During his period in Utrecht he met Anna Maria van Schurman, an extremely gifted and emancipated woman, who lived in a beautiful house at Achter den Dom, where she received celebrities such as Christiaan Huygens and René Descartes. How this elderly lady came to be in touch with the brilliant young student, will remain a mystery. His well-known portrait (previous page, left), where he appears as a self-possessed, possibly even vain person, is attributed to her. There is a second, less known portrait from the time he practiced in Delft (previous page, right). Here he looks older and more serious, but still full of confidence.

Reinier de Graaf became especially famous for his work on the ovary described in his last book on the female reproductive organs, *New Treatise Concerning the Generative Organs of Women*, which was published in Latin, in 1672. Exactly 300 years later, an excellent English translation was published. de Graaf's style of writing is robust and entertaining, and his descriptions reflect an intense fascination with his subject. He systematically interprets function from either anatomy or some fascinating experiments, and in this respect he must be considered the first modern reproductive biologist. His drawings on the female anatomy are meticulous and have an artistic touch.

As the Reinier de Graaf lecture focuses on his remarkable observations on the ovary, I shall focus here on some of his less well known observations, which are not related to the ovary. In his introduction de Graaf almost excuses himself for his realistic and vivid descriptions.

> 'I have described the genital parts, not to encourage seduction, and indulgence in pleasure but to improve man's knowledge of themselves for the benefit of the medical community.'

de Graaf was the first to describe the clitoris in detail. Until that time it was considered to be a small penis, but apart from the similarities de Graaf also stresses the differences. For example, he shows that the clitoris has two instead of three cavernous bodies and stresses the abundant innervation of this subtle organ. His description of the function of the clitoris is quite stunning.

> 'The glans of the clitoris is endowed with such sharp and perceptive sensitivity that it is not without justice called the sweetness of love, the gad-fly of Venus. Indeed, if these parts of the pudendum had not been endowed with such an exquisite sensitivity to pleasure and passion, no woman would be willing to take upon herself the irksome 9-months-long business of gestation, the painful and often fatal process of expelling the fetus and the worrisome and care-ridden task of raising children.'

He is the first to focus on the paraurethral glands which were later described in detail by Skene in 1880; de Graaf calls them the 'female prostate'.

> 'The function of the "female prostate" is to generate a serous juice which makes women more libidinous and lubricates their sexual parts in agreeable fashion during coitus. Here too it should be noted that the discharge of the female "prostate" causes as much pleasure as that does that from the male "prostate" ... I

mean those females who, with lascivious thoughts, frisky fingers or instruments devised contrary to decent morals, wickedly stir themselves up to such a pitch that they eject copious quantities of this kind of matter.'

Indeed, large quantities of fluid from the parurethral glands, resembling an ejaculation, may occur during an orgasm. Certain similarities with the male prostate have also been confirmed. Sexologists teach us that an orgasm provoked by stimulation of the clitoris should be distinguished from an orgasm caused by stimulation of the so-called G-spot, a small area of the vagina just behind the symphysis at the place where the paraurethral glands drain into the vagina. Only an orgasm after stimulation of the G-spot is considered to give rise to the discharge just mentioned. Because of his vivid description of the female 'ejaculation', some sexologists give de Graaf the honour of the discovery of the G-spot, which was first described by Gräfenberg 200 years later. Whether de Graaf's realistic and correct descriptions of these aspects of female sexology were based on personal experience is unknown.

de Graaf describes in detail the anatomy of the vagina. He is probably the first to mention the anastomoses between the hypogastric and ovarian vessels. He marvels about the vagina's function:

'Its function is simply to constrict, when necessary, the part it embraces, particularly at the time of coitus. The woman's vagina in fact is so cleverly constructed that it will accommodate itself to each and every penis; it will go out to meet a short one, retire before a long one, dilate for a fat one, and constrict for a thin one. Nature has taken account of every variety of penis and so there is no need to seek a scabbard the same size as your knife.'

Apart from his work on the ovary, one of his greatest achievements was the discovery of the patency and function of the Fallopian tubes. He performed an experiment:

'Indeed, if air is injected by means of bellows into the cavity of the uterus, the tubes immediately swell (unless phlegm of something abnormal closes their orifices or cavity) and air rushes out through their extremities.'

After an extensive description of their anatomy he continues on their function.

'Having set out all these facts and duly considered them, we give it as our judgement that the real function of the tubes is first, in a fruitful act of coitus, to grant a passage to the finer portion of the male semen making for the female "testicles" and thus to enable the eggs to be made wet; second, when the eggs have been fertilized in this way and expelled from the female "testicles", to receive them into their extremities and to take them down through their inner cavity to the uterus.'

In his honor, an international symposium has been organized every 3 years since 1973, exactly 300 years after his death. Most likely, Reinier de Graaf would have been pleased with this tradition. The 10th Symposium was held in Zeist, the Netherlands, from 9–11 September, 1999, and was dedicated to Female Reproductive Aging. It was on this subject that de Graaf made the following observation on the age-related decline of what he called the 'female testicles':

> 'The size of the female testicle varies not a little according to age. In the pubescent and those in the prime of life they generally weigh 1½ drachms ... In women of advanced age, they become smaller, harder and more dried up, gradually withering more and more, but never entirely disappearing.'

Sonographic studies performed recently confirm de Graaf's account of what is probably the first description of ovarian aging.

ACKNOWLEDGEMENTS

I would like to thank Professor Frits Lammes from the University of Amsterdam for introducing me to the work of Reinier de Graaf.

We gratefully acknowledge the generous support by the main sponsors of the Symposium: Abbott Netherlands BV, Organon Netherlands BV and Serono Benelux BV, and also the additional support by Ferring Nederland BV, Asta Medica BV, Gynotec, Jansen Cilag and Sigma Tau. Without the help of these companies, it would have proved impossible to organize the 10th Reinier de Graaf Symposium.

Reinier de Graaf lecture

Reinier de Graaf and the discovery of the ovary

R.V. Short

Although Reinier de Graaf did not 'discover' the ovaries – he was not the first to describe either their anatomical structure, or their reproductive significance – his amazing *New Treatise Concerning the Generative Organs of Women (De Mulierum Organis Generationi Inservientibus Tractatus Novus*, 1672)[1], and its equally distinguished predecessor, *Treatise Concerning the Generative Organs of Men (Tractatus de Virorum Organis Generationi Inservientibus*, 1668)[2], burst onto the scene of 17th century scientific endeavor like blazing comets. It is no exaggeration to say that they were more brilliant in their breadth and detail than anything that had gone before, and they still repay serious scientific study more than 300 years after publication. None of today's reproductive biologists will be able to claim such lasting distinction. And what makes de Graaf's works even more remarkable is that they were written by a young man in his twenties, as yet unmarried. De Graaf's untimely death in 1673 at the age of 32, possibly from the plague, robbed us of one of the great intellects of the millennium. Delft must have been an amazing place in those days, for it was there, too, that de Graaf's friend, Antoni van Leeuwenhoek, using his home-made microscopic lenses, was able to discover spermatozoa or 'animalcules' in his own semen in 1677[3]. Had de Graaf lived a little longer, he and van Leeuwenhoek might have been the first to discover the mammalian egg, and to witness mammalian fertilization two centuries in advance of the event. Leeuwenhoek even suggested the possibility of fertilization of the egg by the sperm in a letter to the Royal Society in 1683[4]. But there is no need to speculate about what might have been, when we have so much to admire from what de Graaf did accomplish, and even today we still have much to learn from him.

We are fortunate in having an excellent English translation of de Graaf's works by a Latin scholar at the University of Sydney, Dr Jocelyn, with annotations by Professor Setchell, a noted reproductive biologist[5]. This translation is the basis of all the ensuing quotations.

In de Graaf's book on the generative organs of women, after somewhat salacious but nonetheless very informative chapters on the clitoris and the hymen, and a detailed account of the menstrual flow (but no mention of the menopause), he devotes a chapter to 'The testicles of women, or rather their ovaries', and has this to say about them:

> 'The size of the female 'testicle' varies not a little according to age. In the pubescent and those in the prime of life they generally weigh 1½ drachms [= 5.4 g], thus being only about half the size of male testicles, although relatively broader and more full of juice. In women of advanced age and decrepit, they become smaller, harder and more dried up, gradually withering more and more but never entirely disappearing. We have in fact noted that the smallest 'testicles' of old women still weigh a scruple [= 1.2 g]. In infants and the newborn, the 'testicles' weigh from 5 grains to half a scruple [= 300–600 mg].'

Today, few scientists ever do something so mundane as to weigh the ovaries, so it is good to be reminded of what information we may be missing. With the latest ultrasound techniques, it should be possible to record a decrease in ovarian volume with the approach of the menopause, and perhaps this would be a better way of estimating the size of the follicular reserve than by hormone measurements in peripheral blood. Doppler ultrasound also provides a wonderful non-invasive way of visualizing the formation and fate of the corpus luteum.

When discussing the substance of the ovary, de Graaf refers to the numerous vesicles or follicles described by earlier writers. He then goes on to say:

> 'We shall call the vesicles 'eggs' on account of the exact similarity they bear to the eggs which the ovaries of fowls contain. While fowl's eggs are still small they contain nothing except a thin liquid like albumen. The existence of this albumen in women's eggs can also be quite prettily demonstrated by boiling them. The liquid in the eggs of the 'testicles' acquires from being boiled the same colour, flavour and consistency as does the albumen in fowl's eggs.'

It is a brave anatomist indeed who would eat boiled human Graafian follicles from a corpse! No wonder de Graaf died so young.

The first person to state quite clearly that the 'female testicles' should be called ovaries because they contained ova was Bishop Niels Stensen of Denmark, who published his findings in 1667[6]. De Graaf was in contact with Stensen, and had this to say about him:

> 'We asked the distinguished Mr N. Stensen if he would deign to tell us what he had observed concerning the female 'testicles' in various animals (which we did not possess in sufficient quantity or which we did not have the opportunity to dissect at all). He did not disappoint our prayer. Indeed he candidly informed us that he had found eggs of various sizes in fallow deer, guinea pigs, badgers, red deer, wolves, asses and even mules. All these observations combine with our own to confirm abundantly that eggs are found in the females of every species.
>
> If someone asks what eggs are doing in aged animals and in mules, which cannot reproduce, we shall reply that they are doing no more than the uterus, the

'testicles' and the other genital parts which are normally to be observed in these animals as much as in fertile ones.'

Three years after De Graaf's publication, Stensen published his findings in more detail, with an account of the ovaries of two mules that are particularly interesting[7]. In one of these animals, no follicles were visible at all, whereas the other animal had larger ovaries which contained a number of follicles and a corpus luteum. We now know that the infertility of mules can be explained by the difference in chromosome number and karyotypic appearance between the two parental species, resulting in meiotic arrest in the ovary and the testis. However, as Stensen observed, some mules do indeed have a few Graafian follicles which contain oocytes, and these may ovulate, resulting in the formation of a corpus luteum. But even more amazingly, such female mules can sometimes get pregnant and give birth; there are recent genetically proven examples of fertile female mules in the United States, Brazil and China[8]. The only explanation for their unexpected fertility is Ann Chandley's suggestion that non-random association of the two parental chromosome sets at the first meiotic division may result in the production of a few gametes that contain mostly horse or donkey chromosomes and hence are viable, a phenomenon known as affinity[9]. Fertile mules would repay a great deal more scientific investigation, and might cause us to rewrite the rules about the independent segregation of chromosomes at meiosis.

De Graaf was led astray by drawing too close an analogy between the avian and the mammalian ovary. Fabricius had already provided an accurate account of how the large, yolk-filled avian egg was shed from the ovary, to be picked up by the fimbria and transported to the uterus, where it was encased in albumen, a shell membrane and a shell before being laid[10], and de Graaf mistakenly thought that the mammalian follicle was analagous to the avian egg. He even drew a bovine Graafian follicle carefully dissected out of the ovary, ready to enter the ostium of the Fallopian tube (Figures 1 and 2). But he thought that the egg had first to be fertilized in some way by male semen before it left the ovary:

'We give it as our judgement that the real function of the [Fallopian] tubes is first, in a fruitful act of coitus, to grant a passage to the finer portion of the male semen making for the 'testicles' and thus to enable the eggs in the 'testicles' to be made wet; second, when the eggs have been fertilized in this way and expelled from the 'testicles', to receive them into their extremities and to take them down through their inner cavity to the uterus.'

But how the semen could penetrate the thick ovarian capsule to fertilize the eggs baffled de Graaf:

'We state that, for generation, it is not at all essential for semen to ascend to the uterus or the tubes but merely for vapour from it to pass through these places and reach the eggs in the 'testicles'. This will seem more likely if one considers that the semen itself, whether or not it ascends to the uterus and the tubes, cannot reach

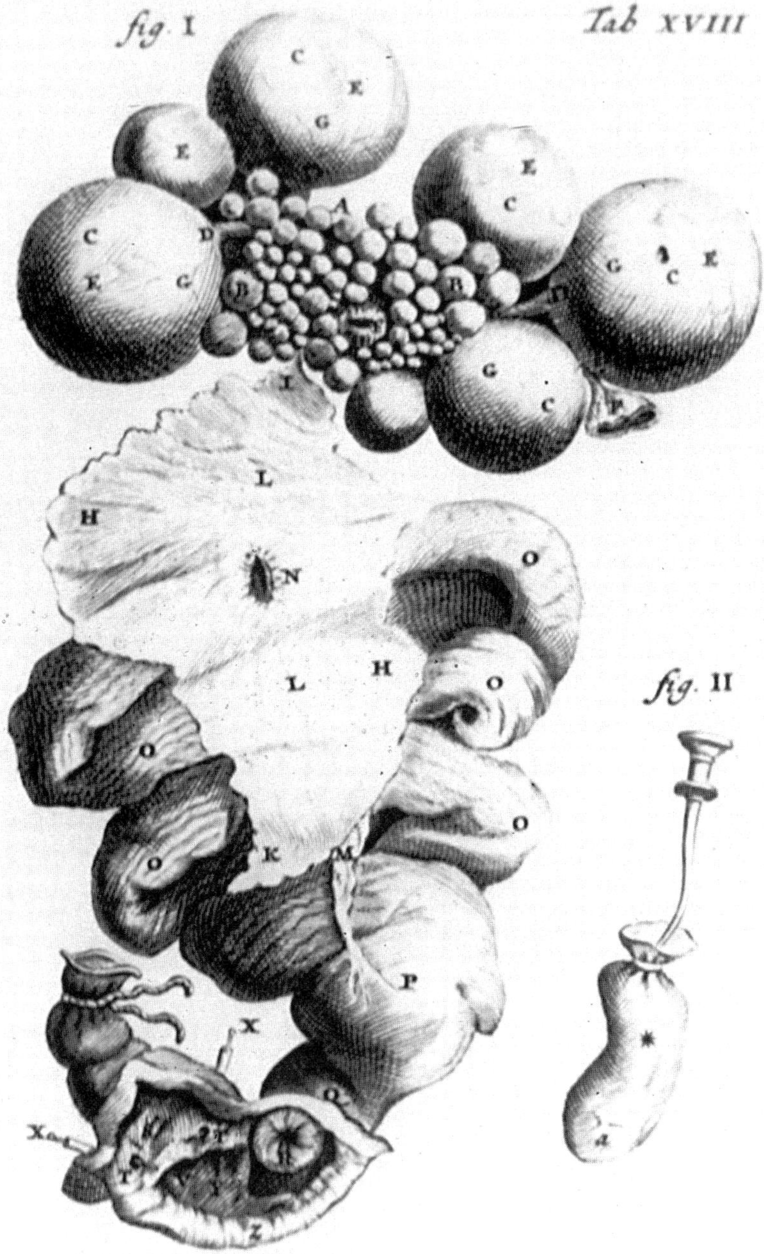

Figure 1 Plate XVIII. *Fig. I* displays the genital parts of a hen.
A, the raceme of yolks or eggs; BB, small yolks around the middle of the raceme; CC, large yolks at the periphery of the raceme; DD, pedicles or peduncles; EE, parts of the large yolks not covered by a calix, i.e. the spaces through which the yolks burst out; FF, calices from which the

the eggs through the very thick tissues of the 'testicles'. Consequently, we must of necessity have recourse to the theory of seminal vapour in order to explain how the eggs are fertilized.'

The fact that the Fallopian tubes were also needed to transport the fertilized egg down into the uterus was evidenced by the occasional reports of tubal pregnancies in women, and he gives a second-hand account of one such case:

'Plate XXI [Figure 3] shows two uteri which were found on 6th January, 1669 by the surgeon Bened. Vassal when he opened up the body of a woman, 32 years of age, of sanguine temperament and masculine appearance. These two uteri were so excellently arranged by the diligent care of Nature that the genuine one conceived eleven times, seven males and four females, all born at the proper time and exactly formed. These were followed by a brother, no more than a fetus, which was conceived in the adjoining uterus. This place was so resistant to being extended that when the fetus sought more room, it caused its mother very severe symptoms for $2^1/_2$ months and finally at about the age of 3 or 4 months loosed the bars that restrained it and found its own grave in that of its mother. A vast out-pouring of blood occurred throughout the abdominal cavity and threw the mother into such violent convulsions for 3 whole days, that she died as the result. The said Vassal preserved the woman's parts in balsam and dissected them one by one over a period of a whole month in his own home in the presence of learned physicians, surgeons, drug-sellers, midwives and natural scientists resident in Paris. He then decided tô record the woman's case by committing it to print along with figure-drawings of the parts under discussion and an explanation which we thought it appropriate to attach here in Latin (see Plate XXI). "It is possible," says the distinguished Oldenburg, the editor of the Philosophical Transactions of the Royal Society from which we have extracted this observation, "that what is thought to be a second uterus by Mr Vassal, the publisher of this report, is only an extension of the true uterus or what is called by anatomists the tube of Falloppia."'

Having achieved fertilization by the improbable medium of seminal vapor (remember that van Leeuwenhoek did not describe spermatozoa until 1677,

---

Figure 1 *Continued*
yolks have escaped; GG, the blood vessels disseminated through the tunics of the calices; HH, the membranous expansion of the oviduct; I, the part of the oviduct joined to the ovary; K, part of the expansion of the oviduct dragged down from the ovary; L, the middle of the expansion of the oviduct joined loosely with the membranous ligament; M, the membranous ligament bound to the uterus; N, the aperture of the oviduct, or infundibulum; OO, the oviduct in its natural position; P, the part of the oviduct, called the uterus, in which the egg is detained for some time and perfected; Q, the part of the oviduct, called the vagina; R, the orifice of the vagina, called the vulva; S, the rectum opened; TT, the outlets of the ureters; V, the aperture of Fabrizzi; XX, styluses inserted in the ureters to reveal their outlets; Y, the common orifice, or cloaca, opened; Z, the upper lip or veil.

Fig. II shows the lower part of the oviduct of a hen no longer breeding and in it the orifice of the vagina (a) so tightly shut by Nature as to deny transit to a very strong injection of air

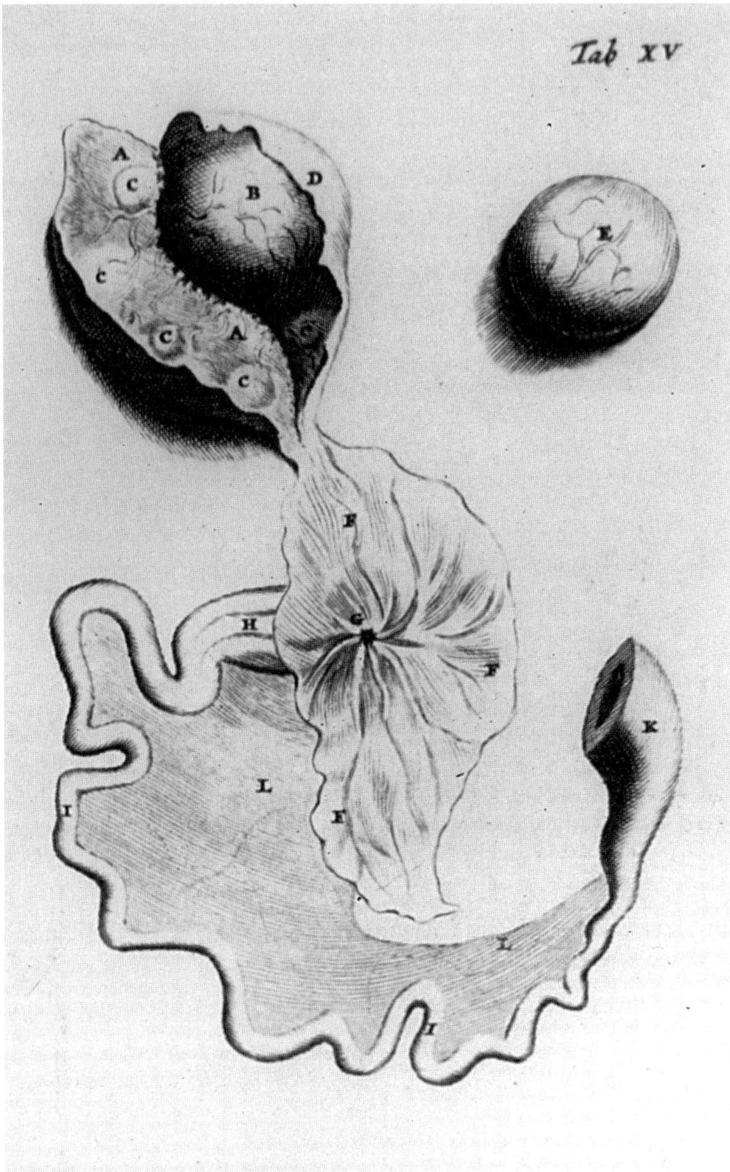

Figure 2 Plate XV displays a cow's 'testicle', or ovary, with the usual appearance before coitus, after being opened.
AA, the 'testicle' opened along its length; B, a very large, i.e. mature, egg still contained in the 'testicle'; CC, small, i.e. immature, eggs embedded in the 'testicle'; DD, the membrane of the 'testicle' called the dartos; E, a very large egg taken from the 'testicle'; F, the membranous expansion of the Fallopian tube; G, the contracted aperture in the extremity of the tube; H, the extremity of the Fallopian tube; II, the remainder of the tube; K, part of the uterine horn cut; L, the ligament of the tube, which in human beings has been likened to a bat's wing

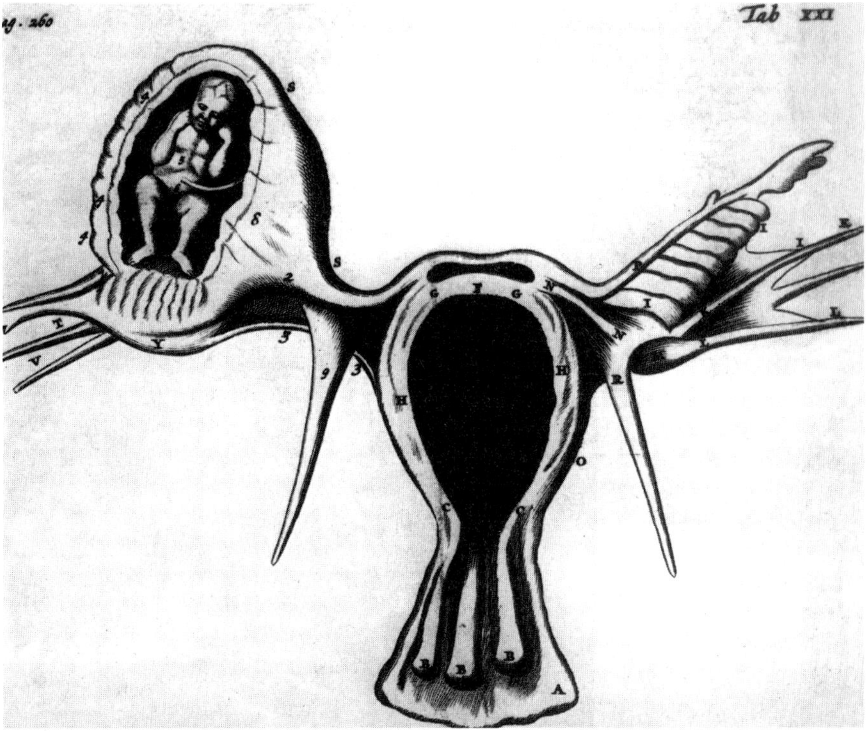

Figure 3 An ectopic pregnancy in the Fallopian tube reprinted by de Graaf from Vassal's report to the Royal Society. Of note is the grossly distended Fallopian tube on the left side (SS), compared to its normal counterpart on the right side (P), the site of rupture and hemorrhage that led to the woman's death (4) and the site of the placental attachment (8). Published in *Philosophical Transactions of the Royal Society*, June 21, 1669; number 48; pages 969–70

five years after de Graaf's work was published), how did the fertilized eggs escape from the ovary? In de Graaf's words:

> 'We said that once they are fertilized the eggs are expelled from the 'testicles'. How this happens is hard to determine, since autopsy is hardly capable of solving our difficulty. Still, so as not to leave the method of expulsion plunged in complete darkness, and for the sake of aiding scientific investigation, we shall gladly communicate to you our thoughts on the matter.
>
> We think that fertilized eggs emerge from the 'testicles' partly through the agency of the 'testicles' and partly because of the peculiar disposition of the eggs themselves. The 'testicles' act by secreting a kind of glandulous matter among their egg-enveloping membranes. Shortly after coitus the tunics of the eggs, previously transparent, become opaque and equipped with a large number of blood vessels. The day after this opacity appears it is possible to observe within the tunics of an egg a glandulous substance enveloping the egg entirely and taking the shape of a globule. This substance gradually grows in quantity and compresses the egg from every side. At length it expels the egg through a hole visible at its

centre. This happens in rabbits on the third day after coitus and later in ewes, cows and other animals which gestate for a longer period.'

Here, de Graaf is giving us a beautiful account of the formation of the corpus luteum, which is a consequence of follicle rupture and ovulation, not its cause, as he wrongly surmised. Being a true experimentalist at heart, de Graaf resorted to autopsies on rabbits killed at different times after copulation in order to study the consequences of ovulation in more detail. He was not to know that rabbits are induced ovulators, so corpora lutea only appear after mating has taken place. He is unquestionably the first person to give a detailed account of the corpora lutea, which he called 'globules':

> 'Bodies, which occur naturally, but only at certain times, in the female 'testicles' are the globules. They resemble conglomerations of glands, each one being composed of a large number of particles running in practically straight lines from the centre to the circumference, and wrapped in its own membrane. The globules in our view do not exist at all times in the female 'testicles'. They can be detected there only after coitus, and there will be one or more according to whether from a particular act of intercourse the animal is to produce one or more fetuses. Nor do they take the same form at all times in all animals or in all animals of the same kind. In cows, they acquire a golden yellow, in sheep a red, in other animals an ashen colour.'

From this account, it is clear that he recognized the relationship between the number of corpora lutea in the ovary and the number of embryos in the uterus. His description of the different color of the 'globules' in different species also explains why he did not call them corpora lutea (yellow bodies), a term first used appropriately a century later by the Italian anatomist, Malpighi, who was studying the ovaries of cows[10].

De Graaf also devotes an entire chapter of his book to the 'semen' of women, weighing up the Aristotelian argument, that attributes procreation exclusively to the semen of the male, against the Hippocratic argument that women, too, produce semen and play a role in procreation. As de Graaf rightly observed:

> 'If a mare receives the semen of an ass, the fetus has the features not of the father alone but those of both parents mixed together; likewise if a goat penetrates a sheep, a sheep with rather coarse wool is produced. Similarly, the offspring of a white man and an Ethiopian woman acquire a mixed colour.
>
> We think that, apart from the eggs described in the previous chapter, women contribute nothing in the way of semen to generation.'

And thus it was that two close neighbors in the little town of Delft, in Holland, between the years 1672 and 1677, unwittingly founded the rival schools of Ovists and Animalculists, and initiated two centuries of fruitless debate about which of the two sexes held the key to reproduction. The argument was only resolved when a German, von Baer, discovered the true mammalian egg lying within the Graafian follicle in 1827, and when a Belgian, van Beneden, ultimately described mammalian fertilization in 1875[10]. If only de Graaf could have lived for a few more years, and collaborated with van Leeuwenhoek! It seems ironic that today we associate de Graaf's name with the follicle, when it should really be called Stensen's follicle, and yet we use the inappropriate Latin epithet 'corpus luteum' to describe what should really be called the globule of de Graaf. But then, you cannot rewrite history!

REFERENCES

1. De Graaf R. *De Mulierum Organis Generationi Inservientibus Tractatus Novus.* Lugduni Batavorum ex Officina Hackiana, 1672
2. De Graaf R. *Tractatus de Virorum Organis Generationi Inservientibus, de Clysteribus et de usu Siphonis in Anatomia*. Lugduni Batavorum et Roterod. ex Officina Hackiana, 1668
3. Van Leeuwenhoek A. Observationes D. Anthonii Leeuwenhoek de Natis e semine genitali Animalculis [Letter dated November 1677]. *Phil Trans R Soc Lond* 1678;12:1040
4. Van Leeuwenhoek A. An abstract of a letter from Mr Anthony Leeuwenhoek of Delft about Generation by an Animalcule of the Male seed. Animals in the seed of a frog. Some other Observables in the parts of a Frog. Digestion, and the motion of the blood in a Feavor. *Phil Trans R Soc Lond* 1683;13:347–55
5. Jocelyn HD, Setchell BP. Reinier de Graaf on the human reproductive organs. *J Reprod Fertil* 1972(suppl 17):222
6. Stensen N. *Elementorum Myologiae Specimen, Seu Musculi Descriptis Geometrica. Cui Accedunt Canis Carchariae Dissectum Caput, et Dissectus Piscis ex Canum Genere*. Florence: 1667
7. Stensen N. Ova viviparorum spectantes observationes. *Thomae Bartholini Acta Medica et Philosophica Hafniensia* 1675;2:219–32
8. Allen WR, Short RV. Interspecific and extraspecific pregnancies in Equids: anything goes. *J Hered* 1997;88:384–92
9. Chandley AC. Does 'affinity' hold the key to fertility in the female mule? *Genet Res* 1981;37:105–9
10. Short RV. The discovery of the ovaries. In Zuckerman S, Weir BJ, eds. *The Ovary* (second edition). New York: Academic Press, 1977:1–39

State-of-the-art lecture

Definition and character of reproductive aging and senescence

R.G. Gosden and C.E. Finch

INTRODUCTION

There is no universal pattern of reproductive senescence in female vertebrates. Rather, there is a spectrum ranging from semelparity – with a single reproductive episode, rapid aging and sudden death – to iteroparity with more than one episode and more gradual senescence. Patterns in iteroparous vertebrates vary enormously. Although in many mammals fertility declines gradually after an early peak, in some species of birds reproductive senescence is negligible, even at advanced ages. The human female has a peculiarly early onset of reproductive senescence considering her longevity, although a state corresponding to the postmenopause can be found in many species, especially in the protected environments of captivity and domestication. Post-reproductive phases will become commoner and longer as animal husbandry improves and lifespans increase. This is because the ovary is endowed with a fixed number of non-renewable germ cells which is depleted by follicular atresia and recruitment for growth. The ovary provides one of the clearest examples of programmed aging, although in laboratory rodents cycle cessation involves refractoriness to positive feedback for release of luteinizing hormone (LH) as a result of chronic exposure to cyclical ovarian hormone secretion. This illustrates the complexity of age changes, which involve multiple loci and are sometimes due to self-limiting physiological processes. In addition, the timing of ovarian failure is affected by heritable factors that probably act at many levels, including the size of the founding follicle population and its rate of attrition. Less often acknowledged are the huge stochastic variations affecting every level and making precise prediction of the timing of cycle cessation impossible. Most germ cells disappear before puberty as a result of programmed cell death (apoptosis), although mice with functional mutations at the *bax* locus have larger numbers surviving to adulthood and old age. Dietary and endocrine manipulations can also slow the pace of ovarian aging, although frozen banking is the only practicable method at present for postponing extinction of primordial follicles. Like other aspects of life history, fecundity and the reproductive lifespan have been shaped by evolutionary selection. In this chapter, we use a number of species and experimental biology to illustrate some principles in reproductive gerontology.

DEFINITION AND MEASUREMENT OF REPRODUCTIVE AGE

According to an old Chinese proverb: 'The Yangtze never runs backwards … man recaptures not his youth'. Aging has often been likened to a thin, exuberant stream widening to a slow, meandering river before it disappears into the sea. The deepest mysteries which science has barely penetrated tempt us to reach for metaphors. Among the more complex aspects of biology none are more perplexing than age changes, but experimental science and comparative biology are gradually making them more intelligible.

For a long time, there was little consistency in definitions of aging. The expression 'age-related' is better reserved for phenomena that are not necessarily adverse to the interests of the organism and where time *per se* is not necessarily a causal factor[1]. There are, of course, plenty of examples of age-related changes that are neutral or even beneficial – witness learned behavior, acquired immunity and even the maturation of a fine red wine! The term 'senescence' is more specific, implying maladaptive or harmful age changes including, *inter alia*, deterioration of memory, postmenopausal osteoporosis and infertility.

We take the fact for granted that the reproductive system becomes senescent because its human manifestations, especially in females, are so striking and familiar. But from a biological perspective, it seems paradoxical that the system responsible for generating new life should be subject to decay. We might argue logically that individuals capable of reproducing for longest and most successfully will contribute more of the genes responsible to the next generation, and this trend would be reinforced in subsequent generations. Additionally, senescence resulting from depletion of the limited store of germ cells sets in train a causal nexus of detrimental age changes. There is, however, a fallacy pointed out many years ago by J.B.S. Haldane and P.B. Medawar that the force of natural selection declines with age; genes are selected for optimal characteristics at young ages irrespective of any harmful actions later in life[2]. This is the basis of George Williams' influential theory of 'antagonistic pleiotropy', although it does not explain all the phenomena of senescence[1]. Nevertheless, it importantly indicates that hundreds, if not thousands, of genes are involved and that it is therefore futile to search for a single pacemaker gene or organ as a universal explanation. More attention is now being given to individual variations that are due to stochastic processes and arise independently of gene programs, producing striking differences in organ cell numbers[3]. In illustrating some of the key points, we take as primary examples the ovarian cycle, follicle dynamics and oocyte quality.

COMPARATIVE RATES OF AGING

Interspecific

The onset and decline of fertility are major transitions in life history and, although modulated by diet and environment, they are sufficiently characteristic of the species that they are presumed to have evolved by natural selection. There is a spectrum of life history strategies. On the one hand, many species of animals (and plants) have a single burst of breeding activity followed by rapid senescence and sudden death. These so-called semelparous species are numerous and include annual plants and many insects but few vertebrates (e.g. Pacific salmon and some marsupial 'mice', but no birds)[1]. As a result of only one reproductive event – albeit explosive – reproductive senescence cannot be said to be gradual, although pronounced changes may occur in the gonads, rendering them inactive even in individuals that survive longer. On the other hand, there are iteroparous species, so called because they have more potential reproductive opportunities and slower senescence. The lifespan is not necessarily longer, and there are some semelparous species, such as bamboo, which have very extended juvenile phases[4]. Human life history lies near the extreme end of the iteroparous spectrum, but the same general pattern prevails in domesticated and laboratory mammals as well as other primates. In a few iteroparous species (e.g. some seabirds) reproductive senescence is negligible – in line with the relatively constant mortality rate doubling time (a general indicator of the rate of somatic senescence)[5].

Where aging occurs slowly there is usually corresponding evidence of reproductive senescence. In mice and rats, for instance, litter sizes decline steadily after a maximum at the second or third litter. In so-called natural fertility societies, such as the Hutterites in North America and where historical populations have been well documented, the decline of fertility has been shown to begin in the middle of the fourth decade of life; some 50% of married women delivered their last baby at 40 years of age – 10 years before the final menses[6]. The French national registry for sperm donation has confirmed that the time to conception starts lengthening when women are still in their early 30s[7].

The long phase of postmenopausal life in our species stands out as a peculiarity, and has stimulated speculation about its biological roots and evolutionary significance. Perhaps the attention has been overblown because a post-reproductive phase is more widespread than has been realized, occurring in some individuals of most species studied, although rarely manifested under natural conditions (Figure 1). Among some of the exceptions are marine pinnepods and certain toothed whales[8], and chimpanzees in Gombe which were occasionally observed to become menopausal.

Otherwise, a post-reproductive phase of life is largely an artifact of domestication in which a protected environment enables a few lucky or hardy individuals to survive to ages that outlast the capacity of the ovarian system.

Since the store of ovarian follicles declines inexorably (see below), we should expect to find more examples and longer phases of sterility as improvements in animal husbandry push up the maximum survival time. For the first time in history, a prolonged period of post-reproductive life has become a dominant experience for the majority of women in this century. Since human life expectancy is rising in most countries of the world, there may come a time when Jeanne Calment, who had been postmenopausal for an estimated 70 years when she died aged 122 years in 1997, is not quite so remarkable.

Intraspecific

Apart from (increasingly) rare data from populations with natural fertility, it is difficult to obtain reliable data about age variations between women. In addition to the confounding effects of pathology in the gonads and genital tract and medical procedures such as hysterectomy, there is the obvious impact of contraception and medical termination of pregnancy on fecundity. Nevertheless, longitudinal data collected in the USA many years ago by the

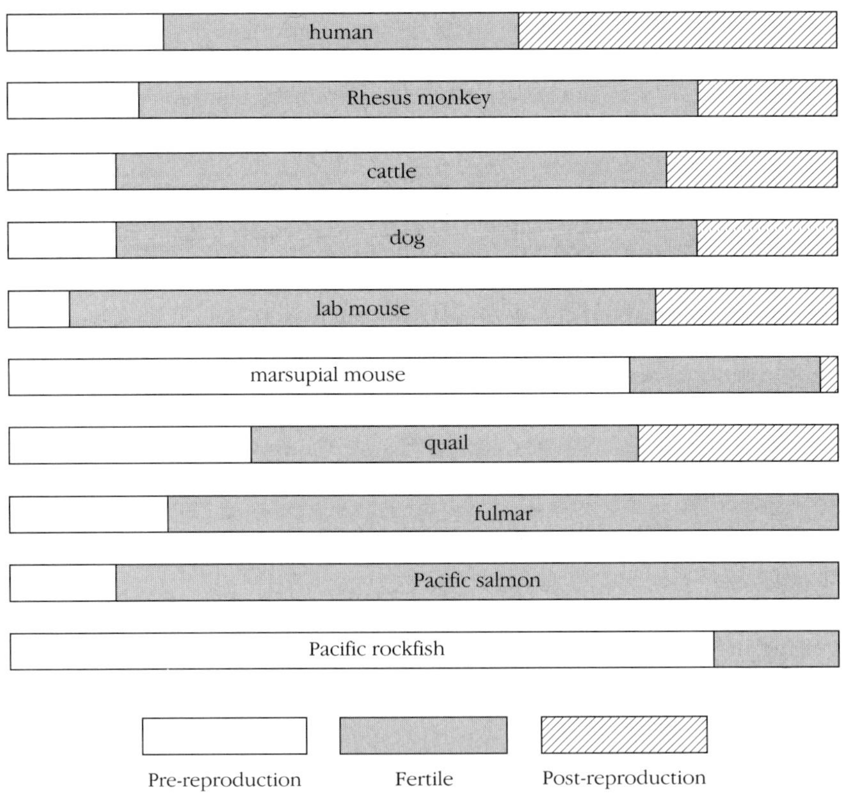

Figure 1 Spectrum of reproductive schedules in female vertebrates

late Alan Treloar, together with a few other sources, indicate huge individual variation in cycle patterns, including differences in onset of menarche, cycle length and cycle characteristics throughout the reproductive lifespan[9]. In addition to these differences, the 5–95% interval for menopausal age is almost a decade long (approximately 45–54 years), and substantial age-specific differences in serum levels of follicle stimulating hormone (FSH) and inhibin have been recorded[10]. Studies on menopause in twins under the family name are being continued by Alan Treloar's grandniece, Susan.

The causes of these differences are, of course, difficult to interpret because, even when the aforementioned factors are controlled, the relative influence of genetics, lifestyle, diet and smoking obscure other factors. On top of these uncertainties, local environmental influences, possibly including human pheromones, may affect menstrual rhythmicity[11]. However, some of the variation may be 'structural' in the sense of being a residue of preceding developmental processes that, for each individual, differentially fix the numbers of stem cells and set the central and peripheral thresholds for reproductive endocrinology. For all these reasons, there are great advantages in studying the cycles of laboratory animals for, although the physiology of estrous and menstrual cycles is distinct, the factors responsible for variation can be better controlled.

Longitudinal studies of mice have demonstrated J- or U-shaped distributions for cycle frequency with respect to age, which is reminiscent of that in humans[12]. There is also striking variability between individuals under uniform conditions and from stocks that have been inbred for scores, if not hundreds, of generations and which are homozygous at virtually all loci. Furthermore, it is obvious from inspecting individual records that there is no strict canonical sequence of age changes. After a phase of relatively regular 4- or 5-day cycles at 5–10 months old (comparable to women aged 25–40 years), some mice pass through a sequence of irregular cycles to the acyclic state of persistent estrus. Some switch early and some later, some abruptly and others gradually. Some have repeated episodes of pseudopregnancy-like cycles associated with pituitary lactotroph tumors. Cycle patterns are not, therefore, highly predictable; nor is the fecundity of individual animals living in the same environment. Such observations are contributing to growing awareness of stochastic processes in life history[2].

Between cells and organs

A question that is seldom asked but nonetheless relevant to this chapter is the extent to which reproductive age changes are correlated, if at all. It is theoretically relevant to the investigation of cause and potentially of practical significance too. For example, the question may be asked: is there a correlation between the chances of aneuploidy in oocytes, the risk of ovarian cancer and the rate of follicle population disappearance?

Clearly, there must be some correspondence between scaling factors that influence the degree of risk of pathology. Some species live fast and die young (*r*-strategists) whilst others (*K*-strategists) have a longer lifespan and a lower age-specific risk of degenerative disease. In the case of our prime example, the ovary, there is not only a larger endowment of follicles in human ovaries[13], but a rate of follicle depletion that is much slower than in mice. In fact, the half-life of the follicle store at ages earlier than 38 years is about 7 years, close to the mortality doubling rate in human populations. If the store of primordial follicles in human ovaries were depleted at the same rate as in mice (i.e. 30 times faster), numbers would fall to the threshold for cyclicity (approximately 1000) by 30 months of age – long before menarcheal age.

We have considered respective indicators of aging for three major parameters in the human ovary – cancer, Down's syndrome and follicle depletion. Fortunately for this exercise, the time constants are approximately exponential but, because they are themselves age-dependent, we have compared the figures as population halvings or doublings only at the transitional ages for fertility (35–50 years). Ovarian cancer rates double every 5 years between 30 years of age and the menopause, levelling out later. Down's syndrome is complicated by a large non-age-dependent component, but the frequency doubles between 31 and 34 years, and afterwards every 2 years[14]. Follicle depletion rates also change, halving every 7.1 years at < 37 years of age but at every 2.9 years after the age of 37 years[15]. The rough correspondence between these factors is interesting and unsurprising. We suspect that these parameters have converged during evolution rather than being part of a common chain of cause and effect.

PACEMAKERS OF BIOLOGICAL DETERIORATION

Genetic

If the reproductive lifespan is an evolved characteristic it follows, *ipso facto*, that genes influence the scheduling of puberty and perhaps also ovarian senescence. There is abundant evidence that hybrids of inbred strains of animals not only live longer but are more fertile. Likewise, it is well-recognized that consanguineous marriages tend to be less fertile and produce more birth defects. Hybrid vigor avoids inbreeding depression of health and fertility by creating heterozygosity at key genetic loci, but it is a large jump from these broad observations to identifying the genes responsible.

The span of menstrual life in women is dictated by the size of the original endowment of follicles and the rate of disappearance. As an illustration of the role of heredity, differences in the numbers of follicles were observed at all ages in a comparative study of mouse strains[16], and when the data were used to construct mathematical models the subtle variations in follicle dynamics became still more apparent[17]. Follicle dynamics were biphasic with a transition around the time of puberty in all strains, and the rates of growth initiation were surprisingly comparable. The chief difference was in the death rates of primordial follicles, which were higher before puberty than afterwards and exceeded the growth rates (Table 1). After puberty, death rates became negligible except in the CBA strain, which is notable because ovarian senescence occurs at the comparatively early age of 16 months. Interestingly, CBA strain mice also have a rate of embryonic aneuploidy that is ten-fold higher than in other strains.

Spontaneous premature menopause (often defined as < 40 years) occurs at a frequency of approximately 1% and is known to have a genetic basis. Although some genes have been identified (see Chapter 11), there is a large number of (mainly unidentified) genes involved in oogenesis and follicle dynamics; the task of revealing their influence on stem cell populations, differentiation and apoptosis has only just begun. Additionally, individuals from inbred strains differ in the number of oocytes (see below).

Since early menopause can be a familial trait, the classical approach of twin studies has been used to gauge the degree of heritability. Several recent studies have demonstrated a closer correlation between the menopausal ages of monozygotic than dizygotic twins, and heritability has been estimated, rather variably, at 31–63%[18,19]. The high upper estimate could be misleading because age at menopause differs by five or more years in 20% of monozygotic twins. This is consistent with the variations in follicle numbers for which there are important non-genetic explanations (see below). Once the genes responsible for early menopause have been identified, screening will become feasible, although it may never be possible to provide a precise forecast. In laboratory mice, it has been shown that alleles in the major histocompatibility complex (MHC) are associated with estrous cycle length and age of onset of reproductive senescence[20], and corresponding influences of the MHC could exist in humans.

Environmental and historical

Some of the clearest evidence of harmful impacts of environmental factors on the reproductive system and fertility is the sterilizing effects of cytotoxic chemotherapy and ionizing radiation. However, whilst these effects can be

Table 1 Growth and death rates for primordial follicles in three inbred strains of mice and an F1 hybrid

Strain	G_1	G_2	D_1	D_2
A	0.0036	0.0047	0.023	0.001
CBA	0.0033	0.0039	0.35	0.011
CBA × A	0.0025	0.0033	0.028	0.001
RIII	0.0070	0.0039	0.028	0

From a mathematical model[17] in which G and D represent respectively the fractions of small follicles that begin growing or dying each day, and at pre- (1) and postpubertal ages (2)

dramatic and irreversible they affect small numbers of patients and, from a demographic perspective, the most widespread ovarian toxicant is smoking. Moderate, regular use of tobacco has been estimated to advance the age of menopause by some 2–3 years. If the loss of 2 years of menstrual life is solely due to ovarian effects, and smoking began at say 20 years of age, it can be calculated that the rate of follicular atresia increased by 7% to account for this[21]. The upsurge in interest in reproductive toxicology will surely reveal many other factors to which humans are exposed during the course of life which reduces fertility and foreshortens the reproductive lifespan.

Reproductive senescence is also influenced by normal physiological processes, and transplantation studies reveal that chronic ovarian hormone exposure of the central apparatus for pituitary gonadotropin secretion can be self-limiting. Reciprocal transplantation of ovaries between young and aging rats revealed that the age of the host was more significant than that of the donor in determining the ability of the grafts to drive estrous cycles[22]. Ovaries from animals in the anovulatory state of persistent estrus were still capable of ovulating in a more youthful environment. Interestingly, the authors also observed that the grafts could function in old hosts that had been deprived of ovarian hormones at an early age by ovariectomy. This intriguing result has been confirmed and extensively investigated in mice[23]. It is consistent with the so-called delayed anovulatory condition in rodents in which small doses of estrogen or aromatizable androgens advance the onset of acyclicity in a dose-dependent manner. Hence, the conclusion has been drawn that cumulative exposure to ovarian steroids causes refractoriness to positive feedback control[24,25]. This hypothesis lays prime responsibility on central neural mechanisms, consistent with the subtle alterations observed in gonadotropin pulses in middle-aged rats *before* their cycles become irregular or cease[26]. There appear to be differences in the balance of responsibility for acyclicity even between species as closely related as rats and mice: in the latter, follicular depletion is a definite contributory factor.

Primacy of ovarian senescence for the etiology of the menopause is more clear-cut in humans, and cycle cessation is associated with a low threshold number of follicles[27]. Nevertheless, there are indications that neuroendocrine changes are occurring in women whilst the ovary is still well-endowed with follicles, paralleling the aforementioned observations in rats[28]. Whether these changes have any significance for cyclicity is unknown, although it is possible that they too are due to the steroidal impact on central mechanisms controlling the release of gonadotropin releasing hormone (GnRH).

Prenatal steroid secretion can have late effects on reproduction, at least in rodents. There are pronounced differences in the numbers of pups per litter and in the timing of the last litter in rats breeding *ad libitum* depending on the sex of the fetal neighbors when the female was still *in utero*[29]. Where there was a male on both sides (2M) the breeding lifespan was shorter than in siblings with only adjacent females (0M). It is supposed that androgen diffusing down a concentration gradient from the amniotic fluid of males to females could affect neuroendocrine thresholds.

By extension, the steroid impact hypothesis could be applied to uterine function, and this is more plausible in rodents than in humans. In the latter, egg donation studies indicate that the age of the oocyte is far more important in determining fertility loss than the uterine environment. To test the hypothesis, inbred mice were ovariectomized at 5 months of age or at 11 months, at which time both groups received ovarian grafts under the renal capsule from young donors. At approximately 1 year of age, fertility was substantially reduced and the animals were mated to make them pseudopregnant; embryos from young donors were transferred to their uteri in attempts to create pregnancy[30]. Pregnancies in animals that had undergone long-term deprivation of ovarian function were much more successful than in intact controls. This is consistent with the evidence of an impact of ovarian hormones on neuroendocrine pacemakers. It was not clear, however, whether differences were due to the pathology of endometrial hyperplasia or to more subtle changes affecting implantation.

The final example is based on observations that the age-dependent increase in aneuploidy in mouse embryos is advanced when mice are unilaterally ovariectomized at young ages[31]. Possibly, this effect is due to accelerated utilization of the follicle store, which is preprogrammed according to the production line hypothesis in which the last formed oocytes are last to be ovulated[32]. There is cytological evidence for this hypothesis, but it should be borne in mind that, because of the exponential character of follicle utilization, oocytes causing aneuploidy in mid-life are a tiny minority of the total (Figure 2). According to a strict interpretation of the hypothesis, they would be represented by the follicles formed in the last hour of the 4-day process of oogenesis in the mouse.

An alternative explanation for the potentiation effect of reducing total follicular mass is that aneuploidy is associated with the onset of irregular cycles and hormonal changes. Whatever the cause, if it applies in humans it would be significant for indicating that aneuploidy is not strictly dependent on chronological age. In a small study of Down's syndrome babies, there was no evidence that the mothers had an earlier menopause[33]. However, two new studies have indicated that elevated FSH is an independent risk factor for a Down's conception[34,35], confirming the original hypothesis of Brook and colleagues[31] that irregularities in follicular maturation resulting from endocrine changes in mid-life could underlie the chromosomal non-disjunction in oocytes.

Stochastic

Whilst most attention on the phenomena of aging has focused on genetic and environmental factors, the huge residual variation has often been overlooked[3]. For example, when inbred roundworms (*Caenorhabditis elegans*) are grown in liquid culture to eliminate environmental differences, individuals still vary three-fold in lifespan. Where a cause cannot be attributed, variation is assumed to be stochastic. In mammals, oogenesis is a good example of a variation-generating process in which the complex effects of survival factors, growth factors and apoptosis each have stochastic components that lead to wide differences in the follicle population at birth. In the new-born human ovary, there is a three-fold variation in follicle numbers[36], and comparable variation exists in inbred mice[16]. In part, these variations arise because individual primordial germ cells have widely differing abilities to divide, as shown in the mouse ovary[37].

There is therefore a sort of biological uncertainty principle in which it is impossible to predict precisely either the initial state of a system or its time course throughout life. Stochastic variation during development is largely beyond our control, which is perhaps why this fundamental aspect of nature has often been ignored.

Another stochastic factor potentially affecting oocytes is reactive oxygen species that are generated continuously during metabolism and which can

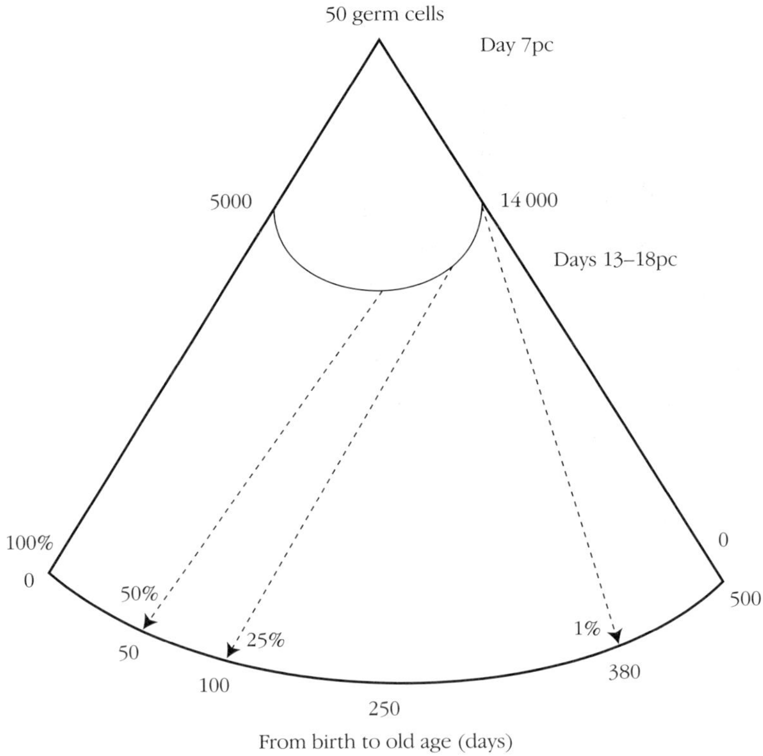

Figure 2 The production line hypothesis of follicle utilization as illustrated by typical numbers of germ cells and follicles in mice. pc, post-coitum

damage DNA. The mitochondrial genome is especially vulnerable, being close to the generation of unpaired electrons, lacking protective histones and having little DNA repair capacity. A decline in human oocyte quality with age could be due in part to defective mitochondria, with consequences for oxidative phosphorylation and intracellular ATP. The 'common' 3977 bp deletion increases in post-mitotic somatic cells with age, and has been detected in spare oocytes from older women[38]. The question of whether mitochondrial dysfunction can explain the early onset of oocyte aging is now a lively area for research.

REPRODUCTIVE SENESCENCE

The pessimistic proverb quoted at the beginning of this chapter asserts the inevitability of the aging process. Once under way, the process may never be put into reverse. Every organism eventually perishes from accidental death, if not from the consequences of senescence itself. Nevertheless, there are some striking examples in which there is negligible biological deterioration of cell lineages or even whole organisms[1]. Nor is the life history of organisms quite as rigid as was once thought: it is possible to extend the lifespan of fruit flies by repeatedly selecting for late fertility under culture conditions[2]. Furthermore, in the field of reproduction, physiological and genetic manipulations that alter the time course of senescence are already practicable under experimental conditions.

The limiting factor in many species, and humans in particular, is the size of the follicle store and its rate of disappearance. Feeding a low-calorie diet to rodents slows the disappearance of ovarian follicles[39], this being *pari passu* with greater resistance to common ailments and extended longevity. The rate of follicle disappearance can also be slowed by hypophysectomy in animals[40]. This has sometimes been attributed to withdrawal of FSH, although the explanation is incompatible with normal rates of follicle depletion in *hpg* mutants and the absence of the FSH receptor in primordial follicles[41]. However, there is some evidence that suppressing gonadotropins using GnRH analogs protects the gonads from cytotoxic drugs, such as cyclophosphamide, and even ionizing radiation[42], although there are conflicting results[43]. The most striking report claimed that follicle wastage was reduced with GnRH agonist treatment in rats[44], but this has not yet been confirmed independently.

In some respects, it would be better if the follicle store could be preserved before puberty to avoid profoundly suppressing estrogen during the reproductive years (and hence requiring hormone replacement therapy). This state can now be produced by targetted mutation of genes affecting germ cell survival and apoptosis. When the death-inducing gene, *bax*, was knocked out, there were 16 300 follicles in young adult mice compared to 5500 in controls[45]. This result indicates that *bax* is involved in the process of eliminating most of the follicles formed initially and provides a numerical advantage for

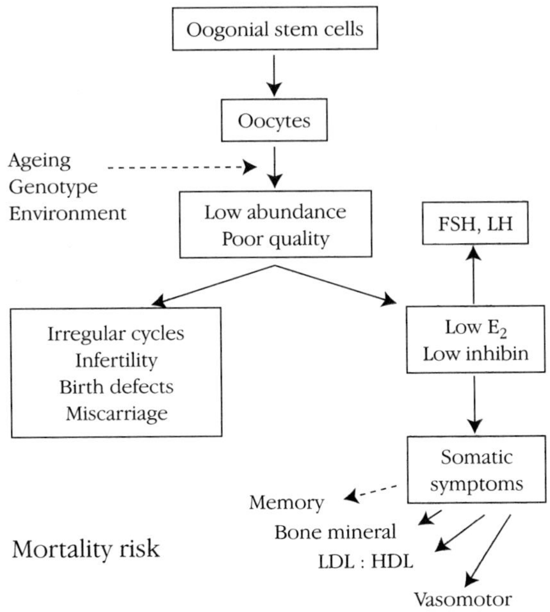

Figure 3 A causal nexus from development of germ cells to pathology in reproduction. FSH, follicle stimulating hormone; LH, luteinizing hormone; E_2, estradiol; LDH, low-density lipoprotein; HDL, high-density lipoprotein

later in life. Interference with *bax* after puberty would be inconsequential, because there is little apoptosis in small follicles. If it is assumed that knockout and wild-type animals have 500 days of cycling, with cycles producing on average ten ovulations in 5-day cycles, it can be calculated that 6% and 18% of the follicles in the two respective groups would be utilized by ovulation. This leads to the paradoxical conclusion that the rate of atresia is lower before puberty in *bax* knockouts and higher afterwards. The anti-apoptotic gene *bcl-2* is also able to increase the numbers of follicles.

At present, the most promising method for conserving ovarian function in humans is by using frozen banking of tissue. This strategy is based on studies showing that, after the freezing of strips of cortical tissue in animals, primordial follicles survive and can restore estrous cycles after autografting[46]. Frozen banking is being developed for conserving fertility in patients undergoing sterilizing chemotherapy, although it could potentially extend fertility and postpone menopause in other women.

EARLY ORIGINS OF SENESCENT CHANGES

This selective survey of reproductive senescence has emphasized the role of factors acting early in development and the key importance of stem cells. In the ovary, the stem cells that produce germ cells disappear before birth in humans and many other species. This fixes an upper limit on the number of potential menstrual/estrous cycles and hence the timing of menopause. The implications are wider still, since ovarian hormones, and particularly estradiol, carry a major health dividend for women. Whether withdrawal of estrogen affects life expectancy is debatable and requires further investigation[47], but the negative somatic effects on cognitive functions, bone mineral density and other health indicators are well known (Figure 3). There is a causal nexus from the formation of stem cells in the fetal ovary to the impact of estrogen withdrawal on health in middle and late life. This emphasizes the importance of taking a broad perspective in understanding and improving the reproductive health and well-being of older women.

ACKNOWLEDGEMENTS

We thank Professors Howard Cuckle and Malcolm Faddy for discussion.

REFERENCES

1. Finch CE. *Longevity, Senescence and the Genome*. Chicago: Chicago University Press, 1990
2. Rose MR. *The Evolutionary Biology of Ageing*. New York: Oxford University Press, 1991
3. Finch CE, Kirkwood TBL. *Chance, Development and Ageing*. Oxford: Oxford University Press, 1999
4. Finch CE. Variations in senescence and longevity include the possibility of negligible senescence. *J Gerontol* 1998;53A:B235–9
5. Finch CE, Pike MC, Witten M. Slow mortality rate accelerations during ageing approximate those of humans. *Science* 1990;249:902–5
6. Tietze C. Reproductive span and rate of reproduction among Hutterite women. *Fertil Steril* 1957;8:89–97
7. Fédération CECOS, Schwartz D, Mayoux NJ. Female fecundity as a function of age. Results of artificial insemination in 2193 nulliparous women with azoospermic husbands. *N Engl J Med* 1982;306:404–6
8. Carey JR, Gruenfelder C. Population biology of the elderly. In Wachter K, Finch CE, eds. *Between Zeus and the Salmon: The Biodemography of Longevity*. Washington DC: National Academy Press, 1997:127–60
9. Treloar AE, Boynton RE, Behn BG, *et al*. Variation of the human menstrual cycle through reproductive life. *Int J Fertil* 1967;12:77–126
10. Welt CK, McNicholl DJ, Taylor AE, *et al*. Female reproductive ageing is marked by decreased secretion of dimeric inhibin. *J Clin Endocrinol Metab* 1999;84:105–11
11. Stern K, McClintock MK. Regulation of ovulation by human pheromones. *Nature (London)* 1998;392:177–9
12. vom Saal FS, Finch CE, Nelson JF. Natural history and mechanisms of reproductive aging in humans, laboratory rodents, and other selected vertebrates. In Knobil E, Neill JD, eds. *The Physiology of Reproduction*. New York: Raven Press, 1994:1213–314
13. Gosden RG, Telfer E. Scaling of follicular sizes in mammalian ovaries. *J Zool* 1987; 211:157–68

14. Cuckle HS, Wald NJ, Thompson SG. Estimating a woman's risk of having a pregnancy associated with Down's syndrome using her age and serum alpha-fetoprotein level. *Br J Obstet Gynaecol* 1987;94:387–402
15. Faddy MJ, Gosden RG, Gougeon A, *et al*. Accelerated disappearance of ovarian follicles in mid-life – implications for forecasting menopause. *Hum Reprod* 1992;7:1342–6
16. Jones EC, Krohn PL. The relationship between age, numbers of oocytes and fertility in virgin and multiparous mice. *J Endocrinol* 1961;21:469–96
17. Faddy MJ, Gosden RG, Edwards RG. Ovarian follicle dynamics in mice: a comparative study of three inbred strains and an F1 hybrid. *J Endocrinol* 1983;96:23–33
18. Snieder H, MacGregor AJ, Spector TD. Genes control the cessation of a woman's reproductive life: a twin study of hysterectomy and age at menopause. *J Clin Endocrinol Metab* 1998;83:1875–80
19. Treloar SA, Do K-A, Martin NG. Genetic influences on the age at menopause. *Lancet* 1998;352:1084–5
20. Lerner SP, Anderson CP, Walford RL, Finch CE. Genotypic influences on reproductive ageing of inbred female mice: effects of H-2 and non-H-2 alleles. *Biol Reprod* 1988;38:1035–43
21. Gosden RG, Faddy MJ. Mathematical models for predicting the timing of menopause. *Prog Reprod Med* 1995;II:95–102
22. Aschheim P Resultats fournis par la greffe heterochrone des ovaries dans l'étude de la regulation hypothalamo-hypophyso-ovarienne de la ratte senile. *Gerontologia* 1965;10:65–75
23. Felicio LS, Nelson JF, Gosden RG, *et al*. Restoration of ovulatory cycles by young ovarian grafts in ageing mice: potentiation by long-term ovariectomy decreases with age. *Proc Natl Acad Sci USA* 1983;80:6076–80
24. Finch CE, Felicio LS, Mobbs CV, *et al*. Ovarian and steroidal influences on neuroendocrine aging processes in female rodents. *Endocr Rev* 1984;5:467–97
25. Kohama SG, Anderson CP, Osterburg HH, *et al*. Oral administration of estradiol to young C57BL/6J mice induces age-like neuroendocrine dysfunctions in the regulation of estrous cycles. *Biol Reprod* 1989;41:227–32
26. Wise PM, Smith MJ, Dubai DB, *et al*. Neuroendocrine influences and repercussions of the menopause. *Endocr Rev* 1999;20:243–8
27. Richardson SJ, Senikas V, Nelson JF. Follicular depletion during the menopausal transition: evidence for accelerated loss and ultimate exhaustion. *J Clin Endocrinol Metab* 1987;65:1231–7
28. Santoro N, Banwell T, Tortoriello D, *et al*. Effects of ageing and gonadal failure on the hypothalamic–pituitary axis in women. *Am J Obstet Gynecol* 1998;178:732–9
29. vom Saal FS, Moyer CL. Prenatal effects on reproductive capacity during ageing in female mice. *Biol Reprod* 1985;32:1116–26
30. Felicio LS, Finch CE, Gosden RG, *et al*. Effects of long-term ovariectomy on the potential for oestrous cyclicity and pregnancy disclosed by ovarian grafts in ageing mice. *J Physiol* 1984;346:122P
31. Brook JD, Gosden RG, Chandley AC. Maternal ageing and aneuploid embryos-evidence from the mouse that biological and not chronological age is the important influence. *Hum Genet* 1984;66:41–5
32. Henderson SA, Edwards RG. Chiasma frequency and maternal age in mammals. *Nature (London)* 1968;218:22–8
33. Phillips OP, Cromwell S, Rivas M, *et al*. Trisomy 21 and maternal age of menopause: does reproductive age rather than chronological age influence risk of non-disjunction? *Hum Genet* 1995;95:117–18

34. van Montfrans JM, Dorland M, Oosterhuis GJE, *et al*. Increased concentrations of follicle-stimulating hormone in mothers of children with Down's syndrome. *Lancet* 1999;353:1853–4
35. Nasseri A, Mukherjee T, Grifo JA, *et al*. Elevated day 3 serum follicle stimulating hormone and/or estradiol may predict fetal aneuploidy. *Fertil Steril* 1999;71:715–18
36. Forabosco A, Sforza C, de Pol A, *et al*. Morphometric study of the human neonatal ovary. *Anat Rec* 1991;231:201–8
37. Ohkubo Y, Shirayoshi Y, Nakatsuji N. Autonomous regulation of proliferation and growth arrest in mouse primordial germ cells studied by mixed and clonal cultures. *Exp Cell Res* 1996;222:291–7
38. Keefe DL, Niven-Fairchild T, Powell S, *et al*. Mitochondrial deoxyribonucleic acid deletions in oocytes and reproductive ageing in women. *Fertil Steril* 1995;64:577–83
39. Nelson JF, Gosden RG, Felicio LS. Effect of dietary restriction on estrous cyclicity and follicular reserves in ageing C57BL/6J mice. *Biol Reprod* 1985;32:515–22
40. Jones EC, Krohn PL. The effect of hypophysectomy on age changes in the ovaries of mice. *J Endocrinol* 1961;21:497–509
41. Oktay K, Briggs D, Gosden RG. Ontogeny of follicle-stimulating hormone receptor gene expression in isolated human ovarian follicles. *J Clin Endocrinol Metab* 1997; 82:3748–51
42. Ataya K, Rao LV, Lawrence E, *et al*. Luteinizing hormone-releasing hormone agonist inhibits cyclophosphamide-induced ovarian follicular depletion in rhesus monkeys. *Biol Reprod* 1995;52:365–72
43. Gosden RG, Wade JC, Fraser HM, *et al*. Impact of congenital or experimental hypogonadotrophism on radiation sensitivity of the mouse ovary. *Hum Reprod* 1997;12: 2483–8
44. Ataya K, Tadros M, Ramahi A. Gonadotropin-releasing hormone agonist inhibits physiologic ovarian follicular loss. *Acta Endocrinol* 1989;121:55–60
45. Perez GI, Robles R, Knudson CM, *et al*. Prolongation of ovarian lifespan into advanced chronological age by *Bax*-deficiency. *Nature Genet* 1999;21:200–3
46. Baird DT, Webb R, Campbell BK, *et al*. Long-term ovarian function in sheep after ovariectomy and transplantation of autografts stored at – 196°C. *Endocrinology* 1999;140:462–71
47. Snowdon DA, Kane RL, Beeson WL, *et al*. Is early natural menopause a biologic marker of health and aging? *Am J Publ Health* 1989;79:709–14

1

Why do women have a mid-life menopause? Grandmothering and the evolution of human longevity

K. Hawkes, J.F. O'Connell and N.G. Blurton Jones

INTRODUCTION

In healthy women, fecundity is statistically zero by age 50, whereas other body processes continue for decades longer at a large fraction of maximum capacity. Among other species in the primate order, the timing and rate of development and ageing vary widely. In all of them, however, the rare females who reach menopause show age-related failure in other physiological processes at the same time. The fact that women experience menopause at mid-life, the ovaries senescing completely, well before the rest of the body, distinguishes humans from other primates and almost all other mammals.

The key to this distinctive mid-life menopause may also be the key to some of the other things that distinguish us and our evolutionary lineage from ancestral and collateral hominids. Our goal here is to explain that assertion, first reviewing evidence against the widely held view that postmenopausal longevity is a recent novelty.

HUMAN LONGEVITY

Historical demography

If demographic statistics are considered for many contemporary human populations, some are surely novel in human experience. Two of the authors live in the state of Utah, where today average life expectancy for a newborn girl is more than 80 years. This pattern is typical of most of the USA, Europe and the rest of the industrial world (Figure 1)[1]. Its consequence is an increasingly 'rectangular' population pyramid, with the fraction of people in the 'golden years' large and growing. This unprecedented pattern is causing enormous changes in the familial, political, commercial and medical dimensions of social life. However, the importance of those changes should not hide the

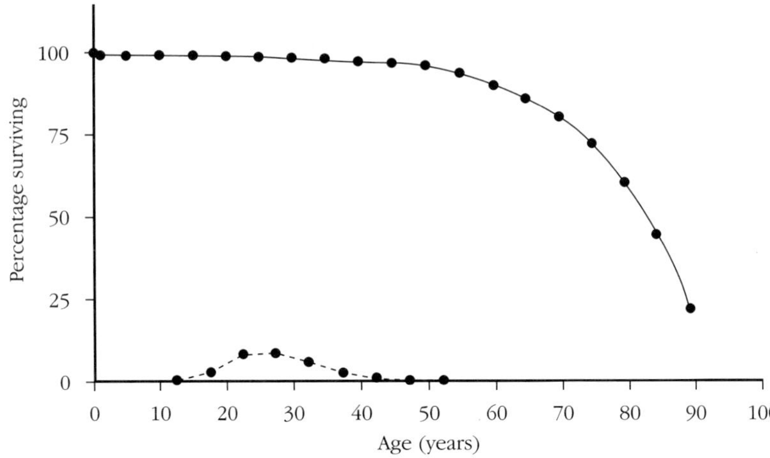

Figure 1 Utah 1990 age-specific fertility (---●---) and survival (–●–). Probability of survival, or annual fecundity (in daughters) indicated on the *y* axis. Data from reference 1

Table 1 Historical demography in France. From references 2 and 3

Year	e_x0	*At maturity, probability of living past 45*	e_x45
1985	79	0.96	36
1950	69	0.92	30
1926	57	0.84	27
1900	48	0.75	25
1850	39	0.72	24

e_x0, life expectancy at birth; e_x45, life expectancy at 45 years

much older pattern of postmenopausal longevity that appears to predate the evolution of *Homo sapiens*.

The older pattern can be obscured when life expectancy, an average, is misinterpreted as something like maximum lifespan. French historical demography illustrates this (Table 1)[2,3]. Life expectancy at birth (e_x0), near 80 in the last few years, was less than half that in 1850. The main determinant of the variation in life expectancy at birth across this time period is infant and juvenile mortality. In the early 19th century those who did not die as children had a good chance of long life ahead. Of those who reached adulthood, 72% lived past the end of their fertility, and those averaged another quarter century of survival (e_x45). The age-specific rates are shown in Figure 2.

Hunter-gatherers

People in 19th-century France were living in an agrarian and just industrializing society, depending on subsistence and economic systems that are

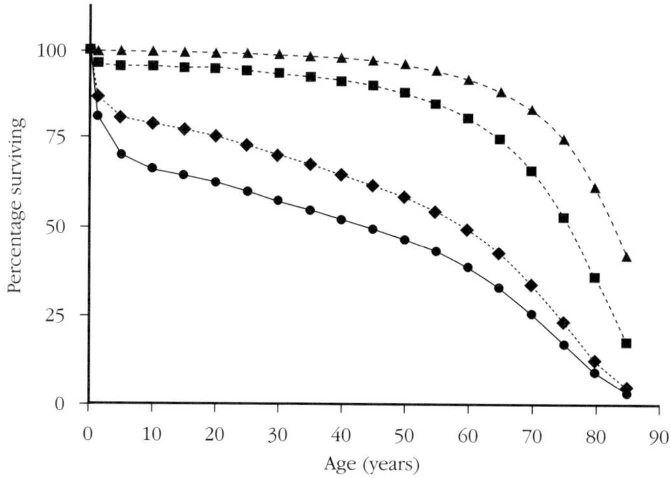

Figure 2 French historical demography. Age-specific probability of survival for 1985 (---▲---), 1950 (---■---), 1900 (---◆---) and 1850 (–●–) indicated on the *y* axis. Data from references 2 and 3

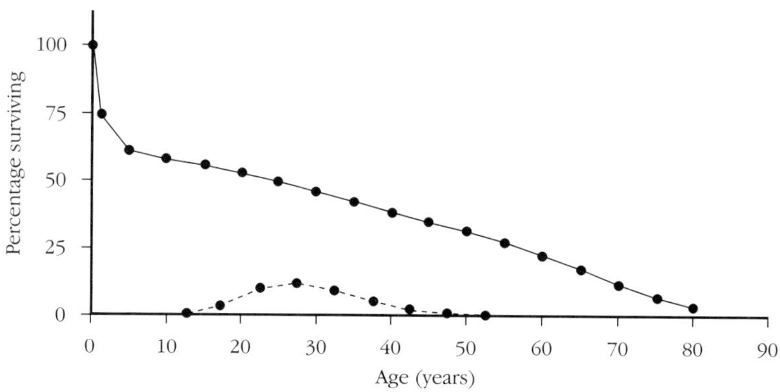

Figure 3 !Kung age-specific fertility (in daughters) (---●---) and survival (–●–). Data from reference 4

quite recent from the perspective of human evolution. Farming and herding are no older than about 10 000 years. However, we can begin to factor out some demographic effects of agriculture by looking at populations in which people live by hunting and gathering, and are largely independent of modern medicine and domesticated foods. Demographic data have now been compiled on a few such populations. We discuss three of the best described cases. They are populations with quite different recent genetic histories, spanning a wide range of ecological circumstances – from South American forests to the arid African tropics. Figure 3 shows age-specific

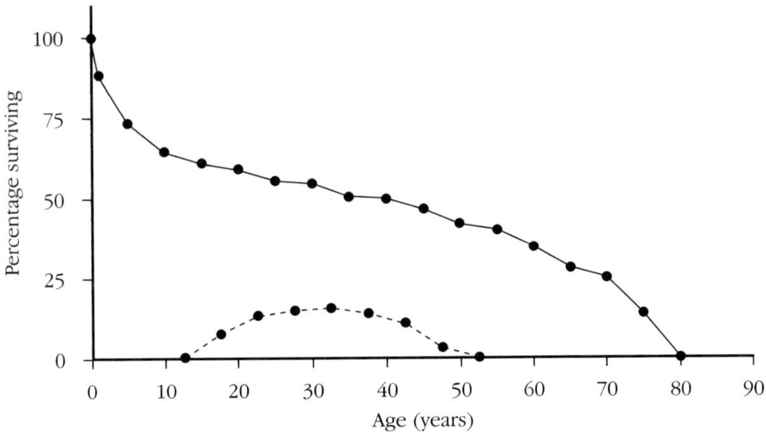

Figure 4 Aché age-specific fertility (in daughters) (---●---) and survival (–●–). Data from reference 5

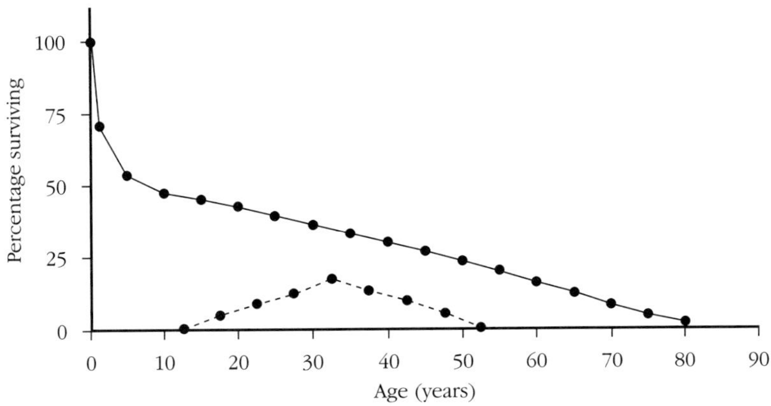

Figure 5 Hadza age-specific fertility (in daughters) (---●---) and survival (–●–). Data from reference 6

fertility (in daughters/year) and survival for the !Kung of Botswana and Namibia in the 1960s, reported by Howell[4]. Figure 4 shows the Aché of Eastern Paraguay before settlement in the 1970s, reported by Hill and Hurtado[5]. Figure 5 shows the Hadza of Northern Tanzania estimated by Blurton Jones and colleagues[6].

In all these populations life expectancy at birth was in the 30s, but anyone who reached adulthood was likely to live past menopause (66–78% did) and those alive at the end of their fertility had an average of two more

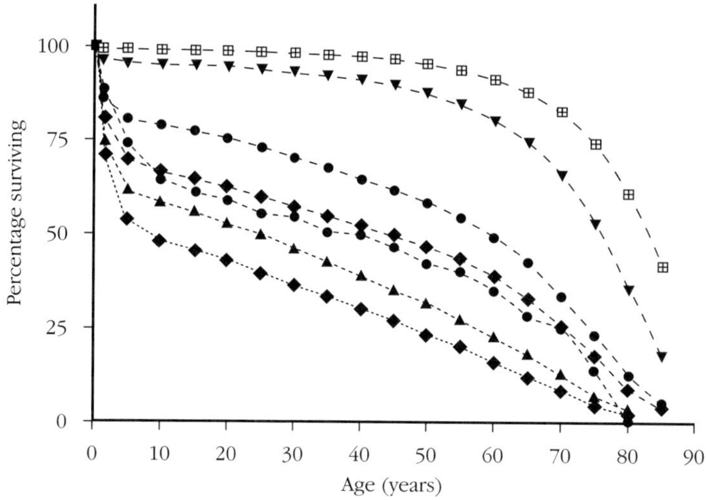

Figure 6 French historical and hunter-gatherer demography. ···◆···, Hadza; ---●---, Aché; ---▲---, !Kung; ---◆---, France 1850; – –●– –, France 1900; – –▼– –, France 1950; – –⊞– –, France 1985. Data reproduced from references 2–6

decades of survival. In these cases, as with other subsistence systems, menopause is not rare, it is the usual human thing (Figure 6).

OTHER SPECIES

The distinctiveness of this human pattern is clear when compared to age-specific fertility and survival in other mammalian species. Chimpanzees (Figure 7) are our nearest living relatives. Data have also been published on baboons (Figure 8)[8] and lions (Figure 9)[8]. It is very rare in all three species for an adult female to live past the end of her fertility.

LIFE HISTORY EVOLUTION

Aging

The aging patterns of other primates are consistent with some general expectations about the evolution of life histories. All aspects of physiology suffer similar age-related declines in performance at about the same time. Evolutionary explanations of aging turn on the proposition that the force of selection weakens with age because, even if the risk of death were constant, cohorts inevitably get smaller over time. Positive age-specific effects are worth

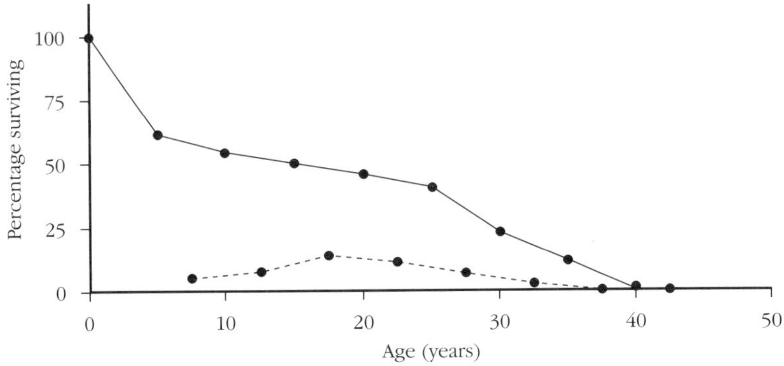

Figure 7 Gombe chimpanzee age-specific fertility (in daughters) (---●---) and survival (–●–). Data from reference 7

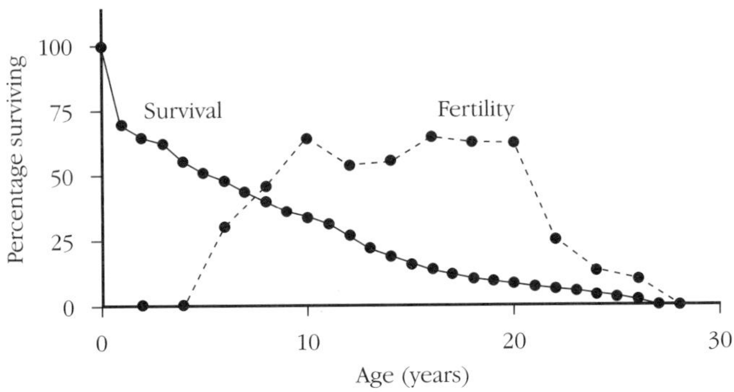

Figure 8 Gombe baboon age-specific fertility (---●---) (in daughters) and survival (–●–). Data from reference 8

more earlier in life, and negative effects less damaging later[9,10]. Moreover, performance declines in all systems at once; for example, longer-lasting kidneys are worthless if everything else fails, but very valuable if other systems are still in working order. This results in selection chipping away at outliers, maintaining general coincidence in the senescence of all aspects of an organism.

Stopping early

What then of mid-life menopause? In a 1957 paper that laid out many of the key ideas in modern life history theory, Williams[9] examined it. He suggested that, in species where maternal care was crucial to offspring survival, mothers who stopped reproducing early might end up with more surviving children. If babies were unlikely to survive their mother's death, and if pregnancy and parturition were more debilitating with age, then older mothers would do better

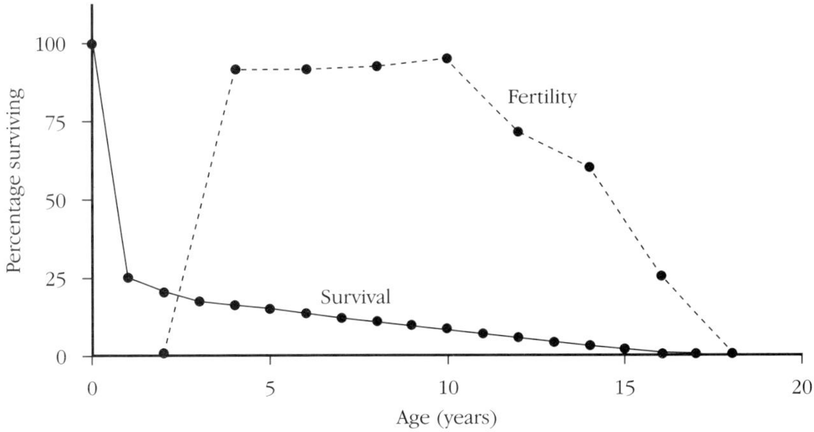

Figure 9 Serengeti lion age-specific fertility (---●---) (in daughters) and survival (–●–). Data from reference 8

to stop giving birth. They would leave more descendants if they allocated their late maternal efforts to increasing the welfare of children already born.

Williams' 'stopping early' hypothesis seems persuasive, and has often been reinvented. However, there are some compelling reasons to reject it and to look at mid-life menopause another way[11–13]. First, primates generally require substantial maternal care for offspring survival. In chimpanzees there is the famous case of Flo, whose life Jane Goodall chronicled at Gombe[14]. Flo was relatively fragile with age when her last baby was born. She died shortly thereafter, and so did the baby. Her previously born son, bereft of his mother, also died soon after. Goodall has since reported other examples of late-born babies dying with their mothers, and sometimes with an older sibling[15]. The examples illustrate the low survival chances of late babies and the cost they impose on a mother's reproductive success. They also show that chimpanzees continue to have them anyway.

A second, and related, reason for skepticism about the 'stopping early' hypothesis is the relatively *short* postnatal period during which human children are directly dependent on their mothers. Hill and Hurtado[5] have shown that, among Aché foragers in eastern Paraguay, a mother's death has no statistically significant effect on the survival of offspring who are over 5 years of age. Nevertheless, among human foragers, women at the age of last birth average about 20 years of additional survival. Moreover, human mothers have the next baby sooner than chimpanzee mothers do, a strong indication that there is more involved than extended maternal care.

A third line of evidence against the 'stopping early' hypothesis is entirely phylogenetic. Compared to our nearest living relatives, the other great apes, humans do not 'stop early'[5]. From a comparative perspective, our fertile spans reflect an ancestral condition that is conserved among all large-bodied

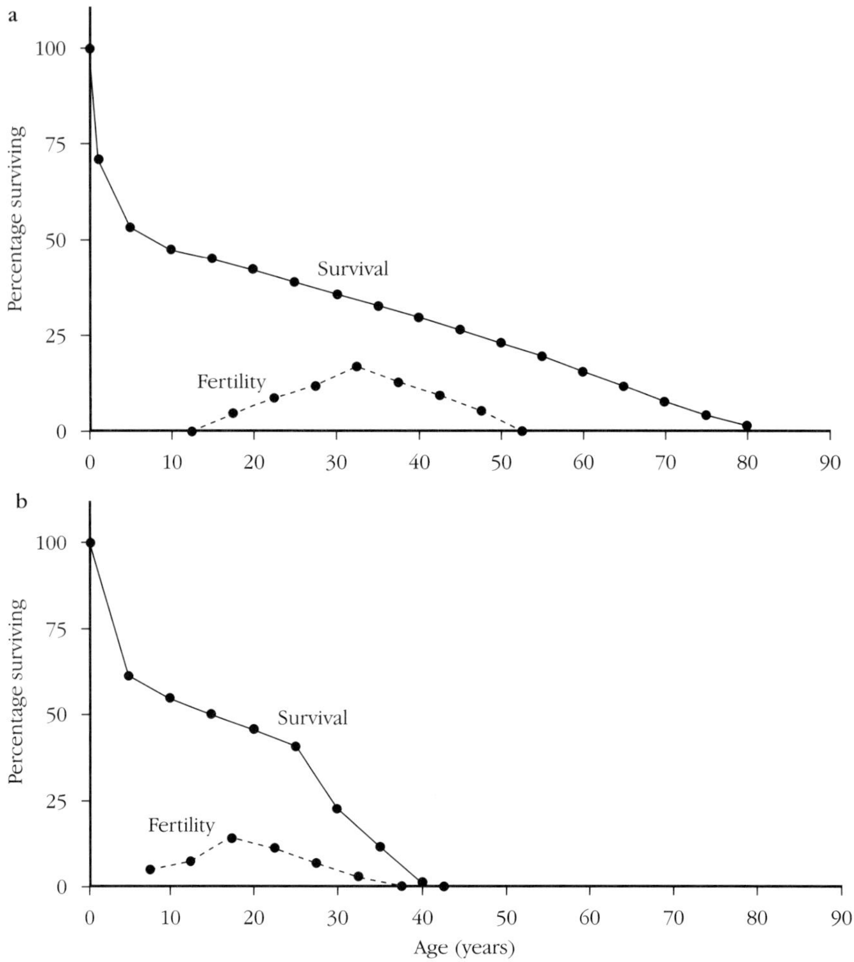

Figure 10 Human (Hadza) (a) and chimpanzee (Gombe) (b) age-specific fertility (---●---) (in daughters) and survival (–●–) on the same age scale. Data from reference 7

apes. Schultz compared life history features across the primate order and drew attention to this 30 years ago[16]. He depicted chimpanzees and humans with childbearing careers of similar duration, but very different postmenopausal lifespans. When the age-specific fertility and survival (under high mortality conditions) of humans[6] and chimpanzees[7] are compared directly (Figure 10), it is the adult survival curves that differ most. The *derived* human feature is this remarkable postmenopausal longevity[11–13].

Living longer

What selection pressures could have slowed senescence in other aspects of physiology without much change in the rate and timing of ovarian senescence? Lessons from hunter-gatherer ethnography provide a promising hypothesis.

Lessons from the Hadza

Among Hadza hunter-gatherers in Northern Tanzania[6,17] men define themselves as hunters and specialize in taking large ungulates[18]. However, successes are very unpredictable and when a hunter *is* successful the meat is widely shared, only a small fraction going to his own family. This makes hunting a poor strategy for supporting the household. People, especially children, need to eat every day. Women attend to the day-to-day business of feeding the children (and themselves) by gathering plant foods. Among the Hadza young children are energetic foragers: in some seasons those as young as 5 years old get half of their nutrient requirements by their own efforts[19]. Mothers take advantage of their children's foraging capacities, choosing to focus on foods the children can handle efficiently when those items are in season[20]. Postmenopausal women are active foragers, spending even more time gathering food than do women of childbearing age[21]. The extra time is largely devoted to digging deeply buried tubers, the year-round diet staple. Digging them requires strength and skill beyond the capacities of young children, but the long-experienced senior women earn rates equivalent to those of younger adults.

The grandmother hypothesis

The seasonal and age-related variation in Hadza foraging highlights some likely causes and consequences of human economic interdependence that have large evolutionary implications. In humans, weaned offspring depend on others to supply a substantial component of their nutrition. A chimpanzee just after weaning gets its own food. In one sense this seems to make human children a greater burden on their mothers. Children require more help with some foods than others. But if human children had to depend on their own foraging, they and their mothers – like chimpanzees – would be tied to foods that the young children could manage themselves. Food sharing allows adults accompanied by young juveniles to exploit resources and invade habitats that they otherwise could not.

Mother–child food sharing also provides a novel opportunity for senior females to have large effects on their own fitness. When a child is not able to feed itself at weaning, a mother who continues to provision it can allocate less effort to preparing for the next baby. This is an opportunity for grandmothers, one that has no parallel in other primates. An ageing female whose fertility is declining can have a large effect on her own fitness by provisioning a just-weaned grandchild, so that her daughter can produce the next grandchild more quickly. More vigorous perimenopausal females can have larger effects on the fertility of younger kin. This would strengthen selection against senescence in older females, lower adult mortality and increase average adult lifespans.

The Hadza again

Interrelationships predicted by this scenario are evident among the Hadza[11]. The foraging effort of a mother who is not nursing has a measurable effect on the nutritional welfare of her weaned children. At the birth of a newborn her foraging effort declines (at the same time, her own nutritional needs go up with lactation) and the link between her work and the nutritional welfare of her weaned children disappears. Now the weight gains of those children depend on the foraging effort of their grandmother.

The evolution of grandmothers

Here is the scenario: imagine ancestral populations with a chimpanzee-like life history. Ecological changes constrict the forests and the availability of fruits that young juveniles can handle. Increasing aridity and seasonality favor plants that cope well with dry seasons, for example, by holding starches in underground storage organs. Such resources can give high return rates, but only to those with the strength and skill to extract and process them. Young juveniles cannot do it. To rely on these resources and succeed in these environments mothers must provision offspring who are still too young to extract and process the tubers for themselves. Older females whose own fertility is declining are less likely to have weanlings of their own needing help. If they feed their just-weaned grandchildren, their daughters can have shorter interbirth intervals without reductions in offspring survivorship. The more vigorous elders will thus leave more descendants. In this scenario there is no pressure to lengthen fertile spans. Older females who continued to have babies themselves could not contribute to the increased fertility of young adults, which would erase the selective advantage for vigorous adaptive performance late in life – collapsing life histories back towards the chimpanzee-like pattern.

LIFE HISTORY INVARIANTS

This verbal argument about grandmothering is generally consistent with evolutionary theories of senescence, and some initial population genetic modelling supports it[22]. Combining it with recent life history theory developed by Charnov and colleagues[23–26] allows some actual tests. The tests in turn reveal previously unappreciated relationships among human life history traits, displaying them as systematic adjustments to a basic primate pattern.

Mortality and maturity

Charnov's assembly rules for mammalian life histories highlight relationships between variables that remain constant over transformations in the values of the individual variables. They provide a framework predicting life history consequences that would follow the evolution of grandmothering. His theory begins with a simple growth model. From weaning to maturity, growth is an allometric function of juvenile size. At maturity females redirect this production from their own growth into babies. Selection sets the age at maturity to maximize lifetime reproduction, given that growing longer means getting larger and so having more productive effort to put into babies, but waiting also means running the risk of dying before reproducing at all. If mortality rates around this age are high and lifespans are short, then the optimal age at maturity will be relatively early. If mortality rates are low and lifespans are long, then growing longer before maturing will be worthwhile. There will be time for the gains to pay off.

Among mammals generally (including primates), the relationship between average adult lifespans (the inverse of the instantaneous adult mortality rate (M) and age at maturity (α) is positive. The product αM is approximately invariant (Figure 11)[23].

If, as postulated in the grandmother hypothesis, the postmenopausal component of human lifespans is spent contributing to reproduction, then survival after menopause adds to the time over which the gains of growing longer will pay off. Grandmothering should therefore favor delaying maturity. Our long lifespans (low adult mortality rate (M)) should be associated with a late age at maturity (high α). We are in fact very late maturers, another aspect of human life histories that Schultz depicted in his classic treatment[16]. He picked out both late maturity and long postmenopausal survival as distinctively human.

If longer human adult lifespans are paying off in reproduction, and the tradeoffs captured in Charnov's model apply, then as M goes down, α goes up. Their product remains more or less invariant. Our αM should be about the same as that of other hominoids, and it is (Table 2)[27]. Our late maturity and long childhoods are as predicted by a combination of the grandmother hypothesis and Charnov's assembly rules.

Maturity and fertility

There is another systematic effect that can be expected if the grandmother hypothesis is correct and these assembly rules capture basic tradeoffs that apply to all mammals. At maturity, longer lived mothers have more to gain from future reproduction and so allocate relatively more to their own maintenence and less to current fertility. Charnov's theory deals with the *inverse* relationship between age at maturity and annual fecundity – the average number of babies produced each year (b) – through the growth allometry.

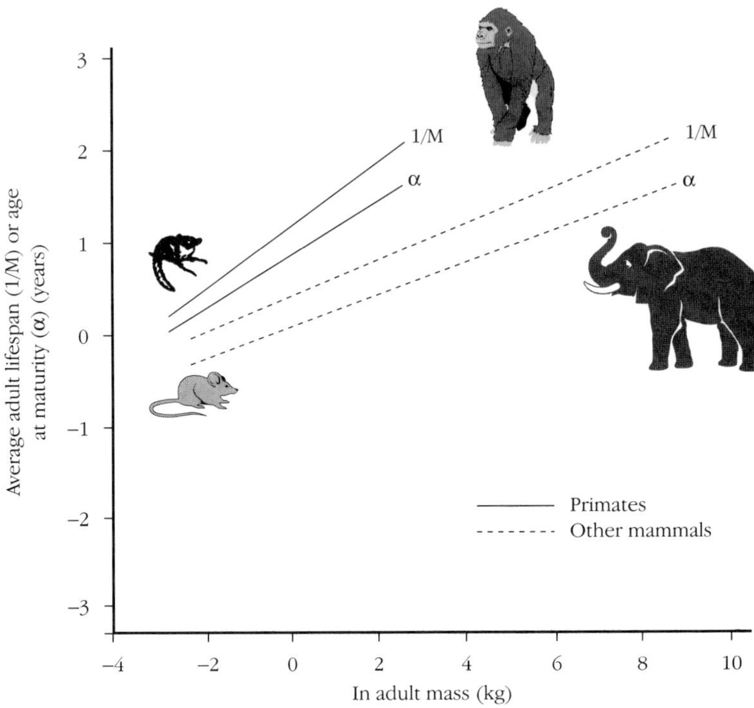

Figure 11 Age at maturity and average adult lifespan in primates and other mammals. Figure reproduced from reference 26 with permission of Wiley-Liss, Inc., a subsidiary of John Wiley & Sons, Inc

Table 2 Average adult lifespan (1/M) and period from weaning to maturity (α) for four modern hominoids. From reference 27, using data from references 4–6 and 28–31

	Average adult lifespan (1/M)	*Weaning to maturity (α)*	*αM*
Orangutans	17.9	8.3	0.46
Gorillas	13.9	6.3	0.45
Chimpanzees	17.9	8.2	0.46
Humans	32.9	14.5	0.44

Later maturity means a longer growing period, so larger mothers. While larger mothers have more production to put into babies, they also make babies that are larger. So they make them at a slower rate (Figure 12)[26]. Consequently the product of α and b is another invariant.

If human longevity evolved because of grandmothering, then the fertility of childbearing-aged women should reflect the grandmothers' help. Human fertilities should be substantially higher than the fertilities of a grandmotherless primate, because the baby production of a whole lifespan is concentrated in the premenopausal years. Table 3[26] shows this to be the case – one thing Schultz was wrong about. He assumed a general lengthening of

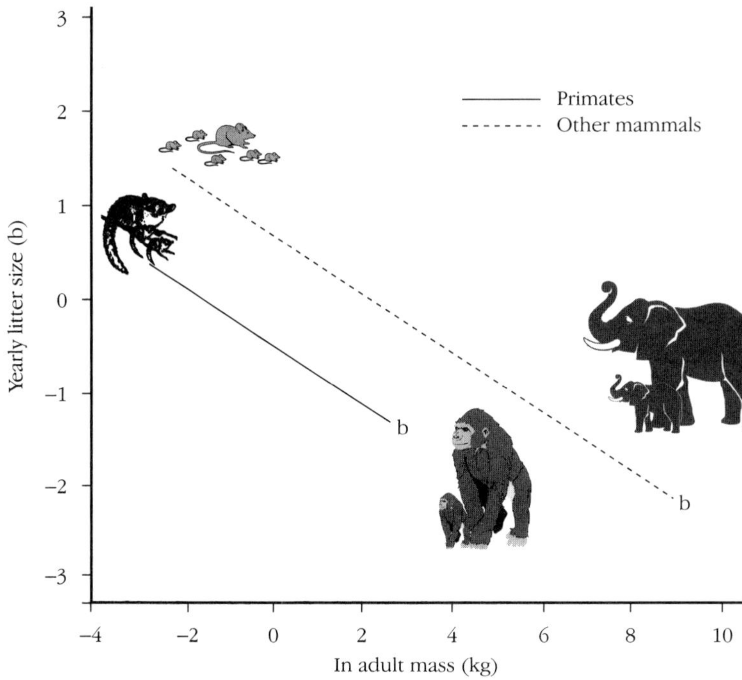

Figure 12 Annual fertility in daughters (b) and adult body size in primates and other mammals. Figure reproduced from reference 26 with permission of Wiley-Liss, Inc., a subsidiary of John Wiley & Sons, Inc

Table 3 Period from weaning to maturity and annual fertility in daughters for four modern hominoids. From reference 27, using data from references 4–6 and 28–31

	Weaning to maturity (α)	*Daughters per year (b)*	*αb*
Orangutans	8.3	0.063	0.52
Gorillas	6.3	0.126	0.79
Chimpanzees	8.2	0.087	0.71
Humans	14.5	0.142	2.05

all growth stages, so depicted our weaning ages as higher than those of chimpanzees, but they are not. Instead we have interbirth intervals that are quite short, and so fertilities that are extremely high for our age at maturity (Table 3), exactly the results predicted of grandmothers.

PALEOANTHROPOLOGY

These comparative lines of evidence show that distinctively human life history features are consistent with predictions of the grandmother hypothesis. The hypothesis also makes predictions about the ecological circumstances, timing and sequence of specific evolutionary transitions in our ancestral past. Only the partial record of paleoanthropology preserves direct evidence of those transitions. Now there are fossil specimens from more than a dozen other species of hominid in three or four genera over the past 5 million years. Initial exploration of this fragmentary but increasingly richer record finds paleontological, paleoecological and archeological evidence generally consistent with the hypothesis that grandmothering was the key adaptation distinguishing the first widely successful member of our genus from ancestral and collateral hominids[32]. This hypothesis is a radical departure from the popular view that hunting and paternal provisioning are the foundations of human evolution. One of the things it explains is our mid-life menopause. A wide array of corollary hypotheses await testing.

ACKNOWLEDGEMENT

The authors wish to thank Ursula Hanly for drafting the figures.

REFERENCES

1. State of Utah Governor's Office of Planning and Budget. *Demographic and Economic Analysis*. http://www.governor.state.ut.us/dsa/demographics
2. Keyfitz N, Flieger W. *World Population: An Analysis of Vital Data*. Chicago: University of Chicago Press, 1968
3. Keyfitz N, Flieger W. *World Population Growth and Ageing: Demographic Trends in the Late Twentieth Century*. Chicago: University of Chicago Press, 1990
4. Howell N. *Demography of the Dobe !Kung*. New York: Academic Press, 1979
5. Hill K, Hurtado AM. *Ache Life History: The Ecology and Demography of a Foraging People*. Hawthorne, NY: Aldine de Gruyter, 1996
6. Blurton Jones NG, Smith LC, O'Connell JF, *et al*. Demography of the Hadza, an increasing and high density population of savanna foragers. *Am J Phys Anthropol* 1992;89:159–81
7. McElreath R. *Why Menopause Indeed?* Department of Anthropology, UCLA, LA. Unpublished manuscript
8. Packer C, Tatar M, Collins A. Reproductive cessation in female mammals. *Nature (London)* 1998;392:807–11
9. Williams GC. Pleiotropy, natural selection, and the evolution of senescence. *Evolution* 1957;11:398–411
10. Kirkwood TL, Rose MR. Evolution of senescence: late survival sacrificed for reproduction. *Philos Trans R Soc B* 1991;332:15–34
11. Hawkes K, O'Connell JF, Blurton Jones NG. Hadza women's time allocation, offspring production, and the evolution of long postmenopausal life spans. *Curr Anthropol* 1997;38:551–77
12. Kaplan H. The evolution of the human life course. In Wachter K, Finch C, eds. *Between Zeus and the Salmon: The Biodemography of Ageing*. Washington, DC: National Academy of Sciences, 1997:175–211
13. Hill K, Hurtado AM. Parker and colleagues' model of menopause in humans. *Hum Nature* 1999;10:199–204

14. Goodall J. *The Chimpanzees of Gombe: Patterns of Behavior*. Cambridge: Harvard University Press, 1986
15. Goodall J. Gombe: highlights and current research. In Heltne P, Marquardt L, eds. *Understanding Chimpanzees*. Cambridge: Harvard University Press, 1989:2–21
16. Schultz AH. *The Life of Primates*. New York: Universe Books, 1969
17. Woodburn J. An introduction to Hadza ecology. In Lee R, DeVore I, eds. *Man the Hunter*. Chicago: Aldine, 1968:49–55
18. Hawkes K, O'Connell JF, Blurton Jones NG. Hunting income patterns among the Hadza: big game, common goods, foraging goals, and the evolution of the human diet. *Philos Trans R Soc B* 1991;334:243–51
19. Blurton Jones NG, Hawkes K, O'Connell JF. Studying costs of children in two foraging societies: implications for schedules of reproduction. In Standon V, Foley R, eds. *Comparative Socioecology of Mammals and Man*. London: Blackwell, 1989:365–90
20. Hawkes K, O'Connell JF, Blurton Jones NG. Hadza children's foraging: juvenile dependency, social arrangements and mobility among hunter-gatherers. *Curr Anthropol* 1995;36:688–700
21. Hawkes K, O'Connell JF, Blurton Jones NG. Hardworking Hadza grandmothers. In Standon V, Foley R, eds. *Comparative Socioecology of Mammals and Man*. London: Blackwell, 1989:341–65
22. Jones JH. A life-cycle approach to the problem of post-reproductive survival. Presented at *HBES Meetings*, Salt Lake City, UT, June 1999
23. Charnov EL. Evolution of life history variation in female mammals. *Proc Natl Acad Sci USA* 1991;88:1134–7
24. Charnov EL. *Life History Invariants: Some Explorations of Symmetry in Evolutionary Ecology*. Oxford: Oxford University Press, 1993
25. Charnov EL, Berrigan D. Dimensionless numbers and the assembly rules for life histories. *Philos Trans R Soc B* 1991;33:241–8
26. Charnov EL, Berrigan D. Why do female primates have such long lifespans and so few babies? or life in the slow lane. *Evolut Anthropol* 1993;1:191–4
27. Hawkes K, O'Connell JF, Blurton Jones NG, *et al*. Grandmothering, menopause, and the evolution of human life histories. *Proc Natl Acad Sci USA* 1998;95:1336–9
28. Galdikis B, Wood J. Birth spacing patterns in humans and apes. *Am J Phys Anthropol* 1990;63:185–91
29. Leighton M, Seal US, Soemarna K, *et al*. Orangutan life history and VORTEX analysis. In Nadler RD, Galdikas BFM, Sheeran LK, *et al*., eds. *The Neglected Ape*. New York: Plenum, 1995:97–107
30. Nishida T, Takasaki H, Takahata Y. Demography and reproductive profiles. In Nishida T, ed. *The Chimpanzees of the Mahale Mountains: Sexual and Life History Strategies*. Tokyo: University of Tokyo Press, 1990:63–97
31. Stewart KJ, Harcourt AH, Watts DP. Determinants of fertility in wild gorillas and other primates. In Diggory P, Potts M, Teper S, eds. *Natural Human Fertility: Social and Biological Determinants*. Hampshire: MacMillian Press, 1988:22–38
32. O'Connell JF, Hawkes K, Blurton Jones N. Grandmothering and the evolution of *Homo erectus*. *J Hum Evolut* 1999;36:461–85

2

Similarities of general and reproductive aging

T.B.L. Kirkwood

INTRODUCTION

This symposium fittingly celebrates the pioneering work of Reinier de Graaf on female reproductive biology. Another pioneer deserving acknowledgement in the field of reproductive aging is August Weismann, who in the late 19th century recognized the fundamental distinction between germline and somatic cells and quickly saw the relevance of this distinction for the science of cellular aging[1]. The germ cell lineage must, in a sense, be immortal, in order to transmit genes through future generations. Somatic cells have no such requirement, since they die with the organism. From this distinction has grown the concept of the 'disposable soma theory' that offers an explanation of why and how we age[2]. This paper discusses some implications of the disposable soma theory and reviews two examples of recent work on the cellular basis of aging and longevity as a background to considering similarities between general aging and female reproductive aging in mammals.

THE DISPOSABLE SOMA CONCEPT

The disposable soma theory recognizes that, under pressure of natural selection, organisms can afford only limited investments in the maintenance and repair of somatic cells and tissues. Maintenance systems are often costly and a significant fraction of basal metabolism is concerned with various aspects of maintenance and repair. In the wild, death usually occurs from extrinsic causes (accident, cold, starvation, etc.). The organism requires only enough maintenance to keep somatic cells in good condition through the typical survival period, plus perhaps some 'reserve'. For example, few wild mice survive beyond a year and probably none reach the 3 years of which they are capable in protected conditions. There would be no evolutionary advantage for the mouse, in its existing ecological niche, in having somatic maintenance systems that could provide longer survival, and to do so would incur extra energy costs that might reduce reproductive fitness. On this basis it is predicted that intrinsic aging is caused by progressive accumulation of unrepaired cellular damage, resulting eventually in frailty, disease and finally death.

This concept leads to several testable predictions[3]. Aging is not programmed in the sense that there exists any active mechanism to cause death; instead, lifespan is influenced by 'longevity assurance' genes that control somatic maintenance and repair. There are many maintenance mechanisms, so aging and longevity are likely to be under highly polygenic control. Individual mechanisms may be more or less important in different tissues, e.g. dividing or post-mitotic cells. The levels at which individual genes are set will influence the *average* rate at which damage accumulates or is repaired. However, at a fine scale the process is intrinsically stochastic. Therefore, chance, as well as genetic and environmental factors, may play a significant role[4].

There is growing evidence supporting the concept that aging results from intrinsic trade-offs of the kind suggested by the disposable soma theory, as well as considerable scope for further testing and refinement of these predictions. In addition to trade-offs between maintenance and reproduction, other genetic factors may contribute to the aging phenotype. These include genes that trade advantage to the young organism against survival of the old[5], or there may simply be accumulation within the genome of late-acting deleterious genes that escape the force of natural selection[6].

MOLECULAR AND CELLULAR BASIS OF AGING AND LONGEVITY

The disposable soma theory predicts that the longevity of different species is determined by optimizing the level of somatic maintenance according to the degree of extrinsic hazard in the species' ecological niche. An adaptation that reduces hazard should result in selection pressure to increase maintenance. This might explain the greater longevity of animals that have evolved flight (birds, bats) compared with those that must remain on the ground. It is also likely that the evolution of human longevity can be explained through the reduction in extrinsic mortality resulting from increased brain size and associated developments such as social living. Several comparative studies have tested the corollary that long-lived species have evolved higher intrinsic capacity for repair and stress resistance at the cell level.

One recent study[7] compared the resistance of primary skin fibroblasts from different mammalian species to a range of stressors applied *in vitro*. Cells were mostly grown from a standard biopsy site (inside forelimb) of young donor animals and tested at early passage levels for their resistance to a range of oxidative and non-oxidative stressors (paraquat, hydrogen peroxide, sodium arsenite, sodium hydroxide, *tert*-butyl hydroperoxide). It was found that cell stress resistance, expressed in terms of the dose of the stressor required to kill 90% of the cell population, correlated positively with species' lifespans.

Several maintenance and stress response systems combine to protect cells and tissues from accumulation of damage, and there is a correspondingly large variety of kinds of molecular damage that may contribute to aging. These mechanisms can act in parallel, presenting opportunities for significant interaction and synergy. Network models of biochemical reactions contributing to cellular aging confirm that taking these interactions explicitly into account can explain more of the data on cellular changes associated with aging than can treating individual processes alone[8]. For example, there may be interactions between somatic mutations, oxidative damage caused by reactive oxygen species, aberrant proteins caused by errors in synthesis or post-translational modifications, or damage to subcellular organelles such as mitochondria. Furthermore, the balance between these various candidate mechanisms is likely to be influenced by mitotic activity (or its absence). Dividing cells need to duplicate cell components between successive divisions and are less prone than post-mitotic cells to suffer accumulation of protease-resistant abnormal proteins and defective mitochondria, but more likely to suffer accumulation of somatic mutations through repeated rounds of DNA replication.

Organs and tissues such as the brain, comprising mainly post-mitotic cells, will experience cumulative losses or disruption of irreplaceable cells, leading eventually to impaired function. Tissues comprising mainly dividing cells, such as fibroblasts, may experience reduced rates of cell renewal and turnover. Many dividing cells exhibit a process of cell replicative senescence when cultured *in vitro*. Even though there is scant evidence for limited cell division contributing directly to senescent changes *in vivo*, there is growing interest in the hypothesis that small numbers of senescent cells or small losses in cell division rates may alter proliferative homeostasis of the cell population. A mechanism of special interest in relation to cell replicative senescence is telomere reduction, caused by inactivation of telomerase in most somatic cells. Reactivation of telomerase in cell cultures extends replicative lifespans[9]. However, the extent to which telomere reduction contributes to aging *in vivo* remains uncertain. Telomerase knockout mice do not show accelerated senescence[10].

The effect of age on tissue stem cells is of great interest, since some stem cells must sustain steady proliferation throughout life and any impairment in their function will affect homeostasis. For example, the epithelium lining the gut is continually renewed from proliferation of stem cells located near the base of the intestinal crypts. Although the intestinal epithelium continues to replace its cells without obvious decline, recent evidence indicates that progressive alterations in tissue morphology occur, and are possibly related to intrinsic age changes detected in stem cells[11,12]. A key aspect of the maintenance of integrity of the intestinal epithelium is the propensity of the stem cells to undergo apoptosis following challenge with low doses of stressors. It makes excellent sense teleologically that stem cells, which if damaged would pose a significant risk of cancer, should be subject to stringent 'quality assurance'. The small intestines of old mice show twice the level of apoptosis following low-dose gamma irradiation than that seen in young and middle-aged animals.

RELEVANCE FOR REPRODUCTIVE AGING

Age changes in the reproductive system are most obvious in the case of female ovarian aging, where not only does the finite oocyte store become exhausted but also there is a clear increase in genetic abnormalities with maternal age. Faced with the fact of intrinsic ovarian aging, the intriguing question is how the germline avoids progressive deterioration from generation to generation.

Apart from the increased risk of genetic abnormalities, babies formed from old oocytes are born as young as babies formed from younger oocytes. Two factors that must, at some level, be involved are first, the use of special maintenance systems to protect the germline from damage that accumulates in somatic cell lineages; and second, the action of selection at all stages in the reproductive cycle. One maintenance system that is a prerequisite in germ cells is the action of telomerase. Without telomerase, telomeres would shorten from generation to generation. The telomerase knockout mouse, although unaffected within a single generation, shows abnormalities due to telomere reduction after a number of generations have passed. The existence of special maintenance systems in germ cells was predicted in the original version of the disposable soma theory[13].

The finite nature of the oocyte store and the fact that in humans this store is depleted well before the onset of general senescence are central to the evolutionary puzzle of menopause. This interesting question is discussed elsewhere in this volume (Chapter 12), but it may be noted that there is no reason related to general mechanisms of aging for oocytes not to last longer than 50 years. Human neurons, for example, can function twice as long as this. Furthermore, the comparative analysis cited above shows that cells from long-lived species are endowed with greater maintenance and stress resistance than cells from short-lived species, indicating that natural selection is quite capable in the right circumstances of evolving better long-term repair.

Selection is the most likely explanation for both the high rate of follicular atresia and the significant numbers of spontaneous abortions that occur in early embryogenesis. Selection of this kind is a powerful way of eliminating potential germline defects. Just as tissue stem cells appear to be subject to stringent quality assurance, resulting in activation of the cell death pathway following low-level stresses that would not kill most other cell types, quality checks of ovarian follicles are likely to be of at least equal importance.

The acceleration in the rate of decline of oocyte reserves after a woman has reached her late 30s may reflect the fact that damage of the kind associated with general senescence begins to build up around this time. Models of biochemical mechanisms of cell aging suggest that change is gradual for long periods but accelerates as the terminal stage is reached. If this is indeed the explanation of why ooctye loss accelerates in the decade before menopause, it raises the interesting question of why oocytes undergo a terminal drop earlier than other non-dividing cells, such as neurons. One possibility is that the quality assurance on oocytes is necessarily much stricter. Another is that the factors responsible for the evolution of the menopause have removed any force of selection for better long-term oocyte maintenance. Whichever reason is correct, better understanding of the similarities and differences between general and reproductive aging will be essential in assessing possible interventions to extend the female reproductive span.

REFERENCES

1. Kirkwood TBL, Cremer T. Cytogerontology since 1881: a reappraisal of August Weismann and a review of modern progress. *Hum Genet* 1982;60:101–21
2. Kirkwood TBL. The origins of human ageing. *Phil Trans R Soc Lond B* 1997;352: 1765–72
3. Kirkwood TBL. Human senescence. *BioEssays* 1996;18:1009–16
4. Finch CE, Kirkwood TBL. *Chance, Development and Ageing.* New York: Oxford University Press, 2000
5. Williams GC. Pleiotropy, natural selection and the evolution of senescence. *Evolution* 1957;11:398–411
6. Medawar PB. *An Unsolved Problem of Biology*. London: Lewis, 1952
7. Kapahi P, Boulton ME, Kirkwood TBL. Enhanced resistance to multiple cellular stresses in long-lived mammalian species. *Free Radical Biol Med* 1999;26:495–500
8. Kowald A, Kirkwood TBL. A network theory of ageing: the interactions of defective mitochondria, aberrant proteins, free radicals and scavengers in the ageing process. *Mutat Res* 1996;315:209–36
9. Bodnar AG, Ouellette M, Frolkis M, *et al.* Extension of life-span by introduction of telomerase into normal human cells. *Science* 1998;279:349–52
10. Rudolph KL, Chang S, Lee H-W, *et al*. Longevity, stress response and cancer in aging telomerase-deficient mice. *Cell* 1999;96:701–12
11. Martin K, Kirkwood TBL, Potten CS. Age changes in stem cells of murine small intestinal crypts. *Exp Cell Res* 1998;241:316–23
12. Martin K, Potten CS, Roberts SA, *et al*. Altered stem cell regeneration in irradiated intestinal crypts of senescent mice. *J Cell Sci* 1998;111:2297–303
13. Kirkwood TBL. Evolution of ageing. *Nature (London)* 1977;270:301–4

3

Concepts in female reproductive aging

E.R. te Velde

INTRODUCTION

Concepts in biological sciences often change or disappear. After scientific debate, new concepts arise on top of the old ones, which gradually become covered by the dust of time. Nevertheless, they were necessary for the development of the new concepts that better explain reality. This movement marks the progress of science. Let us remember, for example, that Reinier de Graaf considered the entire dominant follicle as being the actual egg. This concept turned out to be incorrect, but it contributed to progress in reproductive biology.

The concepts presented here do not have the pretension of being outstanding or reflecting the truth. The main reason for presenting them is to stimulate discussion. Such a debate may give rise to the formulation of new concepts.

CONCEPT I: REPRODUCTIVE AGING IS OVARIAN AGING

Reproductive aging is dictated by the decreasing quantity and quality of the pool of primordial or resting follicles established during fetal life. The famous 'Faddy curve' published by Faddy and others in 1992, has greatly influenced this concept[1]. In Figure 1 their work is summarized schematically and related to the important reproductive events in a woman's life. There is a large body of clinical and demographic data about the time sequence of reproductive events such as the beginning of subfertility, the beginning of infertility, the increasing abortion rate, the increased chance of chromosomal aberrations, the transition of cycle regularity to irregularity and finally the age at menopause (for review see reference 2). The heart of this concept is that the timing of these events is regulated by the decreasing quantity and quality of the primordial follicle pool. Although this concept is highly plausible and in line with many clinical and experimental observations, its ultimate proof is impossible to provide, because total numbers of primordial follicles can be reliably assessed only following removal of the entire ovary. Moreover, the degree of fertility and subfertility and the timing of infertility cannot be assessed in individual women.

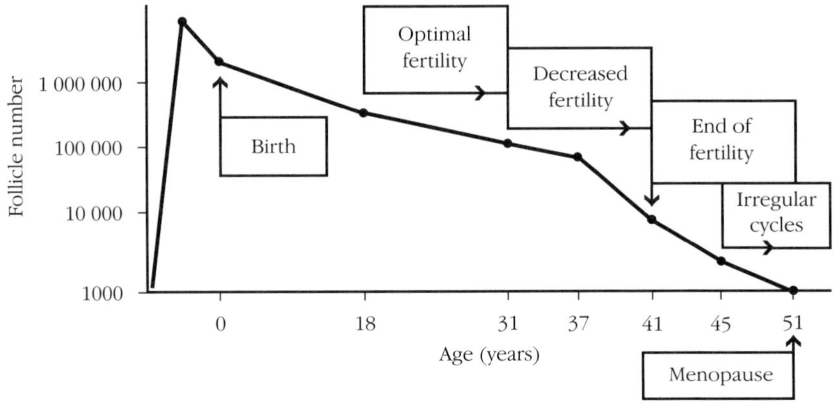

Figure 1 The age-dependent decline of the log-transformed primordial follicle number is related to the main reproductive events

CONCEPT II: AGE AT MENOPAUSE IS A RELIABLE MARKER OF THE PRECEDING REPRODUCTIVE EVENTS

We distinguish four components of this concept.

Component 1: The preceding reproductive events show a similar age variation to age at menopause, and the differences in time between these events are more or less constant

Menopause is the final reproductive event and marks the definite exhaustion of the primordial follicle pool. Moreover, it is the only reproductive event for which the age can be clearly recognized in individuals; the ages and periods of the other reproductive events are retrospective abstractions from large groups of individuals which are always related to mean or median ages (Figure 1). The mean age of menopause is about 50–51 years in all Western countries, but shows a remarkable variation, from 40 to 60 years. Our concept assumes that the preceding reproductive events show a similar age variation and that the time differences between these events and age at menopause are more or less fixed.

In Figure 2 this concept is visualized. On the right of the figure, the 40–60-year variation of age at menopause is presented in a cumulative fashion; this is based on the data of Treloar[3]. The second curve from the right presents the age of transition from cycle regularity to irregularity. Isolde den Tonkelaar from our group demonstrated that our concept is correct for this particular reproductive event[4]. The third line from the right depicts the end of fertility. In natural populations where the timing of having children is not influenced by contraception, the age at last childbirth marks the end of fertility. In Figure 3, the left curve presents the variation of age at last delivery in a natural population of

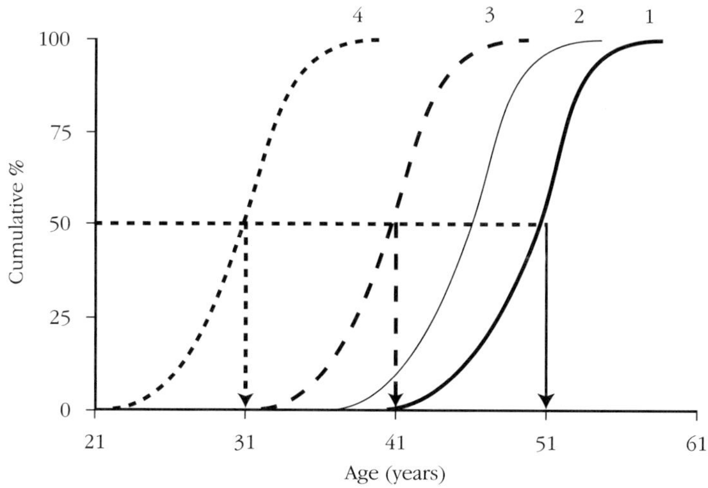

Figure 2 The age variations of the main reproductive events show parallel distribution. 1, menopause (mean 51 years); 2, transition from cycle regularity to irregularity (mean 45 years); 3, beginning of infertility (mean 41 years); 4, beginning of subfertility (mean 31 years)

women living in Canada in the 19th century (unpublished data). The right curve depicts the variation of age at menopause[3]. The striking parallelism of both curves is suggestive, although not a proof, of the correctness of our concept. The course of the left curve of Figure 2, depicting the beginning of subfertility, cannot be corroborated, because markers defining the beginning of subfertility do not yet exist.

Although the ultimate proof of component 1 cannot be provided, in our opinion it is both clinically and biologically plausible.

Component 2: The same factors that determine age at menopause are also involved in the timing of the preceding reproductive events

Various determinants of age at menopause have been related to lifestyle (such as cigarette smoking, food consumption, malnutrition, social economic class and the use of oral contraceptives) and fertility (including parity, age at first delivery, mothers of dizygotic twins and cycle characteristics) (for review see reference 5). It is striking in this respect that conditions in which levels of follicle stimulating hormone (FSH) are relatively high, such as in mothers of dizygotic twins, or in those with short menstrual cycles, are associated with an earlier menopause. In contrast, when FSH levels are relatively low for longer periods (such as high parity, long-lasting use of oral contraceptives, long menstrual cycles), menopause tends to come later.

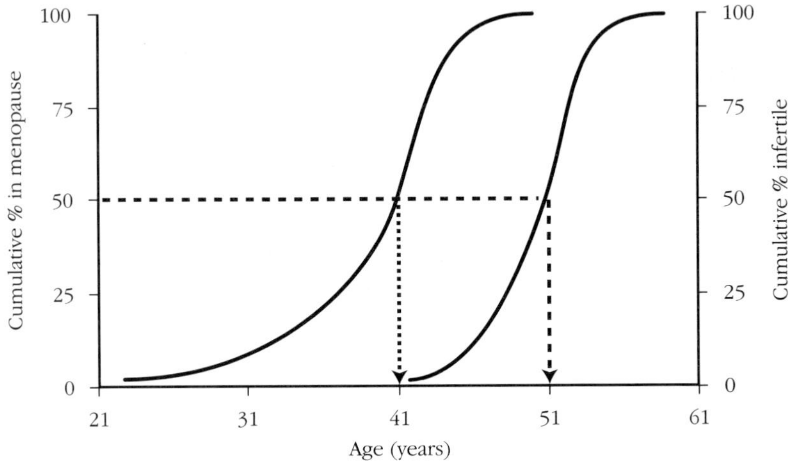

Figure 3 The distributions of age at menopause of a 20th-century population (right) and of age at last childbirth of a 19th-century population (left) are almost parallel

There is growing evidence suggesting that FSH, although not *sine qua non*, may facilitate the initiation of follicular growth and stimulate early follicular development, thereby accelerating depletion of the resting follicle pool, and advancing the occurrence of reproductive events including menopause[2].

Component 3: In spite of the fact that most of the factors just mentioned have a highly significant correlation with age at menopause, they explain only about 3% of its age variation

Paul van Noord of our group demonstrated this 2 years ago in a large study[6]. Another important mechanism must be involved and, like everybody else, we thought of genes.

Component 4: More than 80% of the observed differences in the age of menopause have a genetic origin commonly referred to as heritability

We demonstrated this in a study of 361 sisters of a random population, who had all experienced menopause. While we were writing up our results, two studies on menopausal ages in identical twins were published[7,8], with very similar results to ours.

CONCEPT II: SUMMARY

Concept II can be summarised as follows; the process of follicle loss regulating the time sequence of reproductive events, including age at menopause, is mainly genetically determined.

CONCEPT III: THE NUMBER OF SONOGRAPHICALLY DETECTABLE ANTRAL FOLLICLES RELIABLY REFLECTS THE PROCESS OF REPRODUCTIVE AGING

Faddy and Gosden constructed a mathematical model of follicle dynamics, providing estimates of the average daily number of primordial follicles entering the growth phase[9]. They showed that, from ages 25 to 45, this number dramatically drops. Concept III is based on the assumption that after many months of growth a minor but proportional number of these follicles reach the beginning of a menstrual cycle and are rescued and stimulated to further growth by the FSH rise at the beginning of the follicular phase. From this cohort the dominant follicle will be selected during the following week. If our assumption is correct, the number of antral follicles should reliably reflect the primordial follicle pool, thus being a measure of reproductive age. Since there is no *in vivo* method of measuring numbers of resting and growing follicles, our concept cannot be assessed directly.

We investigated a large group of regularly cycling, normal women who had proven their fertility in the past and whose ages varied from 25 to 46 years. The age-dependent changes in such women are likely to reflect the physiological decline of fertility and, hence, their chronological age can be considered to approximate their reproductive age. In Figure 4 the results are summarized. We conclude that the antral follicle count and reproductive age are highly correlated[10].

We reanalyzed the data of Faddy and colleagues[1], limiting the age range to 25–46, as if it concerned a new data set (Figure 5, upper curve). As in the curve including all ages, a biphasic pattern gave the best fit. The turning point was at 37–38 years, as in the original analysis by Faddy and co-workers[1]. The lower curve presents the age-dependent decline of the log-transformed antral follicle numbers, shown in Figure 4. Also for antral follicles, a biphasic curve gave a significantly better fit of the age-dependent loss than a straight line. The turning point was again at 37 years. Until the turning point the mean age-dependent loss of follicles was 4–5% per year for both primordial and antral follicles. After the turning point the yearly loss of primordial follicles was about twice that of antral follicles, which might be related to the rescuing effect of rising FSH levels. The striking analogy of both curves, in our opinion, is an additional argument to accept the concept that loss of primordial follicles and loss of antral follicles reflect the same process of reproductive aging.

CONCEPT IV: EVEN IF REPRODUCTIVE AGING IS PRIMARILY OVARIAN, IT IS POSSIBLE THAT OTHER ORGANS ARE ALSO INVOLVED; THE MOST LIKELY CANDIDATE IS THE HYPOTHALAMUS

The neuroendocrine concept of reproductive aging considers the hypothalamus as the main initiator of a cascade of events leading to menopause.

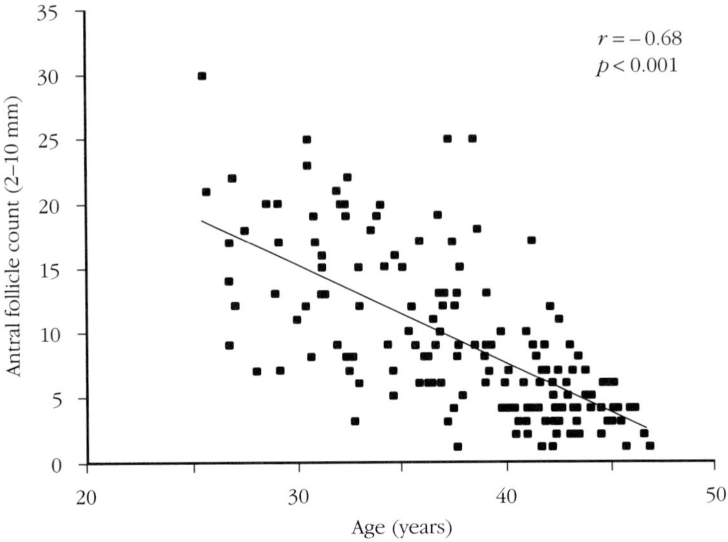

Figure 4 The relationship between antral follicle numbers and chronological age in a population of fertile, regularly cycling women

Reproductive aging is considered as a dysregulation of the gonadotropin releasing hormone (GnRH) pulse generator by a progressive lack of neurochemical control from other brain centers[11]. One of the first signs of this transition is the monotropic risc of FSII during the early follicular phase. Until recently, I was opposed to the neuroendocrine hypothesis, because, in my opinion, everything could be explained from the ovarian point of view. Especially after it became possible to distinguish inhibin A from inhibin B, ovarian feedback seemed to be able to explain everything. The group of Michael Soules carried out a great deal of research to explain the monotropic FSH rise, and I felt supported by the fact that they came to the same conclusion[12]. However, lately, three observations have created some doubts. First, how can one explain why menopausal complaints such as hot flushes and night sweating quite often already become apparent in regularly cycling women between 35 and 40 years old, when estradiol levels are still completely normal?[13] Second, in a recent study by Matt and colleagues[14], changes in pulse patterns of luteinizing hormone (LH) were demonstrated in regularly cycling women of 39 years or older, as compared to a younger age group. These alterations may well be the first sign of hypothalamic aging. Third, in our own study of normal women, the age-dependent variation of FSH levels could only be explained for a small fraction by the ovarian feedback of inhibin B or the combination of inhibin B, inhibin A and estradiol (unpublished data). The mysterious monotropic FSH rise cannot be explained by ovarian

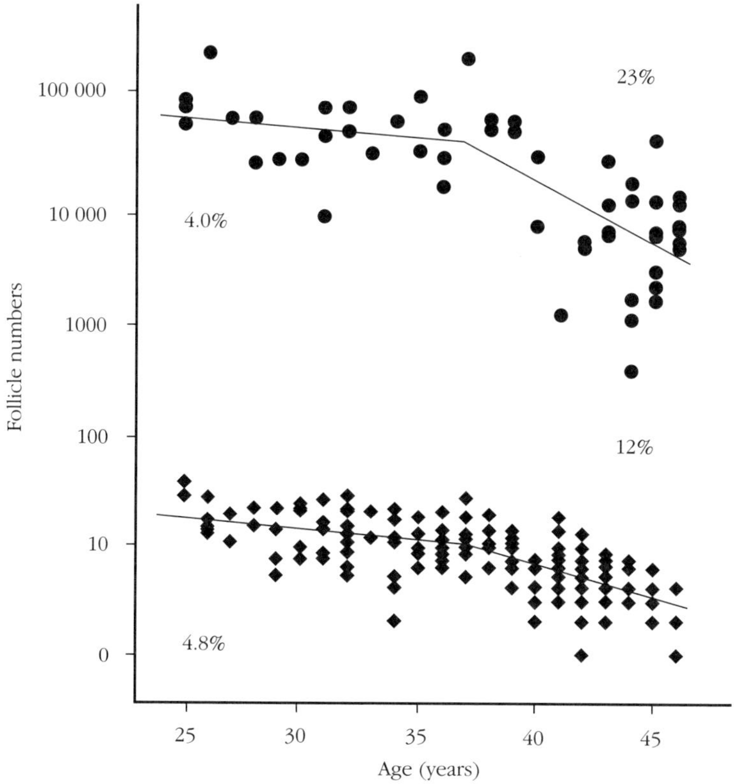

Figure 5 Upper curve: the age-dependent decline of the log-transformed primordial follicle numbers of women between the ages of 25 and 46. Lower curve: the age-dependent decline of the log-transformed antral follicle numbers of women between the ages of 25 and 46. Percentages represent the yearly follicle loss before and after the turning point at about age 37

feedback alone. There must be another mechanism and it is quite possible that, in addition to the ovary, the hypothalamus is involved.

CONCEPT V: HIGH FERTILITY PREDISPOSES TO A LONGER LIFE

The literature on this subject is controversial. On one side, early menopause was found to be associated with earlier age at death[15,16]. Moreover, recently evidence has been published suggesting that the ability to have children after age 40 is a marker of slower aging and consequently of a longer life[17].

In contrast, the disposable soma theory on the evolution of aging argues that a long life requires investments in somatic maintenance at the expense of resources for reproduction. Thus, high fertility predisposes to a shorter life (indeed, the opposite of our concept). The disposable soma theory appears to be true for the fruit fly[18]. In a fascinating piece of work based on records of British nobility since the Middle Ages, Westendorp and Kirkwood claim that the same trade-off between fertility and duration of life also applies to the human[19]. However, analyzing the same dataset, we found that the negative correlation between fertility and duration of life disappeared when corrections were made for age at marriage, a factor apparently not considered in the publication by Westendorp and Kirkwood. In former times, age at marriage marked the beginning of procreation, and it is completely in line with what we know about reproductive aging, that late marriage is associated with a larger proportion of sterility or a reduced number of children. Why late marriage apparently predisposed to a longer life cannot be readily explained, but may be related to the complex customs among the aristocracy of those days with regard to marrying off one's daughter and finding a suitable partner.

We studied a population of about 1200 married women born in the 19th century, in the Saguenay region of Quebec. These data are part of a famous demographic dataset, the so-called Balsac data. For cultural reasons, members of this community explored their reproductive potential to its utmost limits. Three measures of fertility – the time until first conception, the number of children and the age at last childbirth – were considered.

After adjustments for all possible confounders, age at last childbirth appeared to have a direct and highly significant correlation with age at death (unpublished data). Age at last childbirth may be a more direct reflection of female reproductive potential than age at menopause and, consequently, may better correlate with duration of life.

CONCLUDING CONCEPT

These findings indicate that some of the genes regulating ovarian follicle reserve and consequently reproductive aging are also involved in general aging.

ACKNOWLEDGEMENTS

The concepts presented in this chapter are the results of discussions with many people, including Frank Broekmans, Rien Dorland, Peter Pearson, Laszlo Bancsi, Gabriëlle Scheffer, Jan-Peter de Bruin, Piet van Zonneveld, Roger Gosden, Malcolm Faddy, Alain Gougeon, Michael Soules, Ursula Eichenlaub-Ritter, Niels Lambalk, Herjan Coelingh Bennink, Isolde den Tonkelaar, Paul van Noord, Frank de Jong, Rein Blankestein, René Eijkemans, Dik Habbema and Bart Fauser. Whether you like it or not, all of you, in some way or other, contributed to these concepts.

REFERENCES

1. Faddy MJ, Gosden RG, Gougeon A, *et al*. Accelerated disappearance of ovarian follicles in midlife: implications for forecasting menopause. *Hum Reprod* 1992;7:1342–6
2. Te Velde ER, Scheffer GJ, Dorland M, *et al*. Developmental and endocrine aspects of normal ovarian ageing. *Mol Cell Endocrinol* 1998;145:67–73
3. Treloar AE. Menstrual cyclicity and the premenopause. *Maturitas* 1981;3:49–64
4. Den Tonkelaar I, te Velde ER, Looman CWN. Menstrual cycle length preceding menopause in relation to age at menopause. *Maturitas* 1998;29:115–23
5. Te Velde ER, Dorland M, Broekmans FJ. Age at menopause as a marker of reproductive ageing. *Maturitas* 1998;30:119–25
6. Van Noord PAH, Dubas JS, Dorland M, *et al*. Age at natural menopause in a population based screening cohort: the role of menarche, fecundity, and lifestyle factors. *Fertil Steril* 1997;68:95–102
7. Snieder H, MacGregor AJ, Spector TD. Genes control the cessation of a woman's reproductive life: a twin study of hysterectomy and age at menopause. *J Clin Endocrinol Metab* 1998;83:1875–80
8. Treloar SA, Do KA, Martin NG. Genetic influences on the age at menopause. *Lancet* 1998;352:1084–5
9. Faddy MJ, Gosden RG. A mathematical model of follicle dynamics in the human ovary. *Hum Reprod* 1995;10:770–5
10. Scheffer GJ, Broekmans FJM, Dorland M, *et al*. Antral follicle counts by transvaginal sonography are related to age in women with proven natural fertility. *Fertil Steril* 1999; 72:845–51
11. Wise PM, Krajnak KM, Kashon ML. Menopause: the ageing of multiple pacemakers. *Science* 1996;273:67–70
12. Soules MR, Battaglia DE, Klein NA. Inhibin and reproductive ageing in women. *Maturitas* 1998;30:193–206
13. Oldenhave A, Jaszmann LJB, Haspels AA, *et al*. Impact of climacteric on well being. *Am J Obstet Gynecol* 1993;168:772–80
14. Matt DW, Kauma SW, Pincus SM, *et al*. Characteristics of luteinizing hormone secretion in younger versus older premenopausal women. *Am J Obstet Gynecol* 1998;178: 504–10
15. Snowdon DA, Kane RL, Beeson L, *et al*. Is early natural menopause a biologic marker of health and ageing? *Am J Public Health* 1989;79:709–14
16. Cooper GS, Sandler DP. Age at natural menopause and mortality. *Ann Epidemiol* 1998;8:229–35
17. Perls TT, Alpert L, Fretts RC. Mixed blessings for middle-aged mothers. *Nature (London)* 1997;389:133
18. Kirkwood TBL, Rose MR. Evolution of senescence: late survival sacrificed for reproduction. *Phil Trans R Soc Lond* 1991;332:15–24
19. Westendorp RGJ, Kirkwood TBL. Human longevity at the cost of reproductive success. *Nature (London)* 1998;396:743–6

4

Postponement of childbearing and its effect on the prevalence of subfecundity

E.H. Stephen

INTRODUCTION

One of the significant changes in fertility over the past 15–25 years in most European countries, as well as in the USA and other developed countries, has been the increase in the mean age of childbearing. The reasons for delayed childbearing have been discussed elsewhere[1,2]. There are several potential consequences of delayed childbearing, including a greater incidence of late fetal death rates[3], increased risk of lower birth weight[3], increased risk of multiple birth[4] and greater incidence of infertility[5]. This paper focuses on the last mentioned consequence, the relationship between delayed childbearing and infertility. The one variable that has shown consistent association with infertility is age of the woman[5,6].

The potential increase in the number of women with infertility as childbearing is delayed is of concern in Europe and in the USA. Past studies have shown that less than half of all couples who experience infertility seek medical treatment[5,7], but it is advantageous for health-care systems to be able to plan for diagnostic testing and treatment of couples with infertility. To do this, health planners need to have information on the population at risk of needing infertility services.

In this paper, the patterns of fertility decline from 1974 to 1996 and the increasing mean age of childbearing in Europe are discussed first, to determine the long-term fertility changes throughout Europe. Changes in age-specific childbearing patterns for three countries are illustrated as a means of gaining better understanding of the differences between the European pattern of fertility decline and what has been observed in the USA. The number of subfecund women for four European countries and the USA are projected for 1995–2025 so that potential demand for infertility services can be determined.

DATA AND METHODS

Primary sources of data for the analysis of fertility patterns in this paper are Eurostat for European fertility data[8], the National Center for Health Statistics for American fertility data[9] and the United Nations[10].

Projections of the subfecund population are calculated for four representative European countries (France, the Netherlands, Sweden, the UK) and the USA. In each country the number of women with subfecundity is calculated for 5-year cycles beginning in 1995 and ending in 2025. The population base and projections for all countries were provided by the United States Bureau of the Census[11,12]. In each country, three sets of subfecundity projections are made. All three series are based on subfecundity rates from the National Survey of Family Growth (NSFG) conducted by the National Center for Health Statistics in the USA. Documentation of the NSFG is found elsewhere[13]. The first (low) projection series uses the subfecundity rates by broad age group from the 1988 NSFG, the second (medium) projection series uses the age-specific rates from the 1995 NSFG and the third (high) projection series extrapolates from the 1995 NSFG subfecundity rates. The absolute differences between the 1988 and 1995 age-specific rates are added to the 1995 rates for the high series.

FINDINGS

To gain understanding of the patterns of delayed childbearing, it is helpful to examine the overall fertility patterns in Europe and the USA over the past 20–25 years. The total fertility rate (TFR), which indicates the number of children a woman would have if the current fertility rates were to continue over her reproductive years, has decreased in all European countries – with the exceptions of Finland and Luxembourg – as can be seen in Figure 1. For instance, the TFR for the Netherlands was 1.77 in 1974 and was 1.53 in 1996 (a 14% decline). Figure 1 shows that the drop in fertility has been widespread in Western Europe with the decline greatest in Italy, Spain, Portugal, Greece and Ireland. In Italy fertility dropped by nearly half from 2.33 in 1974 to 1.21 in 1996. In comparison, the TFR for the USA was 1.84 in 1974 and was 2.03 in 1996. The lowest TFR in the USA was 1.74 in 1976, and it has increased gradually since then, with values over 2.0 since 1989[4].

At the same time that fertility has been declining in Europe, the mean age of childbearing has been increasing, as can be seen in Figure 2. For instance, the mean age of childbearing in the Netherlands increased by over 2.5 years from 27.4 in 1974 to 30.1 years in 1996. As seen in Figure 2, the trend towards an increased mean age at childbearing was common to virtually all Western European countries. By 1996 the value for the mean age of childbearing for Ireland, the Netherlands and Spain had all exceeded 30 years. Portugal was the only country that experienced a decline in the mean age of childbearing,

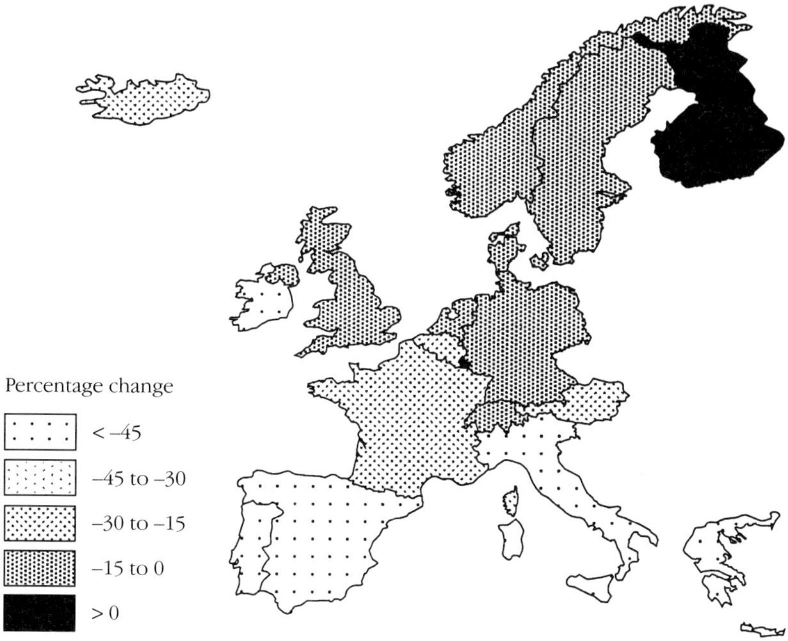

Figure 1 Percentage change in total fertility rates in Europe: 1974–96

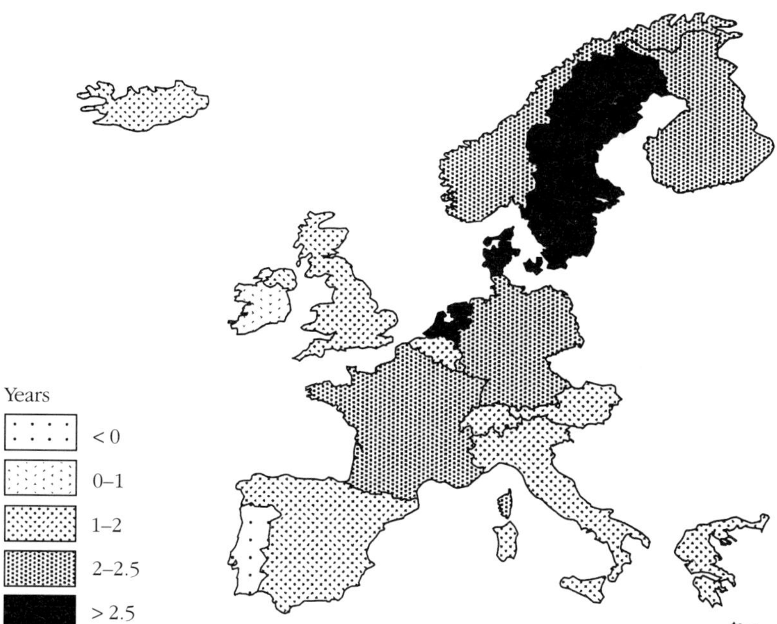

Figure 2 Change in mean age at childbearing in Europe: 1974–96

from 28.7 to 28.2 years. It has lagged behind other European countries in its initial decline to subreplacement fertility levels and postponed childbearing patterns, but has been catching up recently. Portugal's mean age at childbearing bottomed out at 27.1 in the early 1980s and has increased since then, while fertility has declined by 45% from a TFR of 2.6 in 1974 to a value of 1.4 in 1996.

It is helpful to examine age-specific fertility rates over time to determine how the drop in total fertility rates seen in Figure 1 and the increase in mean age at childbearing seen in Figure 2 are affecting childbearing patterns by age for specific countries. Figure 3 shows the age-specific fertility rates for Sweden for 1974 and 1996. Sweden experienced fluctuations in the TFR from 1974 to 1984, and then the TFR increased until 1990 when a peak was reached at 2.13 children per woman. Fertility has declined since then to a level of 1.6 in 1996, which was a 14% decline from 1974. We see here that fertility shifted downward and to the older ages. Fertility for the youngest two age groups was considerably lower in 1996 than in 1974. Peak fertility was still in the 25–29 age group in 1996, although the level was lower in 1996 than in 1974. There was a 'cross-over' with fertility in the oldest three age groups in 1996 exceeding that of 1974.

The age-specific fertility rates for the Netherlands are shown in Figure 4 and again there was a downward shift in fertility from 1974 to 1996 and a shift toward the older ages. As mentioned earlier, overall fertility declined nearly 14% from 1.8 children in 1974 to 1.5 children in 1996. In the Netherlands the peak childbearing age group was 30–34 by 1996, with the 35–39 age group also having higher fertility in 1996 than in 1974.

Age-specific fertility rates for the USA are shown in Figure 5. The pattern in the USA is different in certain respects from that observed in the figures for the Netherlands and Sweden. The primary difference is that fertility increased overall from 1974 to 1996. Although the peak in childbearing shifted from ages 20–24 in 1974 to ages 25–29 in 1996, there has not been a great divergence in fertility rates for the youngest women in the USA over this 22-year period. The steep incline to the peak childbearing ages that was seen in Figures 3 and 4 for Sweden and the Netherlands, respectively, is not as obvious in Figure 5, which reflects much higher levels of teenage childbearing in the USA than in Western Europe. The fertility patterns for older women are quite similar to those observed in the Netherlands and Sweden. Fertility in the USA was 54% higher in 1996 than in 1974 for women aged 30–34. Therefore, patterns of delayed childbearing do indicate a long-term trend across these countries over this time period.

Infertility prevalence

In order to study infertility and subfecundity prevalence and changes over time, we need country-level estimates. There are four major difficulties in

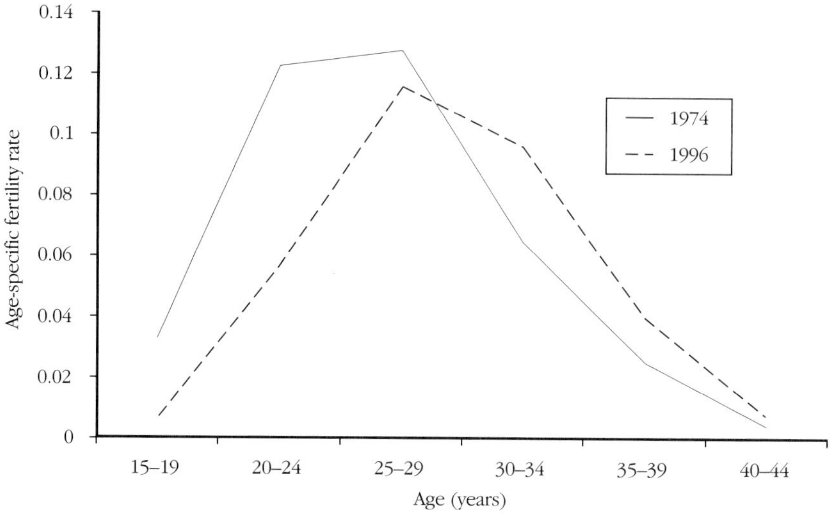

Figure 3 Age-specific fertility rates in Sweden: 1974 and 1996

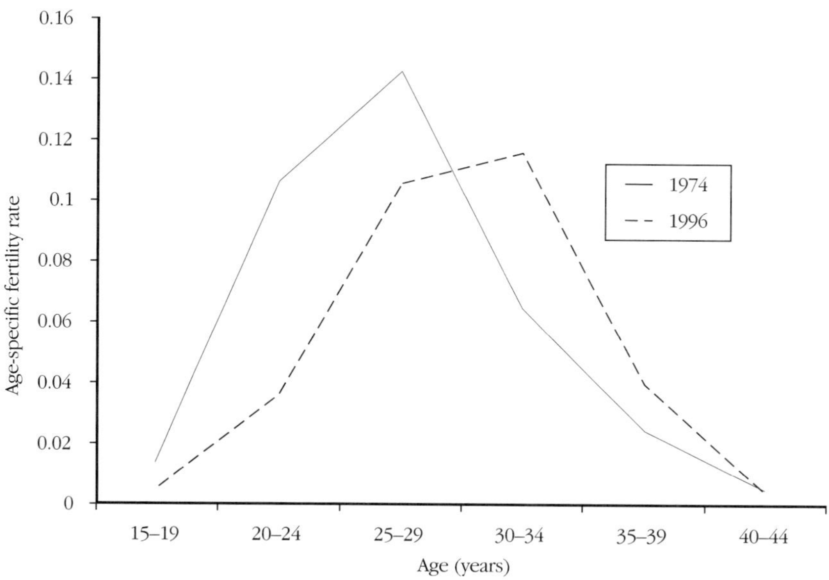

Figure 4 Age-specific fertility rates in the Netherlands: 1974 and 1996

cross-national comparisons of infertility and subfecundity. One is that there is no standard definition of infertility and/or subfecundity. The NSFG in the USA uses a very specific definition of subfecundity. The subfecund population is defined[5] as meeting one of the following conditions:

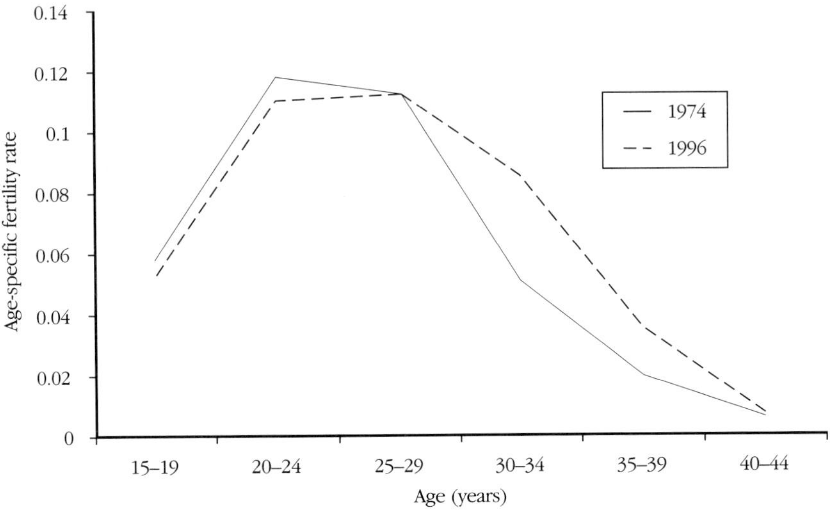

Figure 5 Age-specific fertility rates in the USA: 1974 and 1996

(1) It is physically difficult for the woman to conceive or deliver a baby (again) or for her partner to father a baby;
(2) A doctor has told the woman never to become pregnant (again) because it would pose a danger to her, to her fetus, or both.

Most studies define infertility as the inability to conceive within 12 months[14,15], but it is less clear how subfecundity has been defined. At times it appears that researchers have used the terms infertility and subfecundity interchangeably. For instance, Rachootin and Olsen[16] defined subfecundity as a couple failing to achieve a pregnancy after engaging in sexual activity without contraception for a period of 1 year or longer, which conforms closely to the more universal definition of infertility. Olsen and colleagues[7] refer to subfecundity in the title of their paper, but define subfecundity only as reduced fecundity as measured by questions referring to the longest waiting time to pregnancy.

As a result of the variation in definitions, rates may vary widely. In a MEDLINE search, Schmidt and co-workers[14] found 17 studies of infertility prevalence in industrialized countries. Lifetime prevalence of infertility ranged from 12.5 to 32.6% and current prevalence from 3.6 to 14.3%, but the studies used a variety of definitions.

The second problem in cross-national comparisons is that, because there have been few, if any, national-level surveys in Western Europe that have included questions on infertility, it has been difficult to estimate the prevalence at the country level. Rachootin and Olsen[16] estimated that approximately 16% of all women in Denmark had a history of subfecundity in 1982. Olsen and associates[7] conducted population-based surveys of women seeking medical help for subfecundity in several regions of Denmark, Germany, Italy, Poland and Spain, but did not provide information on country-specific prevalence rates of infertility or subfecundity.

The information that we do have on the prevalence of infertility has largely been for clinics or for relatively small areas. Templeton and colleagues[17] conducted random sample surveys of women 36–40 and 46–50 years old in the Aberdeen city district of the UK and found that infertility (as measured by failure to conceive after trying for more than 2 years) was 9.4% for the younger cohort and 8.9% for the older cohort, leading the authors to conclude that the prevalence of infertility was similar for both cohorts, although there had been an increase in pelvic infections in the community. Templeton and associates[17] did not gather information on the timing of the infertility diagnosis so we are not able to determine whether infertility has been increasing in the older reproductive ages.

A third difficulty in comparing surveys lies in the variation in the ages of women surveyed. Several surveys have used women in the older reproductive ages or women who are past reproductive ages[15,17], while other studies interviewed women spanning more of the reproductive ages[14,16,18].

A fourth problem is that, other than the USA-based NSFG, no survey is representative of an entire country and is repeated over several years. While it is helpful to have information at the county level such as the study of Copenhagen by Schmidt and colleagues[14], or an analysis of a rural population[17], we are unable to make comparisons across entire countries. Because the surveys that have been conducted have not been repeated, we do not know whether overall infertility is rising, is decreasing, or is stable. Our information about infertility prevalence by age is limited, and again no repeat panel surveys have been conducted at the national level to determine change by age over time.

Several of the European analyses have examined primary versus secondary infertility, but very few surveys have focused on subfecundity. We do have data on the subfecund population in the USA over time, and, as can be seen in Table 1, virtually all of the increase in impaired fecundity between 1982 and 1995 in the USA was because of an increase in the subfecund category.

For further detail, Table 2 shows subfecundity rates in the USA by broad age group for this same period of time. Subfecundity rates decreased slightly for ages 25–34 and 35–44 from 1982 to 1988, but all three age groups experienced an increase in subfecundity from 1988 to 1995. Subfecundity increased by 36% for the 15–24 age group, 26% for the 25–34 age group and 46% for the 35–44 age group. Subfecundity rates for all three survey years were highest for the 25–34 age group. The NSFG classifies women hierarchically with sterilization being the first classification category. Because rates of sterilization are highest among the oldest age group of women, there are fewer women at risk of being classified as subfecund among women aged 35–44 than in the younger age groups.

Table 1 Percentage distribution of women aged 15–44 years by fecundity status in the USA: 1982–95

	1982 (n = 7969)	*1988* (n = 8450)	*1995* (n = 10 847)
Surgically sterile	25.3	28.0	27.3
for contraceptive reasons	17.5	23.3	24.2
for non-contraceptive reasons	7.8	4.7	3.1
Impaired fecundity	8.4	8.4	10.2
non-surgically sterile	1.7	1.4	1.7
subfecund	5.6	5.7	7.7
long interval without conception	1.1	1.3	0.9
Fecund	66.3	63.6	62.5
Total	100	100	100

Table 2 Subfecundity rates by age in the USA: 1982–95

Age (years)	*1982*	*1988*	*1995*
15–24	3.5	3.9	5.3
25–34	7.3	7.2	9.1
35–44	6.2	5.7	8.3

Given that we do not have national level estimates of subfecundity rates for European countries and that we do not have standard definitions, I have used the NSFG definition of subfecundity and NSFG age-specific subfecundity rates to project numbers of subfecund women for four countries representative of Europe and for the USA for the period 1995–2025. I used three sets of rates to project the subfecund population in each country in each year. The first set of projections used the 1988 subfecundity rates by broad age group from the NSFG; the second set used the 1995 NSFG rates. Both of these age-specific rates are shown in Table 2. The third set of projections used a linear projection based on the absolute difference between the 1988 and 1995 rates. The age-specific rates for the third series were 0.067 (ages 15–24), 0.110 (ages 25–34) and 0.109 (ages 35–44).

The starting values for 1995 for the USA used the number of subfecund women, since that is a known value. Starting with the 2000 projections, the USA numbers utilized the appropriate projection assumptions for the three series.

These subfecundity rates – referred to as low, medium and high – when applied to population projections indicate the number of women in each country who would be considered subfecund in that given year. This allows us to see the contribution of changes in the age structure over time as well as the effect of an increase in subfecundity that has been observed in the USA.

There are two effects in evidence in Table 3. As indicated in Figure 1, the continued fertility decline in Europe will result in fewer women of childbearing age over the next 30 years in France, the Netherlands, Sweden and the UK. Because the base population is shrinking, the number of subfecund women will decline from 1995 to 2025 even if rates of subfecundity increase

Table 3 Projected number of subfecund women in France, the Netherlands, Sweden, the UK and the USA: 1995–2025

	1995	*2000*	*2005*	*2010*	*2015*	*2020*	*2025*
France							
Low	707 879	695 514	676 014	653 539	632 071	601 606	577 720
Medium	956 405	940 024	915 365	885 780	854 960	813 296	782 150
High	1 204 930	1 184 533	1 154 717	1 118 020	1 077 850	1 024 986	986 580
Netherlands							
Low	197 639	194 001	185 573	175 789	166 457	159 799	154 276
Medium	266 313	262 330	252 264	239 232	225 504	215 621	208 361
High	334 987	330 660	318 954	302 675	284 551	271 443	262 445
Sweden							
Low	97 629	96 612	95 903	94 926	93 827	94 240	93 263
Medium	131 700	130 479	129 977	128 823	126 857	126 903	125 894
High	165 771	164 346	164 052	162 719	159 886	159 567	158 525
UK							
Low	697 016	694 191	677 084	651 194	629 672	618 770	609 354
Medium	937 496	938 686	920 242	883 788	850 263	834 229	823 683
High	1 177 976	1 183 181	1 163 400	1 116 383	1 070 853	1 049 688	1 038 012
USA							
Low	4 571 530	3 355 509	3 312 477	3 322 959	3 402 882	3 519 975	3 627 903
Medium	4 571 530	4 556 528	4 494 168	4 491 828	4 588 671	4 747 154	4 900 878
High	4 571 530	5 757 547	5 675 859	5 660 697	5 774 460	5 974 333	6 173 853

over the time period. For instance, in France the number of subfecund women will drop from 1.2 million in 1995 to just over 986 000 in 2025, using the high rates of subfecundity. That pattern is reflected in the numbers for the Netherlands, Sweden and the UK.

Within these four countries, the range among low, medium and high levels of subfecundity tends to be quite large. Although we can only speculate about the future, there is every reason to believe that subfecundity rates will remain at the 1995 levels or increase. There are two primary reasons for this: sustained levels of delayed childbearing; and delayed effects of sexually transmitted diseases. Thus, it seems that the probable range of subfecundity for the countries shown is within the medium to high series. We can project, then, that by the year 2025 the number of subfecund women of reproductive age in France will range from over three-quarters of a million to nearly a million. In the Netherlands for the same year, the range is from 208 000 to 262 000, in Sweden from 125 000 to 158 000 and in the UK from 824 000 to just over a million. In the USA, the number ranges from 4.9 million to 6.1 million by the year 2025.

The USA is an anomaly, with decreases in the number of subfecund women from 1995 to 2005, but then increases from then on. This is indicative of the 'baby boom' aging out of the reproductive ages through 2005, but the effects of sustained fertility at nearly replacement levels will result in an increase in the number of women of reproductive age in the USA from 2010 until 2025.

CONCLUSIONS

As women in developed countries reach an era in which there is greater control of the timing and the number of children, there is one group – the subfecund – who have difficulty in achieving their desired fertility or who may not be able to have children at all. Any number of factors may cause subfecundity but two primary conditions that have had a direct effect in the past are sexually transmitted diseases and delayed childbearing[19]. Western European countries and the USA have experienced increased postponement of childbearing over the past 25 years and, with that, the risk of higher rates of overall subfecundity.

Although the fertility rates among women in the older reproductive years are very similar in Sweden, the Netherlands and the USA, the historically unprecedented declines in total fertility rates observed in Europe have not yet been seen in the USA. In part, fertility has remained near replacement level in the USA because of high fertility levels in the younger reproductive ages relative to Sweden and the Netherlands. Small decreases in age-specific fertility rates among younger women in the USA have been offset by increases among older women, so that the country's total fertility rate has increased over the past 20 years. This has resulted in nearly replacement level fertility in the USA, whereas many European countries are now beginning to see the effects of 20–25 years of decreasing fertility.

One of the effects of below replacement fertility is that the number of women of reproductive age is decreasing in many European countries. One question we should ask ourselves, though, is how much lower is fertility likely to go? There must be a minimum threshold of fertility. One demographer has suggested that it might be possible for a country to sustain a total fertility rate as low as 0.7 to 0.8 – at least for 20 years or so[20]. If countries were to reach that level and sustain it over a long period of time, we would expect that the number of women in the reproductive ages would eventually stabilize at a level much lower than currently seen in European countries. Childlessness rates would be in the range of 20 to 30%, with the other 70 to 80% of women having only one child.

This is important, as we consider the base population on which to estimate the number of subfecund women. The prevalence of subfecundity is not known for most European countries, and the trends over time are even less evident.

In the USA subfecundity rates increased for women in three broad age groups between 1988 and 1995. The reasons for this increase may include the facts that more women experience the delayed effects of sexually transmitted diseases; fewer women have hysterectomies, thus being more likely to be classified as subfecund (especially women with endometriosis or uterine fibroids); and women may be more likely to report being subfecund as a result of more press coverage of reproductive health issues and, in particular, infertility. Given the likely reasons for the increase observed in the past, there is every reason to believe that rates of subfecundity will continue to increase in the USA and Western European countries.

Even when increased rates of subfecundity are applied to population projections for France, the Netherlands, Sweden and the UK, the numbers of subfecund women will drop over the next 30 years. This does not diminish in any way the concern over delayed childbearing and its effect on subfecundity, but rather indicates the importance of understanding the population base. Most surveys have shown that the percentage of women with infertility who seek treatment has been relatively steady[5], thus enabling health systems to plan for service delivery for subfecund women.

Technological advances within the assisted reproductive field could diminish the concern over delayed childbearing and its effect on subfecundity. When women are able to freeze their own eggs during their young reproductive years and then use those eggs when they are older, delayed childbearing will have only a muted effect on subfecundity. Until that time, we can expect higher rates but fewer numbers of subfecund women in most European countries.

ACKNOWLEDGEMENTS

Cheryl Chriss Sawyer provided expert research and technical expertise. Linda J. Piccinino was invaluable in providing age-specific rates of subfecundity. Ai Yamazaki assisted with graphical expertise.

REFERENCES

1. Rindfuss RR, Morgan SP, Swicegood G. *First Births in America: Changes in the Timing of Parenthood*. Berkeley: University of California Press, 1988
2. Van de Kaa DJ. Europe's second demographic transition. *Popul Bull* 1987;42:1–57
3. Cnattinguis S, Forman MR, Berendes HW, *et al*. Delayed childbearing and risk of adverse perinatal outcome. *J Am Med Assoc* 1992;268:886–90
4. Ventura SJ, Martin JA, Curtin SC, *et al*. Births: final data for 1997. *Natl Vital Stat Rep* 1999;47:1–96
5. Chandra A, Stephen EH. Impaired fecundity in the United States: 1982–1995. *Fam Plann Perspect* 1998;30:34–42
6. Mosher WD, Pratt WF. Fecundity and infertility in the United States: 1965–1988. *Adv Data* 1990;192:1–11
7. Olsen J, Küppers-Chinnow M, Spinelli A. Seeking medical help for subfecundity: a study based upon surveys in five European countries. *Fertil Steril* 1996;66:95–100
8. Eurostat. *New Cronos Database* (CD-ROM). Luxembourg, 1998
9. National Center for Health Statistics. *Natl Vital Stat Rep* 1998;47:9
10. United Nations. *Demographic Yearbook*. New York, USA: UN;1975:580
11. United States Bureau of the Census. *International Database* 1999. Washington, DC: US Bureau of the Census

12. United States Bureau of the Census. Population projections of the United States by age, sex, race, and Hispanic origin: 1995–2050. *Curr Popul Rep* 1996:25–1130
13. Abma JC, Chandra A, Mosher WD, *et al*. Fertility, family planning, and women's health: new data from the 1995 National Survey of Family Growth. *Vital Health Stat* 1997;23:1–3
14. Schmidt L, Münster K, Helm P. Infertility and the seeking of infertility treatment in a representative population. *Br J Obstet Gynaecol* 1995;102:978–84
15. Buckett W, Bentick B. The epidemiology of infertility in a rural population. *Acta Obstet Gynecol Scand* 1997;76:233–7
16. Rachootin P, Olsen J. Prevalence and socioeconomic correlates of subfecundity and spontaneous abortion in Denmark. *Int J Epidemiol* 1982;11:245–9
17. Templeton A, Fraser C, Thompson B. Infertility – epidemiology and referral practice. *Hum Reprod* 1991;6:1391–4
18. Page H. Estimation of the prevalence and incidence of infertility in a population: a pilot study. *Fertil Steril* 1989;51:571–7
19. Menken J. Age and fertility: how late can you wait? *Demography* 1985;22:469–83
20. Golini A. How low can fertility be? An empirical exploration. *Popul Dev Rev* 1998;24:59–73

5

Mathematical models for follicle development and depletion

M.J. Faddy and R.G. Gosden

INTRODUCTION

The stock of ovarian follicles is fixed before birth in human females. Throughout life these follicles grow from the initial or primordial stage through various intermediate stages to mature antral follicles. Not all follicles grow to full maturity, as many become atretic before reaching the antral stages. The purpose of this paper is to model the process of growth and atresia of human ovarian follicles as the ovary ages. Different patterns of development and atresia are identified for different stages of follicle growth, and age-related changes are described.

The data used are those that have already been analyzed using simple 'broken stick'-type mathematical models[1]. Here more mathematically appealing models with continuous, rather than discontinuous, changes in the parameters describing follicle growth and atresia are used.

MODELLING FOLLICLE DYNAMICS

The data describing follicle development as the ovary ages[1] were counts of follicles in the ovaries from 52 women ranging from 19 to 50 years of age. The follicles were classified into three stages of growth: stage I, small unilaminar follicles with a single layer of squamous pregranulosa cells; stage II, unilaminar follicles consisting of one layer of cuboidal granulosa cells, with or without some squamous cells in the same ring; stage III, growing follicles with an enlarged oocyte and two or more layers of granulosa cells. Stage I here is normally regarded as the 'resting' or primordial stage, with stage II an early growing form and stage III containing more advanced stages – both growing and atretic. Figures 1–3 show plots of the numbers of follicles in these stages against age, together with kernel smoothed regressions[2] (dashed lines) of these data.

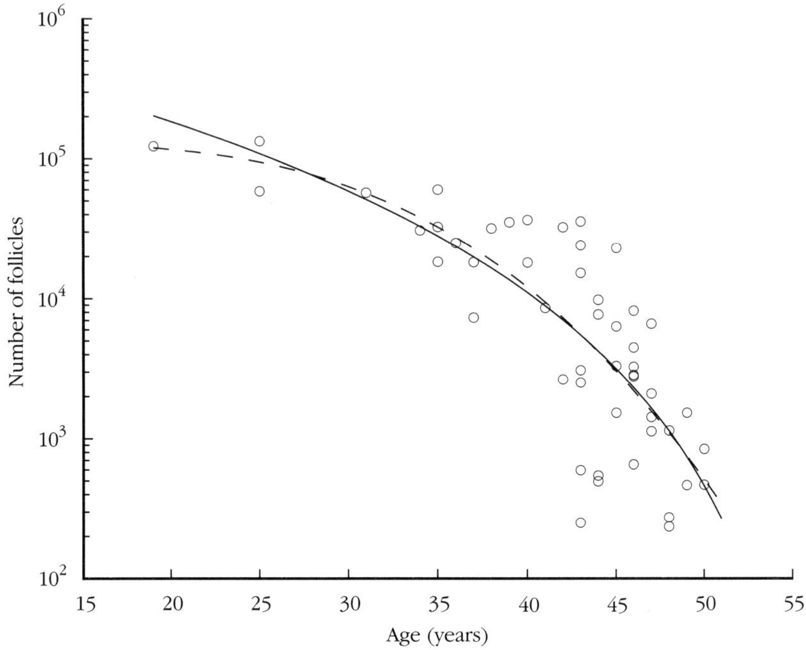

Figure 1 Observed stage I data (circles), kernel smoothed regression (dashed line) and fitted model (unbroken line)

A three-compartment model for the process of growth and atresia of follicles through these stages can be described by the differential equations:

$$\frac{dy_1}{dx} = -b_1 y_1 \tag{1}$$

$$\frac{dy_2}{dx} = b_1 p_1 y_1 - b_2 y_2 \tag{2}$$

$$\frac{dy_3}{dx} = b_2 p_2 y_2 - b_3 y_3 \tag{3}$$

Here, y_1, y_2 and y_3 represent the numbers of follicles in the three stages and x refers to age. The left-hand sides of these equations represent the instantaneous rates of temporal change of numbers of follicles in the three stages. The parameters b_1, b_2 and b_3 on the right-hand sides are the net rates of exponential loss of follicles from the respective stages so that (for example) with b_1 *constant*, numbers of follicles in stage I would exhibit *exponential* decline with increasing age, or *linear* decline in logged numbers. The parameters p_1 and p_2 (on the right-hand sides of equations (2) and (3)) represent the

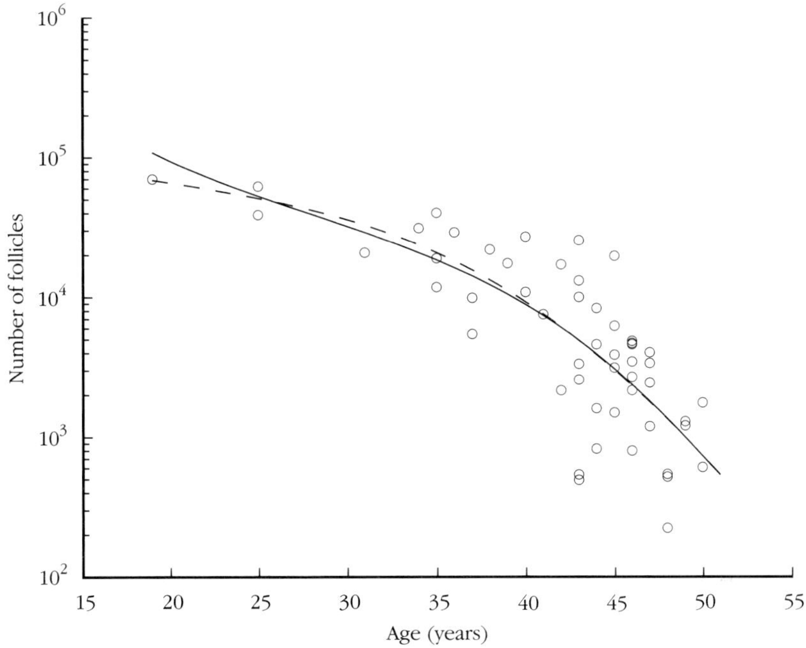

Figure 2 Observed stage II data (circles), kernel smoothed regression (dashed line) and fitted model (unbroken line)

proportions of follicles from one stage (I or II) that grow to the next stage (II or III) with $(1-p_1)$ and $(1-p_2)$ being the proportions lost to atresia. The previous modelling[1] can be formulated in terms of equations (1)–(3) with piece-wise constant forms, with abrupt changes at age 38 years, for these parameters. In this analysis, b_1, b_2 and b_3 will be considered to vary continuously according to:

$$\log b_i = \beta_i + \gamma_i \log y_i, \quad i = 1, 2, 3 \tag{4}$$

and p_1 and p_2:

$$\log\left(\frac{p_i}{1-p_i}\right) = \pi_i + \rho_i \log y_i, \quad i = 1, 2 \tag{5}$$

Here γ_1, γ_2, γ_3, ρ_1 and ρ_2 are *extra* parameters which result in these forms (4) and (5) allowing for changes as the ovary ages, expressed in terms of changing numbers of follicles in the three stages. Indeed, for the purposes of this discussion, aging of the ovary will be characterized by *declining* numbers of follicles.

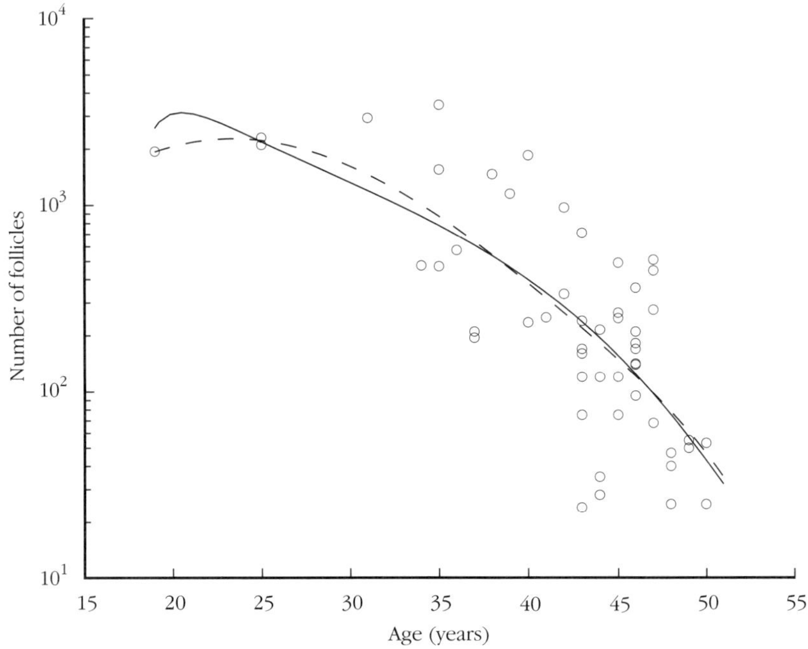

Figure 3 Observed stage III data (circles), kernel smoothed regression (dashed line) and fitted model (unbroken line)

Models of increasing complexity described by equations (1)–(5) were fitted to the data, estimating all the parameters by weighted least squares, with weights given by the residual variances and covariances from the kernel smoothed regressions of the data shown in Figures 1–3.

RESULTS

A model with *constant* b_1, b_2, b_3, p_1 and p_2 resulted in a weighted sum of squares of 160.98. Allowing b_1 to vary according to equation (4) reduced this sum of squares to 156.71, and additionally allowing p_1 to vary according to equation (5) further reduced this sum of squares to 154.26. Shown in Figures 4 and 5 are plots of the resulting estimates b_1 and p_1 as functions of the number of stage I follicles: an increasing net rate of exponential loss of primordial follicles together with a decreasing proportion growing to later stages as the ovary ages are clearly apparent here. Close agreement between the resulting solutions of equations (1)–(3) and the kernel smoothed regressions can be seen in Figures 1–3.

Further effects of the changing numbers of follicles on the parameters b_2, p_2 and b_3 in equations (2) and (3) are more equivocal: allowing these

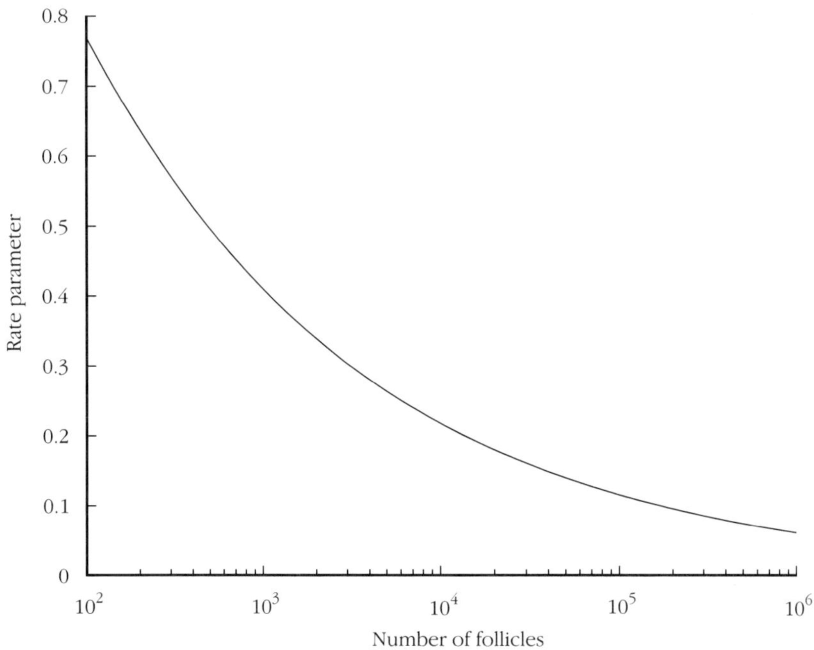

Figure 4 Estimated net rate b_1 of exponential loss of primordial follicles, as the ovary ages

parameters to vary according to equations (4) and (5) reduced the weighted sum of squares by only a small amount equal to 1.09 on three degrees of freedom, so any such effects cannot be considered at all significant, although similar dependence on numbers of follicles to those shown in Figures 4 and 5 was apparent. Moreover, the estimates of *constant* b_2, p_2 and b_3 were very imprecise, exemplified by a 90% confidence interval for p_2 consisting of the range of values between 0.014 and 1. Nevertheless, it is interesting to note that changing b_1 and p_1 according to Figures 4 and 5 as the ovary ages with b_2, p_2 and b_3 constant is sufficient for follicle numbers in *all* three stages to exhibit the *accelerated* decline apparent in Figures 1–3, which is similar to that for *total* follicle numbers[3].

DISCUSSION

It is far from clear what factors might underlie the accelerated net loss of stage I follicles, with high rates of atresia later in life. In adult mice, there is little atresia at stage I in most strains[4] and so it is likely that the follicle-sparing effects of hypophysectomy[5] and dietary restriction[6] are due to partial inhibition of follicle recruitment. On the other hand, evidence obtained in the *bax* knockout mouse demonstrates that preservation of the follicle store can be achieved by disrupting a gene involved in a pathway for apoptosis[7].

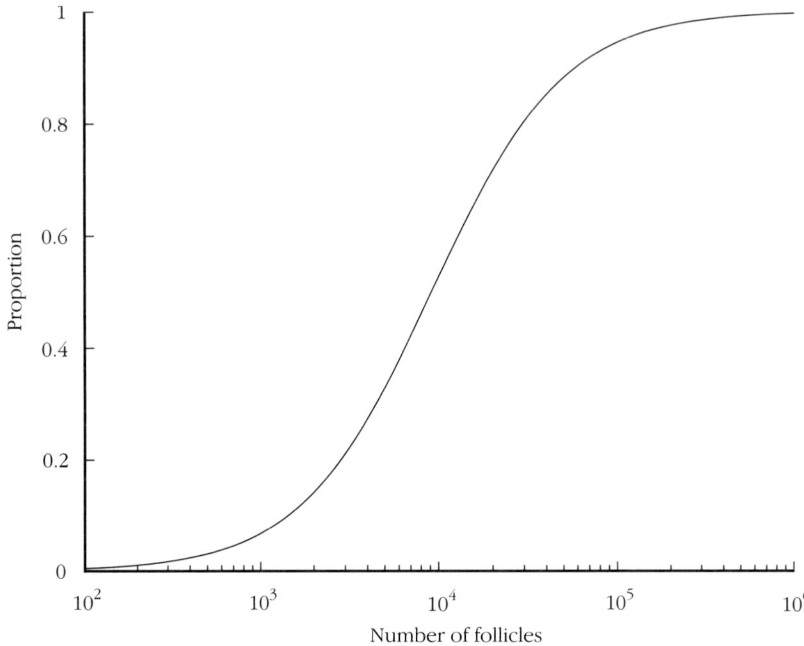

Figure 5 Estimated proportion p_1 of primordial follicles growing to the next stage, as the ovary ages

These analyses illustrate the value of the mathematical approach in gaining inferences that are currently impossible to obtain by direct observation in our species. Morphological changes have been observed in the follicles of old ovaries[8], but it is unclear whether they have any functional significance. Perhaps it will become possible to measure follicular age changes in single follicles on the basis of, for example, telomere length or mitochondrial DNA deletions, or using sophisticated cell culture methods, and progress on these questions is awaited with interest. The causes of oocyte deterioration are still far from clear, although egg donation programs clearly point to the oocyte as opposed to the physiological support system of pregnancy as the primary factor in the decline of human fertility[9]. It is possible that deterioration is related to the chronological age of the cell, this being more likely because the oocyte and pregranulosa cells are quiescent for up to 5 decades. Alternatively, it may be a response to the declining density of follicles or changes in growth factor 'tone' from changes in cell populations in the aging ovary. The least likely hypothesis is the action of follicle stimulating hormone (FSH) for, although plasma hormone levels begin to rise more than a decade before menopause and coincident with accelerated follicle loss, its receptor is not expressed in follicles until they have reached stage II[10].

The increase in FSH levels would, however, be expected to increase the survival of follicles at subsequent stages; our findings indicate that there are no

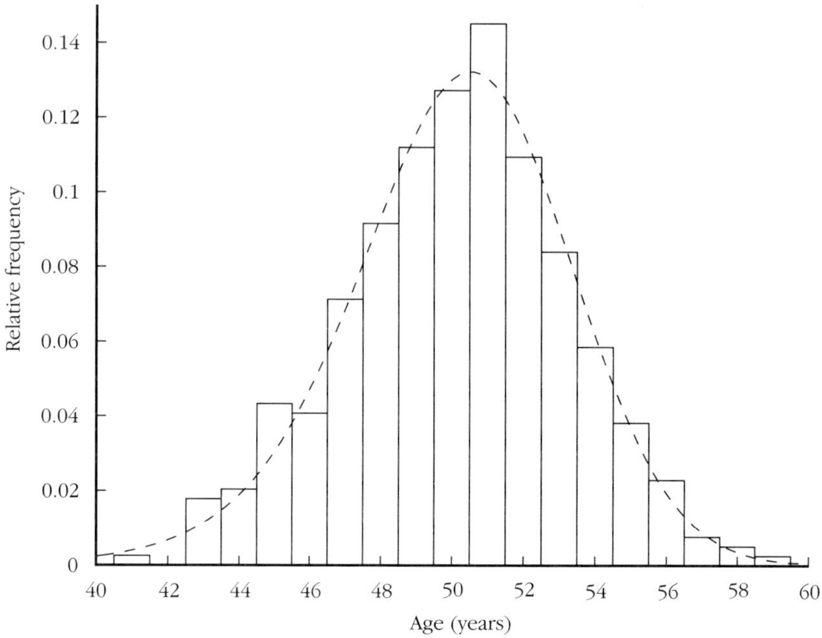

Figure 6 Observed (bars) and model-constructed (dashed lines) distributions of menopausal ages

significant changes in follicle growth or atresia rates at stages beyond the primordial stage. This conclusion is probably an oversimplification, because there may be subtle changes within stage III, which includes all stages after the primary or one-layer follicle stage. Unfortunately, as the numbers at successive stages dwindle and their coefficient of variation rises, it is futile to build a more detailed model without a large amount of data. However, the observation is consistent with the conclusions from morphology and follicle dynamics in rodents, which indicate that the intermediate stages are 'coasting' and that the primordial and small antral follicles are the more vulnerable to apoptosis.

It is interesting to note that follicles in all three stages exhibit a similar accelerated decline as the ovary ages (Figures 1–3). Thus, the declining reserve capacity of the ovary and the timing of ovulatory failure are a reflection of the original store size and attrition of primordial follicles. This is yet another reason for focusing more research effort in the future on this stage. In addition, the decline in stage III numbers could be used correlatively as an indicator of the store size and hence perhaps predict the time of menopause. Indeed, using a threshold number of stage III follicles to trigger menopause, in a way similar to that for total follicle numbers[3], leads to the distribution of menopausal age shown (dashed line) in Figure 6 compared with observed data (bars)[11]. The threshold number of stage III follicles here is 40, which of course is much smaller than that of 1100 for total follicle numbers[3], and more directly related to functional decline. Hence it would be desirable to develop ways of monitoring larger follicle stages, and indeed it is more practical to do this than for total follicles. Once follicles reach the antral stage (approximately 250 μm) they begin to secrete inhibin, which can be detected in plasma[12]; those reaching about 3 mm in diameter become large enough to be measured non-invasively using transvaginal ultrasound[13]. Indeed, there is already evidence that antral follicles can be used as bioindicators of ovarian aging[14] (and G. Scheffer, personal communication), although it remains to be demonstrated how predictive this is of menopause.

REFERENCES

1. Faddy MJ, Gosden RG. A mathematical model of follicle dynamics in the human ovary. *Hum Reprod* 1995;7:1342–6
2. Bowman AW, Azzalini A. *Applied Smoothing Techniques; the Kernel Approach with S-Plus Illustrations*. Oxford: Oxford University Press, 1997:48–52
3. Faddy MJ, Gosden RG. A model conforming the decline in follicle numbers to the age of menopause in women. *Hum Reprod* 1996;11:1484–6
4. Faddy MJ, Gosden RG, Edwards RG. Ovarian follicle dynamics in mice: a comparative study of three inbred strains and an F1 hybrid. *J Endocrinol* 1983;96:23–33
5. Jones EC, Krohn PL. The effect of hypophysectomy on age changes in the ovaries of mice. *J Endocrinol* 1961;21:497–508
6. Nelson JF, Gosden RG, Felicio LS. Effect of dietry restrictions on estrous cyclicity and follicular reserves in ageing C57BL/6J mice. *Biol Reprod* 1985;32:515–22
7. Perez GI, Robles R, Knudson CM, *et al*. Prolongation of ovarian lifespan into advanced chronological age by Bax-deficiency. *Nature Genet* 1999;21:200–3
8. Guraya SS. *Biology of Ovarian Follicles in Mammals*. Berlin: Springer-Verlag, 1985
9. Navot D, Drews MR, Bergh PA, *et al*. Age related decline in female infertility is not due to diminished capacity of the uterus to sustain embryo implantation. *Fertil Steril* 1994; 61:97–101
10. Oktay K, Briggs D, Gosden RG. Ontogeny of follicle-stimulating hormone receptor gene expression in isolated human ovarian follicles. *J Clin Endocrinol Metab* 1997;82: 3748–51
11. Treloar AE. Menstrual cyclicity and the pre-menopause. *Maturitas* 1981;3:249–64
12. Groome NP, Illingworth PJ, O'Brien M, *et al*. Measurement of dimeric inhibin B throughout the human menstrual cycle. *J Clin Endocrinol Metab* 1996;81:1401–5
13. Goswamy R. Ultrasound in assisted conception. In Brinsden PR, ed. *A Textbook of In Vitro Fertilization and Assisted Reproduction*, 2nd edn. Carnforth, UK: Parthenon Publishing, 1999:157–69
14. Ruess ML, Kline J, Santos R, *et al*. Age and the ovarian follicle pool assessed with transvaginal ultrasonography. *Am J Obstet Gynecol* 1996;174:624–7

6

The endocrinology of ovarian (reproductive) aging in women

M.R. Soules, D.E. Battaglia and N.A. Klein

INTRODUCTION

Although follicular depletion within the ovary is the final common pathway of reproductive aging, in reality the entire hypothalamic–pituitary–ovarian (HPO) axis is involved. Aging of an organ system involves a decline in physiological function over time, as the organism experiences an increase in chronologic age. Pathology (e.g. cancer) can also lead to physiological deterioration of an organ system, but aging is a natural process. Although the ovary is the organ that loses all reproductive and endocrine function at menopause, it is necessary to consider the entire HPO axis in describing reproductive aging. In one sense the female reproductive system begins to age (experiences follicular depletion) at a time that even precedes birth. Therefore, anatomic aging goes all the way back to development. If aging is considered more in the context of physiology, then fertility and hormone secretion are the major functions. At puberty the female reproductive system becomes functional; it reaches its zenith in terms of fertility when a woman is in her late 20s.

In terms of deterioration of physiological function secondary to aging, this presentation focuses on the decline in hormone secretion and fertility that women experience in the last two decades of their reproductive life. If the HPO axis represents a precise and sensitive endocrine system, then there will be endocrine changes that occur as part of reproductive aging. The average woman reaches peak fertility by age 30 and has no ovarian function (menopause) by age 50. Therefore, the last 20 years of HPO axis functioning are when the most relevant changes occur. It would be an overstatement to declare that the endocrine system *causes* reproductive aging, but this biological signalling system is intrinsically involved in orchestrating the events that lead to sterility and the menopause. Therefore, this presentation concentrates on the last two decades of HPO axis endocrine function, an interval that represents the decline and demise of reproductive function in the normal female.

Figure 1 indicates that there are dramatic changes in menstrual function, fertility and circulating endocrine levels in a woman's fifth decade. These manifestations of reproductive aging occur in a relatively rapid sequence compared to the absence of any signs in her first 40 years. For the average woman the first indication is a decrease in her relative fertility before she experiences any change in menstrual function. The next step is the monotropic rise in follicle stimulating hormone (FSH), which usually occurs simultaneously with a shortened follicular phase and decreased overall menstrual cycle length. Women often notice this subtle change in their cycle length (usually about 3–5 days). These shorter and more frequent menstrual cycles signal the onset of what has been referred to as both the climacteric and the menopausal transition. The next phase, which is accompanied by a profound decrease in fertility, is a dramatic change in menstrual cyclicity (the perimenopause). The perimenopause is characterized by irregular menstrual periods that occur in a random fashion. This phase is a mixture of ovulatory cycles, anovulatory cycles and ovarian quiescence. These changes are very noticeable and are sometimes accompanied by ancillary symptoms such as vasomotor hot flushes and premenstrual syndrome. The perimenopause tends to last for 3–4 years[1]. The menopause is reached when a woman is 12 months past her last physiological period. Although the average age of menopause is 50–51 years, the 95% confidence interval is relatively large (42–58 years). This age range would indicate that there is moderate variability in the time course of reproductive aging.

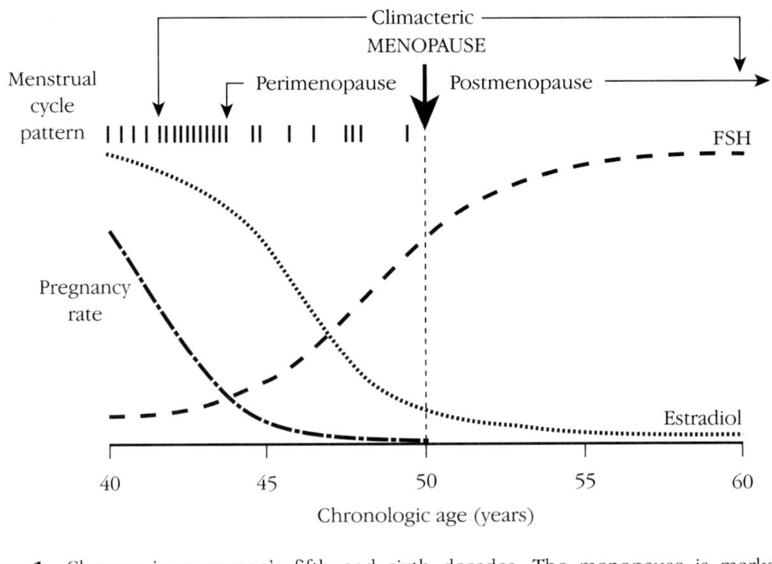

Figure 1 Changes in a woman's fifth and sixth decades. The menopause is marked by the last physiological menstrual period. It is preceded by the perimenopause, which is primarily recognized by gross menstrual cycle irregularity. The beginning of the menopausal transition has been called the climacteric and is heralded by more frequent but regular menstrual cycles. FSH, follicle stimulating hormone

Our group has proposed a six-stage clarification system for reproductive aging that is analogous to the Tanner–Marshall stages of puberty (Figure 2). These proposed stages have not been tested for clinical relevance and are only theoretical at this time. Stage 0 is normal reproductive function. Stage I appears clinically and endocrinologically normal, but a woman has had a subtle but real decrease in her fertility, probably secondary to a mild compromise of oocyte function. In stage II, the menstrual cycles become shorter and the monotropic FSH rise occurs. In stage III, there is a mixture of ovulatory and anovulatory cycles with more cycle irregularity and changes in ovarian steroid (estradiol, progesterone) secretion. In stage IV, there is a nearly complete breakdown of HPO function and the typical woman infrequently secretes significant quantities of estrogen, rarely ovulates and has only infrequent menstrual periods. Stage V is the menopause. Figure 3 illustrates the average woman as entering stage II (shorter cycles and a monotropic FSH rise) at about age 38 which, based on a mathematical model, is the age at which there is an acceleration of primordial follicle loss[2]. It is assumed that women enter stage II when they show a drop below a critical threshold of primordial follicles remaining in the ovary. It is hypothesized that they proceed through the latter stages of reproductive aging subsequent to further follicle loss with successive thresholds followed by further deterioration of function.

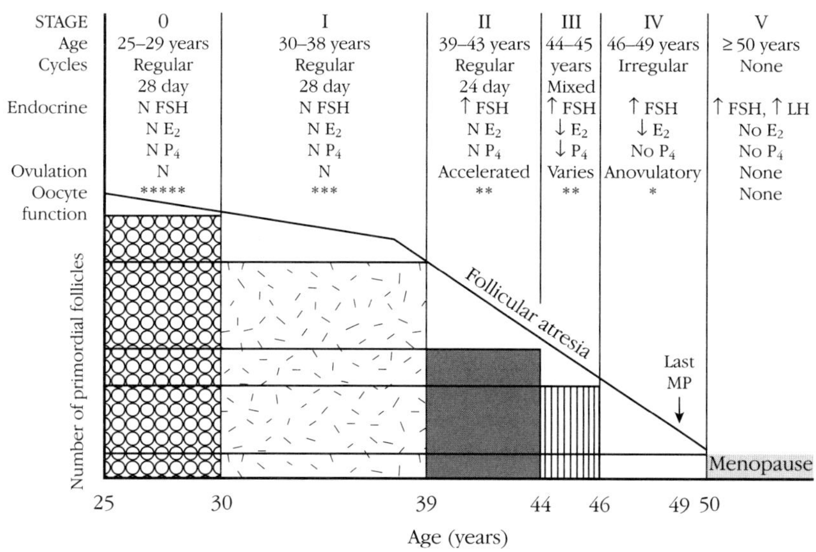

Figure 2 Stages of reproductive aging. Reproductive function has been divided into six stages according to the presence or absence of cycle regularity, changes in specific endocrine hormones (e.g. follicle stimulating hormone (FSH)) and the presence or absence of ovulation and oocyte function as reflected in relative fertility. These changes are depicted as occurring at specific chronologic ages which are hypothetical, based on the average woman reaching menopause at age 50. N, normal; LH, luteinizing hormone; E_2, estradiol; P_4, progesterone; MP, menstrual period

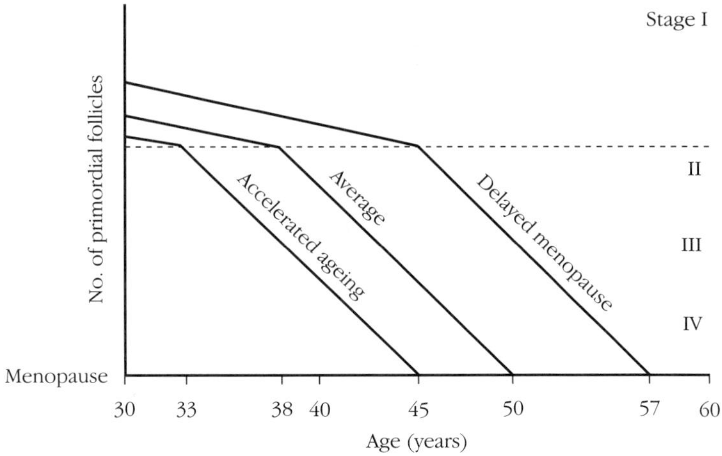

Figure 3 Reproductive aging in a normal woman. She can achieve menopause as early as age 42 or as late as age 58. A woman with an earlier menopause reaches critical thresholds in her reserve of primordial follicles (dotted line) at an earlier chronologic age for each stage of reproductive aging

STAGES I AND II

Early endocrine and menstrual cycle changes

Our initial studies focused on stages I and II of reproductive aging[3–7]. We have considered these stages the most relevant, because these women, while distinctly less fertile, still retain sufficient reproductive function to have a realistic hope for fertility. Considering that the theoretical average woman reaches stage II in her late 30s, we elected to study women aged 40–45 with regular ovulatory menstrual cycles. We considered it important to understand the endocrine changes in normal women as the necessary prerequisite to studying any pathological states. Therefore, our subjects were required to be healthy – normal medical history and physical examination, normal weight for height, taking no medications and no history of infertility or pregnancy wastage. The following screening procedures were required: normal prolactin and testosterone levels and a luteal phase progesterone level that exceeded 3 ng/ml. These women were studied intensively with daily blood drawing and daily assessment of follicle development by ultrasound at mid-cycle. The control group was normal women selected by the same criteria who were 20–25 years old. While group results will be presented, it is important to point out that some of the older women showed no endocrine signs of reproductive aging and were in stage I, while others demonstrated subtle signs and were, in effect, in stage II. The 40–45-year-old group, the women of advanced reproductive age (ARA), had shorter menstrual cycles of the order of 25 days because their follicular phase length was approximately 3 days shorter (Figure 4)[3]. While ARA women did not form larger preovulatory follicles, they demonstrated an

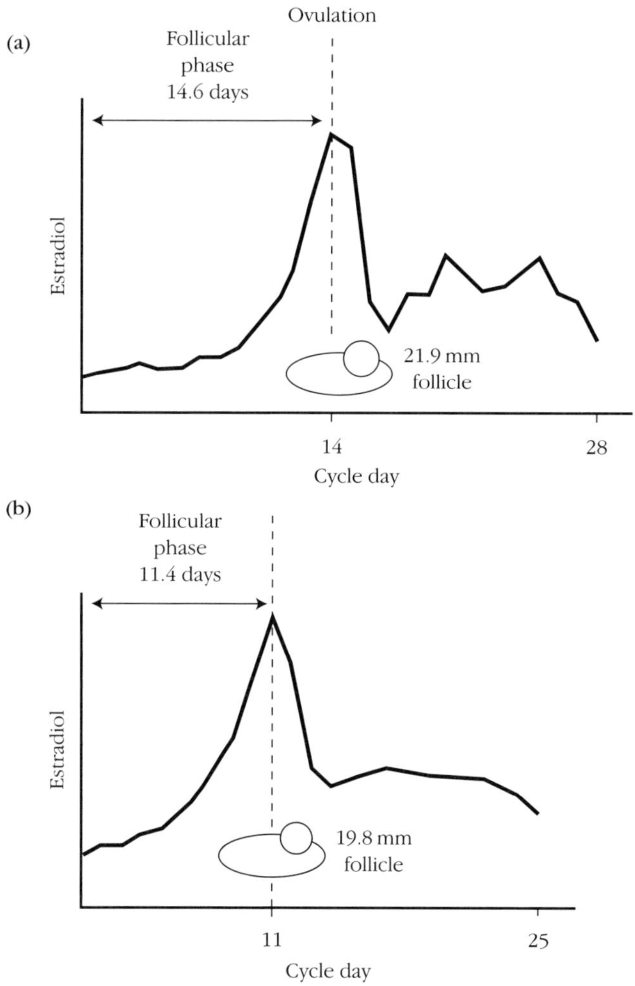

Figure 4 Menstrual cycle duration. The acute rise in estradiol occurred sooner in older ovulatory women (40–45 years (b)), resulting in a follicular phase that was 3 days shorter, subsequently leading to a shorter cycle than in women of 20–25 years (a). The mean preovulatory follicle diameter was slightly smaller in the older women but this difference was not significant

increase in serum estradiol levels beginning on cycle day 4 and continuing until ovulation (Figure 5). When estradiol levels were graphed according to the surge of luteinizing hormone (LH), which compensates for the advanced follicle development experienced by ARA women, estrogen levels were the same or elevated in the older compared to the younger group (Figure 6)[3]. Advanced follicular development in ARA women can be explained by earlier recruitment and selection of the dominant follicle, since there was a significantly earlier FSH rise in the late luteal phase of the preceding cycle.

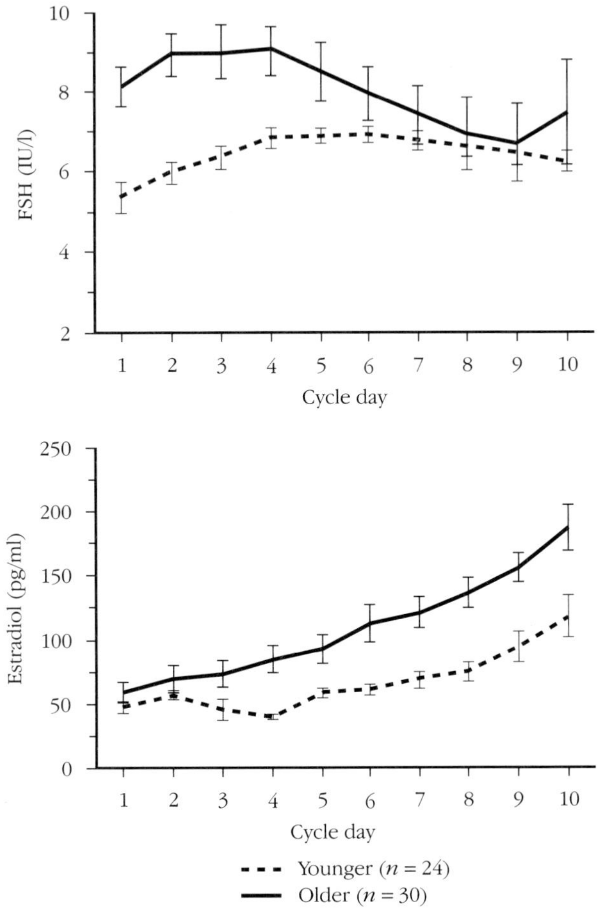

Figure 5 Older ovulatory women (40–45 years) demonstrate elevated FSH levels in the early follicular phase. Older women also demonstrate higher circulating estradiol levels than younger women (20–25 years), beginning on cycle day 4 and continuing through ovulation. Cycle day 1 corresponds to the onset of menses. Figure reproduced with permission from reference 3

While there was a subtle but significant FSH elevation throughout the entire menstrual cycle in the ARA group, there were no changes in circulating LH levels (Figure 7)[3]. Besides the earlier timing of the mid-cycle LH surge in ARA women, there were no changes in the amount or duration of LH secretion. The primary change in moving from stage I to stage II of reproductive aging is an advanced process of follicular development. Follicular development in older ovulatory women appears to be robust and strong by standard endocrine criteria and is followed by normal corpus luteum function (Figure 6)[3]. Normal function of the corpus luteum is a further sign of adequate follicular development.

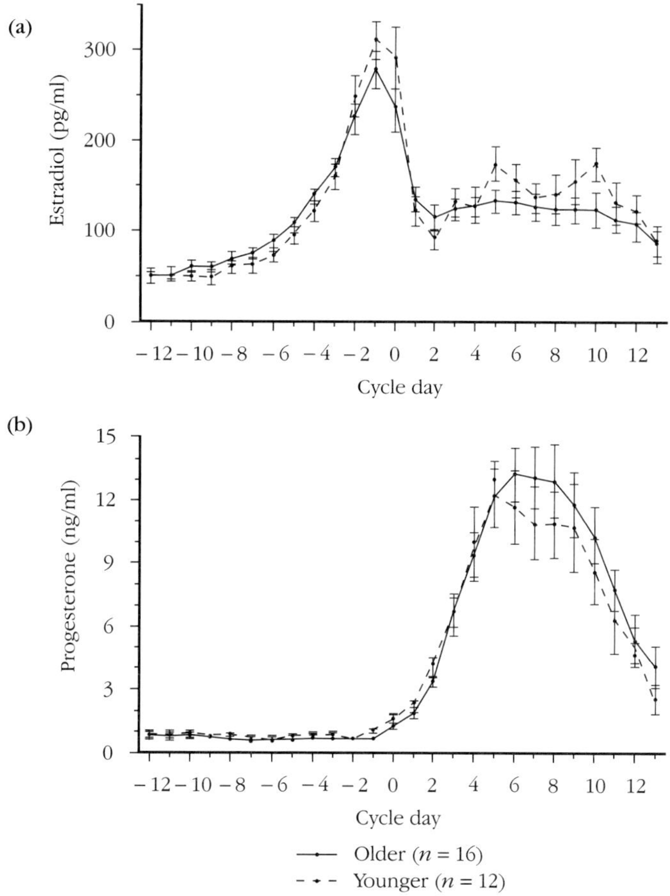

Figure 6 When estradiol levels were graphed according to the day of the luteinizing hormone surge (day 0) the estradiol levels (a) were comparable between younger (20–25 years) and older (40–45 years) women. Likewise, there were no differences in progesterone secretion after ovulation (b). Figure reproduced with permission from reference 3

The monotropic FSH rise is the subtle unilateral increase in serum FSH levels demonstrated by ARA women. This was first described many years ago by Sherman and colleagues[8] and is the sentinel early endocrine sign of reproductive aging. We have performed a series of studies directed at an increased understanding of the physiological basis for the monotropic FSH rise. We theorized that it could occur by several different mechanisms:

(1) Neuroendocrine – a slowing of the gonadotropin releasing hormone (GnRH) pulse generator;
(2) Pituitary – a change in the biopotency of the FSH molecule;
(3) Ovary – a change in the amount or secretion pattern of known FSH-modulating hormones (Figure 8).

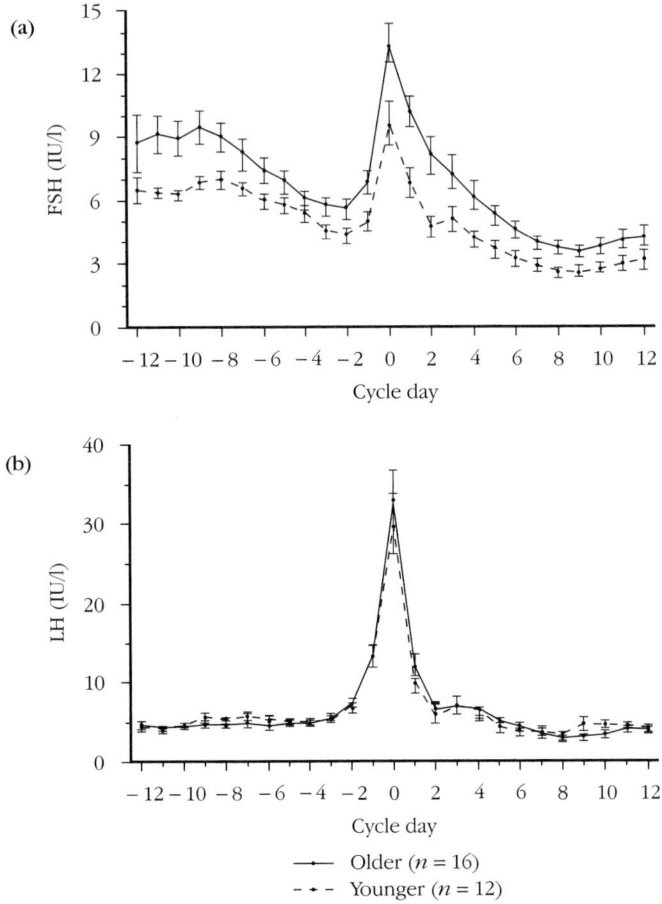

Figure 7 The monotropic rise in follicle stimulating hormone (FSH) (a) in the older group (40–45 years) compared to the younger group (20–25 years) persisted throughout the cycle but was most prominent in the early follicular phase. There were no differences in circulating levels of luteinizing hormone (LH) (b) throughout the cycle between the younger group (20–25 years) and older group (40–45 years) and this included the LH surge. Figure reproduced with permission from reference 3

Early landmark studies in hypothalamically lesioned monkeys clearly demonstrated that the rate of secretion of GnRH by the arcuate nucleus determined the relative levels of circulating FSH[9]. A slowing of the GnRH pulse generator, as occurs normally in the luteal phase, leads to an FSH elevation (the intercycle FSH rise). However, our group and other investigators did not find a change in LH (GnRH) pulse frequency in ovulatory older women of advanced reproductive age in either the early follicular or the mid-luteal phases of their menstrual cycles (Figure 9)[7]. The LH pulse frequency is considered to be reflective of the frequency of GnRH secretion by the hypothalamus. All studies agree that there is not a slowing of the GnRH pulse

Hypothesis	Alteration
Neuroendocrine	Slowing of GnRH pulsegenerator
Pituitary	Biopotency of FSH molecule
Ovarian	Secretion of FSH-modulating hormones (estradiol, inhibin, activin, follistatin)

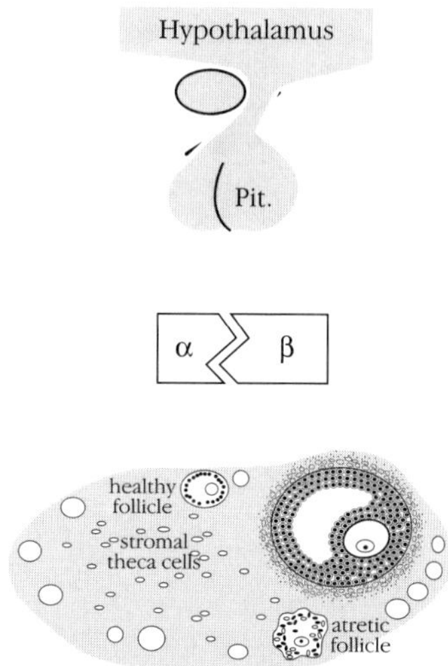

Figure 8 It is hypothesized that the initiation of the monotropic follicle stimulating hormone (FSH) rise could be secondary to alterations at any level of the hypothalamic–pituitary–ovarian axis. GnRH, gonadotropin releasing hormone; Pit., pituitary

generator in association with the monotropic FSH rise. The studies by Reame and co-workers[10] and C.H. de Koning and co-workers (unpublished data) did find an increase in FSH pulse amplitude which would indicate that the increased FSH secretion with early reproductive aging is intrinsic to the pituitary. This finding is compatible with estradiol, inhibin and/or activin potentiating the secretory capability of the pituitary gonadotrope. Additional studies found no change in the biopotency of the FSH molecule across the menstrual cycle in ARA women (Figure 10)[3]. We currently subscribe to the theory that the monotropic FSH rise occurs because of changes to the secretory pattern of FSH-modulating proteins from the ovary (Figure 11). Note that it has been demonstrated that estradiol secretion from the dominant follicle is not reduced in ARA women. Recent research has appropriately focused on the inhibin–activin–follistatin family of FSH-modulating proteins. These investigations have only recently been feasible with the development of sensitive and specific assays for inhibin A, inhibin B, activin A and follistatin. With *in situ* hybridization, Roberts and colleagues[11] elegantly demonstrated that granulosa cells in small antral follicles preferentially synthesized the β_B subunit of inhibin. Likewise, the granulosa cells of dominant follicles demonstrated a dominance of β_A subunit production. It was subsequently shown that inhibin B is the dominant form of inhibin secreted early in the follicular phase while inhibin A is the dominant inhibin molecule secreted by the mature follicle[12]. We hypothesized and demonstrated that women with a monotropic FSH rise had a decrease in circulating inhibin B levels in the early follicular phase of their cycles (Figure 12)[6]. Since this initial publication of the finding of an inhibin B deficiency in ARA women, this has been confirmed by

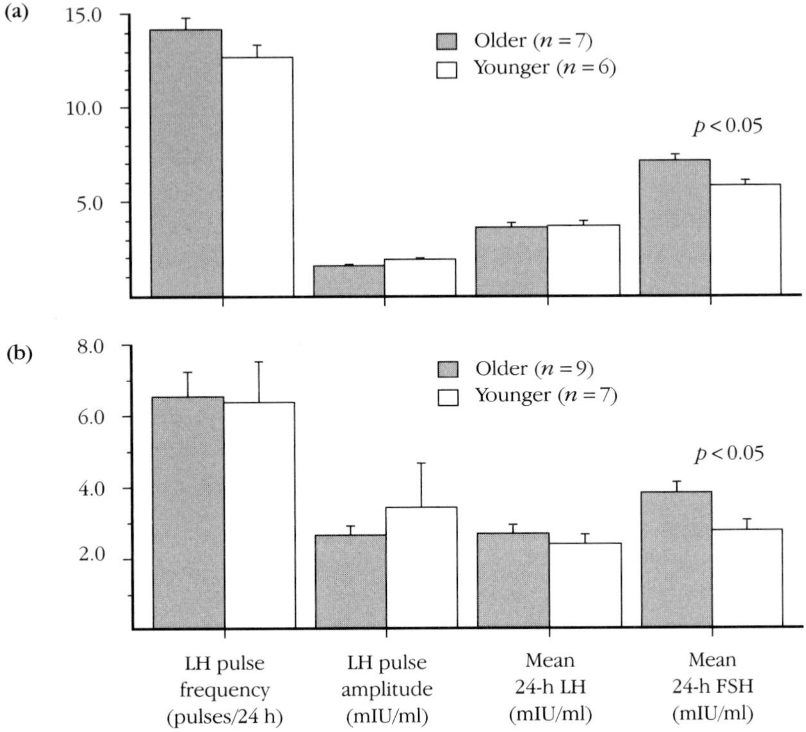

Figure 9 The luteinizing hormone (LH) pulse frequency, pulse amplitude and mean 24-h level was not different between younger (20–25 years) and older (40–45 years) ovulatory women in either the early follicular (a) or the mid-luteal (b) phase of normal menstrual cycles

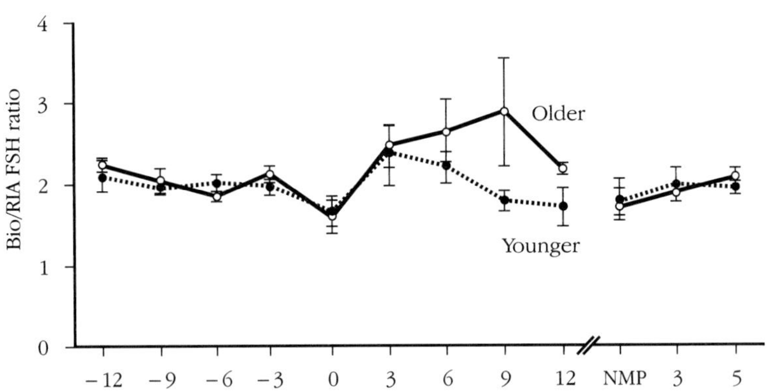

Figure 10 The biological/immunological (Bio/RIA) ratio for the follicle stimulating hormone (FSH) molecule was found not to be significantly different across the menstrual cycles between the older women (40–45 years) and the younger women (20–25 years). NMP, normal menstrual period. Figure reproduced with permission from reference 3

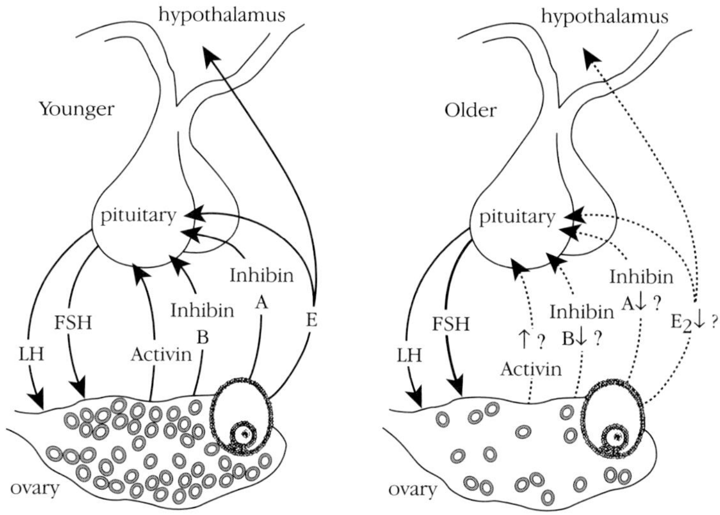

Figure 11 The stimulation–feedback mechanisms between the ovary and the brain are complex. An alteration in estradiol, inhibin A, inhibin B, and/or activin levels could account for the monotropic follicle stimulating hormone (FSH) rise. LH, luteinizing hormone

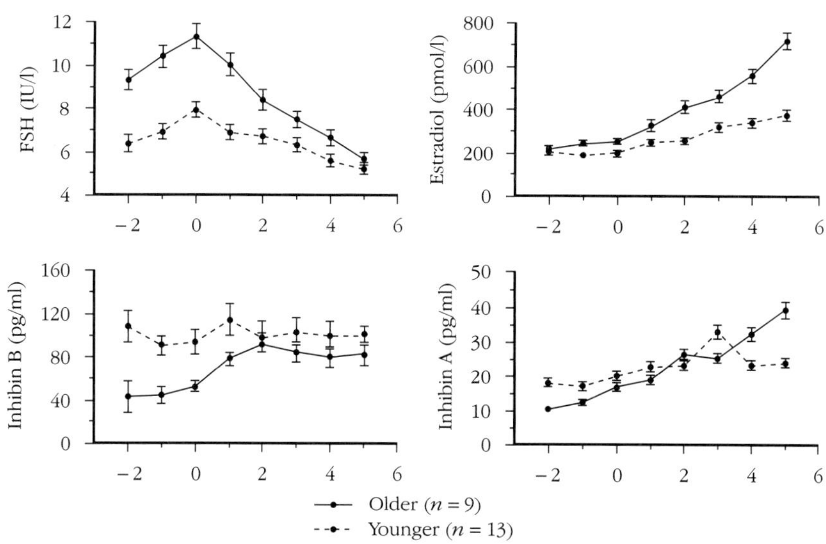

Figure 12 Early follicular levels of follicle stimulating hormone (FSH) in relation to dimeric inhibin A and B. The data are arranged around the day of the early follicular peak FSH level in each subject (day 0). There was a significant increase in the FSH levels on days – 2 to + 2 in the older group along with a simultaneous decrease in inhibin B but not inhibin A. Reproduced with permission from reference 6

five separate investigators throughout the world[13–17]. In 1998, Reame and colleagues proposed that the monotropic FSH rise may be secondary not only to a deficiency of inhibin B but also to increased circulating levels of activin A[13]. This contention has not been well supported by subsequent studies from other groups and is highly doubtful in the context of the endocrinology of follistatin. Follistatin is the carrier/binding protein of activin; a molecule of follistatin binds to each of the homodimers of activin. This binding completely blocks the biological function of activin. While it has been shown that both activin A and follistatin levels increase with age in both men and women[18,19], the dominant and consistent finding has been that there is a large excess of circulating follistatin in relation to activin A[20]. It is not then surprising that total activin A was demonstrated to be increased in ARA women, but the concomitant increase in follistatin negates its physiologic significance. Therefore, if activin A has a role in the monotropic FSH rise it would have to be on an autocrine/paracrine level (Figure 13). The monotropic FSH rise advances follicular development and perhaps is the primary antecedent to accelerated follicular depletion.

Growth hormone (GH) has been investigated as a potential determinant of reproductive aging in women. A decrease in circulating GH and insulin-like growth factor (IGF)-I has been well described to occur in conjunction with increased chronologic age in both men and women[21]. GH levels are also modulated by estrogen, and circulating GH levels increase with estrogen replacement after the menopause[22]. Numerous studies have shown that both IGF-I and IGF-II potentiate FSH stimulation of granulosa cells and follicle

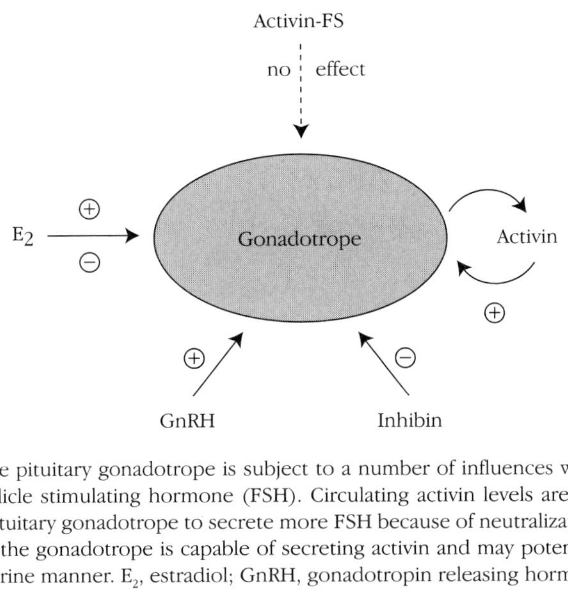

Figure 13 The pituitary gonadotrope is subject to a number of influences with regard to its secretion of follicle stimulating hormone (FSH). Circulating activin levels are not believed to influence the pituitary gonadotrope to secrete more FSH because of neutralization by follistatin (FS). However, the gonadotrope is capable of secreting activin and may potentiate FSH secretion in an autocrine manner. E_2, estradiol; GnRH, gonadotropin releasing hormone

development. IGF-II is considered to be the dominant secretory product of human granulosa cells as opposed to IGF-I[23]. GH has been described as an adjunct medication to gonadotropins and has been used to enhance ovulation induction. Taking these relationships into consideration, it was hypothesized that GH secretion may regulate and influence reproductive aging. In 1995, Wilshire and colleagues[24] reported that the 12-h integrated daytime GH concentrations were lower in ARA women as compared to a younger control group. Subsequently, our group published a similar study in which we found no significant changes in GH pulse frequency, nor integrated GH levels in our somewhat younger ARA ovulatory women (Figure 14)[5]. We did find significantly lower serum IGF-I levels in the older group. However, since a decrease in circulating IGF-I appears to be a general phenomenon of aging, we were most interested in the relative IGF levels in the dominant follicles of ARA women. While IGF-I levels were decreased in the follicular fluid of dominant follicles in ARA women, the IGF-II levels (considered to be more significant) were not different (Figure 15)[4]. Without a consistent change in GH secretion and no change in IGF-II within the follicle, it does not appear that GH is a major contributor to reproductive aging.

STAGES III AND IV

The more advanced stages of reproductive aging are commonly referred to as the perimenopause. The perimenopause is characterized by cycle irregularity which is secondary to erratic steroid hormone secretion from the ovary. A typical woman in the perimenopausal period will have regular (albeit short) menstrual cycles for several months followed by irregular menses or amenorrhea or some other variation of menstrual cyclicity. Cycle irregularity, erratic hormone secretion and repressed reproductive function is the norm for this stage of HPO axis function. The hormonal dynamics of this period were well described and illustrated by Santoro and colleagues[25] in 1996. Figure 16 encompasses a 6-month period of time and illustrates the erratic nature of ovarian function in the perimenopause. The subject had presumably normal follicular development on two occasions during this 180-day interval, as shown by normal estrogen secretion, and on a third occasion she had high levels of estrogen secretion which appeared to be supraphysiological. Each episode of estrogen secretion was followed by ovulation and progesterone secretion. This steroid secretion suppressed gonadotropin levels into the normal range. Between these episodes of ovarian function there were 30- to 60-day episodes where the ovary demonstrated only minimal function and gonadotropin levels were elevated into the early menopausal range with the hypothalamus/pituitary responding in normal fashion to ovarian feedback. Based on the landmark study of Richardson and co-workers[26], it is assumed that the ovaries from this woman contained only a few hundred remaining primordial follicles.

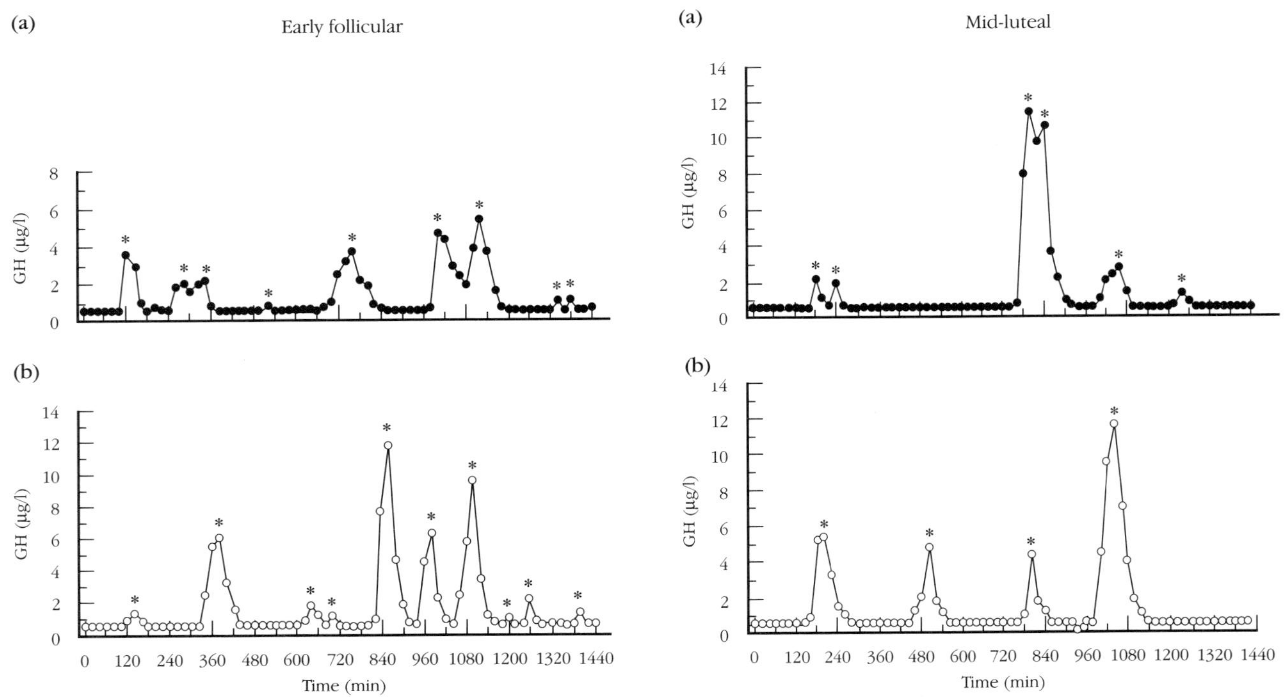

Figure 14 Representative growth hormone (GH) secretory profiles over a 24-h admission in the early follicular and mid-luteal phases of selected cycles in representative older (a) and younger (b) subjects. The asterisks represent a recognized secretory pulse. Reproduced with permission from reference 5

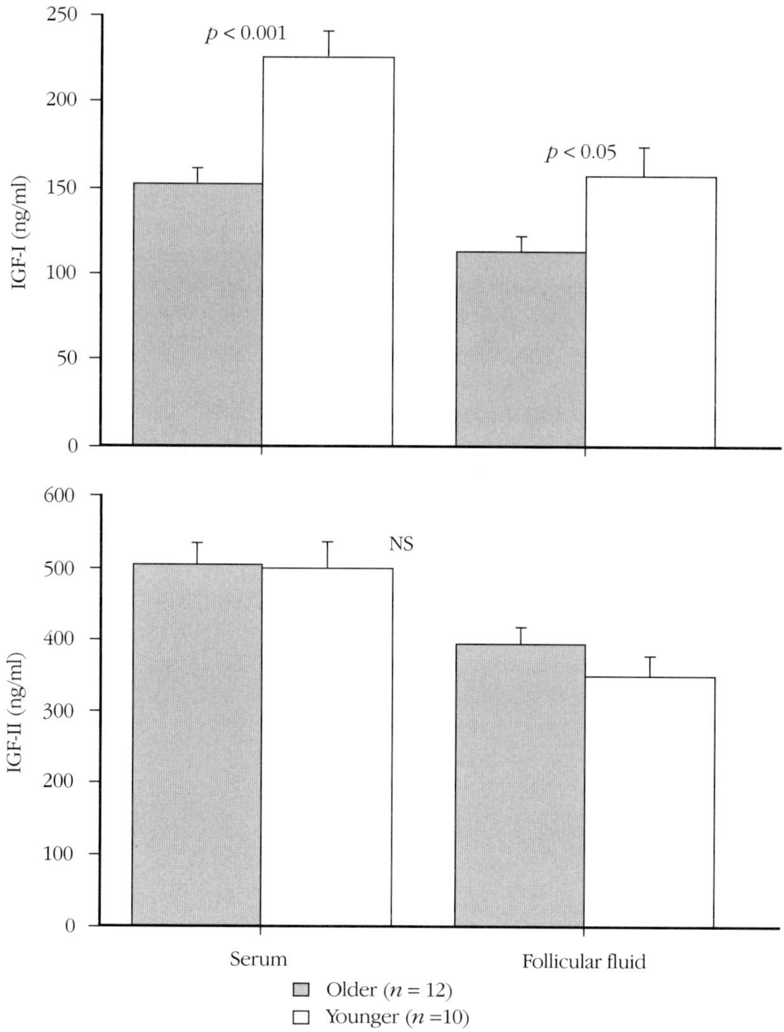

Figure 15 Insulin-like growth factor (IGF)-I levels were significantly lower in the follicular fluid of older (40–45 years) ovulatory women than younger (20–25 years) women, appearing to reflect the general decrease in circulating IGF-I levels. IGF-II levels were not decreased in the serum or follicular fluid when the two groups were compared. Reproduced with permission from reference 4

A cross-sectional analysis of a prospective longitudinal study from Melbourne, Australia illustrates the decline of HPO axis function as women approach the menopause (Figure 17)[14]. In that study, women who were in the early perimenopause (a menstrual period within the past 3 months) had a subtle monotropic FSH rise associated with a decrease in inhibin B, but otherwise had normal ovarian function in terms of estradiol and inhibin A

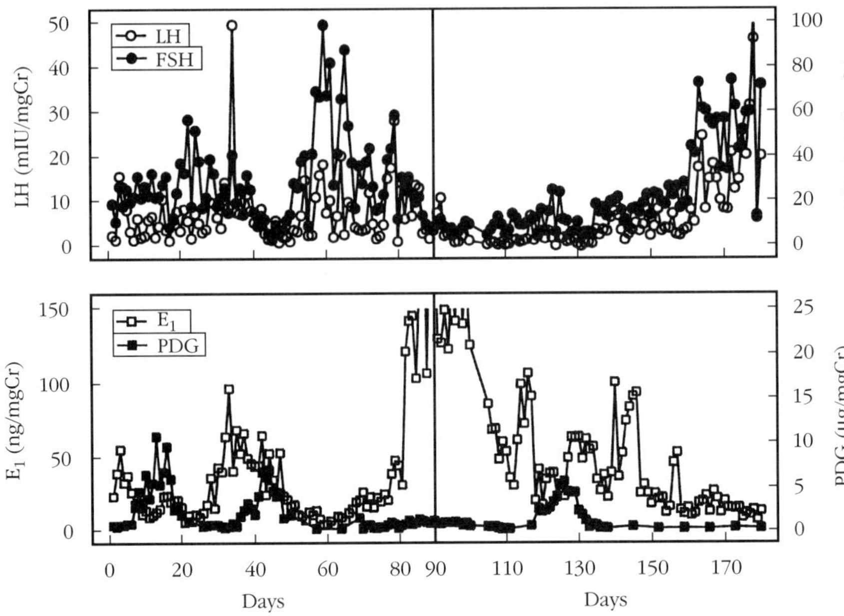

Figure 16 A representative pattern of hormonal secretion in a perimenopausal woman. Episodes of hypergonadotropism with no ovarian function are followed by hyperestrogenism without ovulation and later by estrogen secretion with ovulation. LH, luteinizing hormone; FSH, follicle stimulating hormone; E_1, estrone; PDG, pregnanediol glucutonide. Reproduced with permission from reference 25

levels. Later in the perimenopause, in women who had not had a menstrual period for 3 months, the findings were significantly different. Not only were inhibin B levels decreased and FSH levels higher but both estradiol and inhibin A levels were significantly decreased as well. It was concluded that the monotropic FSH rise was initially due to a decrease in inhibin B, but was subsequently further accentuated by decreased inhibin A and estradiol.

Summary of changes in circulating hormones

The endocrine changes in the last 10 years of a woman's reproductive life are subtle but substantial (Table 1). The early changes could be described as compensatory; they consist of a robust and advanced follicular development followed by ovulation and normal corpus luteum function. An early intercycle FSH rise is the immediate antecedent to this advanced follicle development and is part of the overall monotropic FSH rise. A decrease in levels of inhibin B that emanates from small antral follicles is the initial cause of the monotropic FSH rise. Circulating activin levels are not considered to have a role in this FSH elevation, because it is bound and inactivated by follistatin. As a woman approaches the menopause, the ability of the follicles to produce

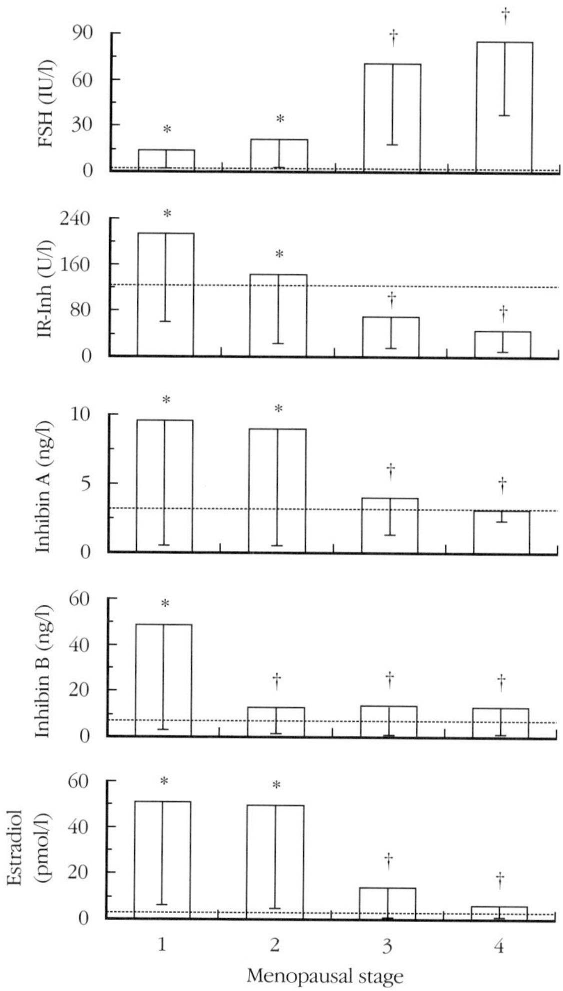

Figure 17 In this cross-sectional analysis, 110 women were divided into four arbitrary stages: stage 1, premenopausal; stage 2, early perimenopause with menstrual bleeding within 3 months; stage 3, late perimenopause with amenorrhea for 3–11 months; stage 4, postmenopause (more than 12 months of amenorrhea). The geometric means are illustrated for the hormones indicated. IR-Inh, immunoreactive inhibin. Different symbols indicate significant differences ($p < 0.05$). Reproduced with permission from reference 14

normal levels of estradiol and the corpus luteum to produce normal levels of progesterone are compromised. At this stage the cycles become more irregular and fertility is virtually nil. Altogether the circulating endocrine changes associated with the latter stages of reproductive aging are predictable if one assumes that there are very few follicles remaining in the ovary and that these remaining follicles are compromised and prone to erratic function.

Table 1 Major changes in circulating hormones that accompany early and late reproductive aging. Mean levels are described as increased (↑), normal or decreased (↓) when the older group was contrasted with the younger controls

Intercycle FSH rise, E_2 rise and ovulation occurs earlier in cycle
Early aging
↑ FSH
↓ inhibin B
E_2 ↑ or normal
P_4 normal
Late aging
↓ E_2
↓ inhibin A
LPD
↑ Activin but complexed with follistatin (inactive)

FSH, follicle stimulating hormone; E_2, estradiol; P_4, progesterone; LPD, luteal phase deficiency

The follicular fluid hormone environment in reproductive aging

To attempt to understand the endocrinology of reproductive aging further, our group has also investigated the follicular fluid (FF) hormonal environment in normal women of advanced reproductive age[4,27]. The women were selected in the same manner as in our earlier studies. The FF was aspirated from the developing dominant follicle by transvaginal ultrasound techniques when the follicle had reached a diameter of 16 mm and/or achieved a serum estradiol level of 150 pg/ml. A total of 36 ARA women have been studied in this manner. Essentially the same hormones that were assayed in the circulation were measured in FF. In addition, we measured FF levels of IGF binding protein (IGFBP)-2 and IGFBP-3 as well as vascular endothelial growth factor (VEGF)[27]. When FF levels of these hormones were compared between the older ovulatory women and the control group we found many hormones to be normal while others were increased; only IGF-I was decreased (Figure 18). As illustrated, the estrogen/androgen ratio, activin A, follistatin and VEGF levels were increased in the FF of the ARA group. The levels of estradiol, testosterone, androstenedione, progesterone, free follistatin, inhibin A and B, IGF-II, IGFBP-2 and IGFBP-3 were normal. These findings led us to the concept of follicular development being either compensated or compromised in older ovulatory women. For instance, the increase in the estradiol/androgen ratio would appear to be a compensatory mechanism for follicular development, since a higher estrogen/androgen ratio is considered to reflect a healthier follicle. On the other hand, if the increased levels of VEGF represent relative hypoxia then this would indicate follicle compromise. Altogether, the endocrine environment of the mature follicle in older ovulatory women appears to exhibit elements of both compensation and compromise (Table 2).

In older ovulatory women the FF steroid environment appears to be healthy. Inhibin A is noted to be the dominant form of inhibin in the mature

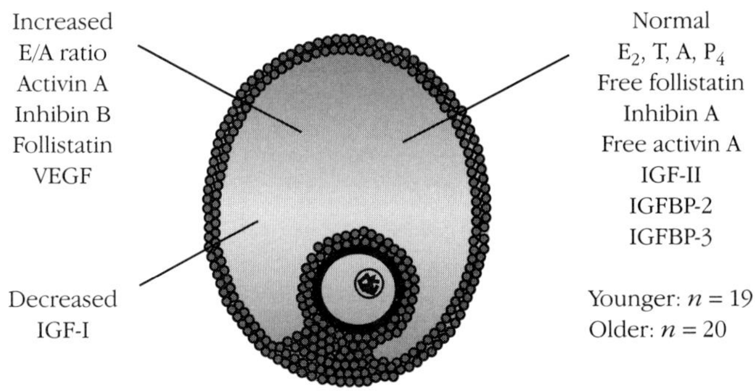

Figure 18 The key follicular fluid hormones and growth factors involved in reproductive aging, measured in women of advanced reproductive age (40–45 years) versus controls (20–25 years). E/A, estrogen/androgen; VEGF, vascular endothelial growth factor; E_2, estradiol; T, testosterone; A, androstenedione; P_4, progesterone; IGF, insulin-like growth factor; IGFBP, IGF binding protein

Table 2 Key follicular fluid hormones and growth factors involved in reproductive aging, in women of advanced reproductive age

	Findings
Steroid environment	compensated slightly (↑ E/A)
Inhibin A and B	no significant change
Activin A	↑ but neutralized by follistatin
IGF-I	reflects ↓ in serum (not biologically important)
IGF-II	no change
Activin → IGFBP-2	pathway present but not altered
VEGF	↑ but? physiologic significance

E/A, estradiol/androstenedione ratio; IGF, insulin-like growth factor; IGFBP, IGF binding protein; VEGF, vascular endothelial growth factor

follicle and there is no difference between younger and older subjects in this regard, further indicating a healthy dominant follicle in ARA women. Based on studies in rodents and monkeys, an increase in activin in the dominant follicle promotes oocyte degeneration and earlier ovulation[28–30]. Activin has also been shown to increase the levels of IGFBP-2, which in turn binds increased levels of IGF-II, decreasing the overall tropic stimulus to the follicle[31]. While we found elevated activin A levels in the FF, the follistatin levels were also elevated, and free activin A levels were not increased. Altogether, this would indicate that the higher levels of activin A are probably neutralized by follistatin and do not necessarily cause any follicular compromise in older women who ovulate regularly. The growth hormone axis does not appear to be active in follicular compromise, since IGF-II levels were not decreased in the ARA group. The decreased levels of FF IGF-I are considered to reflect decreased serum levels and are not as pertinent as IGF-II in human follicles. The higher VEGF levels in FF of older ovulatory women could be interpreted in two ways: as a sign of follicular hypoxia (compromise) or a sign of more robust granulosa cells that can secrete more of this particular growth factor (compensated)[32].

The primary function of the HPO axis in women is reproduction. The health and function of the HPO axis can be appropriately judged in terms of its efficiency as reflected in the ability to conceive healthy pregnancies. As women age into their 30s and 40s their fertility goes from mildly to severely compromised. The endocrine changes (both in the circulation and in the dominant follicle) that accompany this decrease in fertility potential are quite subtle until the very late stages of reproductive aging. In an ovulatory woman in her early 40s the loss of fertility is much more dramatic than the endocrine changes. In many ways the endocrine function of the HPO axis early in a woman's fifth decade can be viewed as compensating for the decrease in fertility, until compensation is no longer feasible, owing to almost complete follicular depletion. Our current thinking considers the oocyte as the major cause of decreased reproductive efficiency as women age. The oocyte does not function well, as reflected in the increase in aneuploid embryos, chromosome abnormalities in pregnancy and a dramatic increase in spontaneous abortions. These major changes occur when there are only minor changes in the endocrine environment. While further studies of the endocrine aspects of reproductive aging are warranted, it is recommended that future studies seeking a better understanding of compromised fertility with aging should focus on the oocyte.

REFERENCES

1. McKinlay S, Brambilla D, Posner J. The normal menopause transition. *Maturitias* 1992;14:103–15
2. Faddy M, Gosden R. A model conforming the decline in follicle numbers to the age of menopause in women. *Hum Reprod* 1996;11:1484–6
3. Klein N, Battaglia D, Fujimoto V, *et al*. Reproductive ageing: accelerated ovarian follicular development associated with a monotropic follicle-stimulating hormone rise in normal older women. *J Clin Endocrinol Metab* 1996;81:1038–45
4. Klein N, Battaglia D, Miller P, *et al*. Ovarian follicular development and the follicular fluid hormones and growth factors in normal women of advanced reproductive age. *J Clin Endocrinol Metab* 1996;81:1946–51
5. Klein N, Battaglia D, Miller P, Soules M. Circulating levels of growth hormone, insulin-like growth factor-I and growth hormone binding protein in normal women of advanced reproductive age. *Clin Endocrinol* 1996;44:285–92
6. Klein N, Illingworth P, Groome N, *et al*. Decreased inhibin B secretion is associated with the monotropic FSH rise in older, ovulatory women: a study of serum and follicular fluid levels of dimeric inhibin A and B in spontaneous menstrual cycles. *J Clin Endocrinol Metab* 1996;81:2742–5
7. Klein N, Battaglia D, Clifton D, *et al*. The gonadotropin secretion pattern in normal women of advanced reproductive age in relation to the monotropic FSH rise. *J Soc Gynecol Invest* 1996;3:27–32

8. Sherman B, West J, Korenman S. The menopausal transition: analysis of LH, FSH, estradiol, and progesterone concentrations during menstrual cycles of older women. *J Clin Endocrinol Metab* 1976;42:629–36
9. Wildt L, Hausler A, Marshall G. Frequency and amplitude of gonadotropin-releasing hormone stimulation and gonadotropin secretion in the rhesus monkey. *Endocrinology* 1981;109:376–85
10. Reame N, Kelch R, Beitins I, *et al*. Age effects on follicle-stimulating hormone and pulsatile luteinizing hormone secretion across the menstrual cycle of premenopausal women. *J Clin Endocrinol Metab* 1996;81:1512–18.
11. Roberts V, Barth S, El-Roeiy A, Yen S. Expression of inhibin/activin subunits and follistatin messenger ribonucleic acids and proteins in ovarian follicles and the corpus luteum during the human menstrual cycle. *J Clin Endocrinol Metab* 1993;77:1402–10
12. Groome N, Illingworth P, O'Brien M, *et al*. Measurement of dimeric inhibin B throughout the human menstrual cycle. *J Clin Endocrinol Metab* 1996;81:1401–5
13. Reame N, Wyman TL, Phillips D, *et al*. Net increase in stimulatory input resulting from a decrease in inhibin B and an increase in activin A may contribute in part to the rise in follicular phase follicle-stimulating hormone of ageing cycling women. *J Clin Endocrinol Metab* 1998;83:3302–7
14. Burger H, Cahir N, Robertson D, *et al*. Serum inhibins A and B fall differentially as FSH rises in perimenopausal women. *Clin Endocrinol* 1998;48:809–13
15. Hoffman G, Danforth DR, Seifer DB. Inhibin-B: the physiologic basis of the clomiphene citrate challenge test for ovarian reserve screening. *Fertil Steril* 1998;69:474–81
16. Welt C, McNicholl D, Taylor A, Hall J. Female reproductive ageing is marked by decreased secretion of dimeric inhibin. *J Clin Endocrinol Metab* 1999;84:105–11
17. Santoro N, Adel T, Skurnick J. Decreased inhibin tone and increased activin A secretion characterize reproductive ageing in women. *Fertil Steril* 1999;71:658–62
18. Harada K, Shintani Y, Sakamoto Y, *et al*. Serum immunoreactive activin A levels in normal subjects and patients with various diseases. *J Clin Endocrinol Metab* 1996;81:2125–30
19. Wakatsuki J, Shintani YM, Liu Z, *et al*. Immunoradiometric assay for follistatin: serum immunoreactive follistatin levels in normal adults and pregnant women. *J Clin Endocrinol Metab* 1996;81:630–4
20. McConnell D, Wang Q, Sluss PM. A two-site solid phase immunochemiluminescent assay for activin-free follistatin reveals that most follistatin circulating in men and normal cycling women is in an activin-bound state. *J Clin Endocrinol Metab* 1998; 83:851–8
21. Weltman A, Weltman J, Hartman M, *et al*. Relationship between age, percentage body fat, fitness, and 24-hour growth hormone release in healthy young adults: effects of gender. *J Clin Endocrinol Metab* 1994;78:543–8
22. Ho K, Evans W, Blizzard R, *et al*. Effects of sex and age on the 24-hour profile of growth hormone secretion in man: importance of endogenous estradiol concentrations. *J Clin Endocrinol Metab* 1987;51:51–8
23. Giudice L, Chandrasekher Y, Cataldo N. The potential roles of intraovarian peptides in normal and abnormal mechanisms of reproductive physiology. *Curr Opin Obstet Gynecol* 1993;5:350–9
24. Wilshire G, Loughlin J, Brown J, *et al*. Diminished function of the somatotropic axis in older reproductive-aged women. *J Clin Endocrinol Metab* 1995;80:608–13
25. Santoro N, Brown J, Adel T, Skurnick J. Characterization of reproductive hormonal dynamics in the perimenopause. *J Clin Endocrinol Metab* 1996;81:1495–501

26. Richardson S, Senikas V, Nelson J. Follicular depletion during the menopausal transition: evidence for accelerated loss and ultimate exhaustion. *J Clin Endocrinol Metab* 1987;65:1231–7
27. Klein N, Battaglia D, Woodruff T, *et al*. Ovarian follicular concentrations of activin, follistatin, inhibin, IGF-I, IGF-II, IGFBP-2, IBFBP-3, and VEGF in spontaneous menstrual cycles of normal women of advanced reproductive age. *J Clin Endocrinol Metab* 2000;in press
28. Woodruff T, Lyon R, Hansen S, *et al*. Inhibin and activin locally regulate rat ovarian folliculogenesis. *Endocrinology* 1990;127:1237–42
29. Stouffer R, Woodruff T, Dahl K, *et al*. Human recombinant activin-A alters pituitary luteinizing hormone and follicle-stimulating hormone secretion, follicular development, and steroidogenesis during the menstural cycle in rhesus monkeys. *J Clin Endocrinol Metab* 1993;77:241–8
30. Erickson G, Kokka S, Rivier C. Activin causes premature superovulation. *Endocrinology* 1995;136:4804–13
31. Cataldo N, Fujimuto V, Jaffe R. Interferon-gamma and activin A promote insulin-like growth factor-binding protein-2 and -4 accumulation by human luteinizing granulosa cells, and interferon-gamma promotes their apoptosis. *J Clin Endocrinol Metab* 1998;83:179–86
32. Van Blerkom J, Schrader R, Antczak M. The developmental potential of the human oocyte is related to the dissolved oxygen content of follicular fluid: association with vascular endothelial growth factor levels and perifollicular blood flow characteristics. *Hum Reprod* 1997;12:1047–55

7

Ultrasound and ovarian reserve

F.J. Broekmans, G.J. Scheffer, L.F.J.M.M. Bancsi, I.A.J. van Rooy and E.R. te Velde

INTRODUCTION

As a woman ages, thousands and thousands of follicles per year are lost due to atresia. At the same time, after a period of optimal fertility in her 20s, a woman's fertility decreases in her 30s and comes to an end at the beginning of her 40s. One should, however, bear in mind that this pattern of fertility decline represents the mean for the population and may show a high degree of variation. Therefore, if a woman pursues her career and only attempts to achieve pregnancy for the first time after the age of 30, she may have a residual fecundity of about half of the mean for her age group. She may then be confronted with the problem of infertility.

Age-related fertility decline is mainly caused by a decrease in oocyte quality[1,2]. Direct data on oocyte quality in *in vivo* situations are yet lacking for obvious reasons, or are derived from assisted reproduction treatment. During the process of aging, the total number of follicles left in the ovary declines[3], as does the number of antral follicles available in the late luteal phase of the menstrual cycle for delivery of the dominant follicle[4,5]. Related to this reduction in the cohort size is the decline in the production of inhibin B from the small antral follicles[6], thereby causing follicle stimulating hormone (FSH) levels to rise more profoundly in the late luteal and early follicular phases.

OVARIAN RESERVE TESTS

In the studies on ovarian reserve testing, most attention has been paid to parameters related to the number of antral follicles present at the onset of the cycle. Tests such as early follicular FSH[7], inhibin B[8] and estradiol, and the endocrine response to exogenous stimuli (clomiphene citrate test[9], gonadotropin releasing hormone agonist test[10] and the FSH stimulation test[11]), indirectly express the size of the antral follicle cohort.

Ultrasound-based antral follicle counts and ovarian volume measurements[12,13] are considered a more direct quantitative approach towards the assessment of the cohort size. The factor that all tests have in common is that they aim to predict a more advanced stage of aging of the ovary. It is, however, clear that a gold standard assessment of the condition 'advanced aged ovary' is lacking at the moment. Therefore, ovarian reserve tests are frequently evaluated by using the probability of pregnancy or the ovarian response to hyperstimulation as the outcome parameter. It should be stressed here that, when performing and evaluating these tests, one may actually test a woman's ovarian function without knowing if ovarian aging *per se*, subtle ovarian dysfunction by other causes or a combination of both is the underlying problem. Moreover, predicting pregnancy from a test system that is assumed to be related to ovarian reserve, but may well be far removed from the numerous unknown factors that determine the occurrence of pregnancy, seems a difficult task.

In the following, an overview is given of the current status of the most prominent ovarian reserve test currently used, basal FSH, in the management of infertility patients. In addition, the prospects of the use of antral follicle counts in the prediction of *in vitro* fertilization (IVF) outcome are discussed.

When reviewing the performance of an ovarian reserve test, the prognostic value of the test is best expressed by calculating the positive likelihood ratio (representing the relationship between sensitivity and specificity, and indicating the probability of finding an abnormal test in a couple that does not become pregnant or will experience a bad response to ovarian hyperstimulation over the probability of having a normal test in a couple that will become pregnant or perform adequately to ovarian hyperstimulation). From the literature, it appears that the positive likelihood ratio of the test should reach at least the level of 5–10 to be clinically relevant. Moreover, the pretest and post-test probabilities of the outcome parameter, as well as the proportion of patients with an abnormal test, should be calculated to be able to interpret the overall impact of the test for screening in a large population.

BASAL FSH

FSH levels in the early follicular phase of the cycle will become increased with advancing age, presumably due to a reduced inhibin B-mediated feedback towards the pituitary. The decrease in inhibin B production is assumed to be an expression of the reduction in the size of the early follicular antral follicle cohort. Therefore, FSH may indirectly represent cohort size and hence the degree of ovarian reserve, as antral follicle cohort size is clearly related to chronological age[5].

From the literature, we extracted 11 studies dealing with FSH in IVF populations. Studies addressing the predictive value of basal FSH in the general infertility population are lacking at the moment. The IVF studies identified were screened and selected according to the following criteria:

(1) Only one cycle per couple was allowed for analysis in order to prevent the overrepresentation of certain cases in the evaluation of treatment outcome;

(2) Pregnancy rates should have been expressed as the number of pregnancies per started cycle;

(3) Selection bias with regard to the role of ovarian aging in the population under study should have been avoided.

In only five of the 11 studies were the above-mentioned criteria met, and these studies were further analyzed. From the data in the original publications, cross-tabulations could be constructed to calculate likelihood ratios and the pre- and post-test probabilities. In Table 1, the studies are summarized with regard to the outcome variable pregnancy[7,14–18]. Ten per cent of the tests were abnormal. The likelihood ratio of a positive test was between 2 and 5, indicating that FSH as a test has only a moderate performance in the prediction of pregnancy after IVF. Cut-off values are chosen at a very high level in order to limit the number of false positives. By applying the test, one can estimate a greatly reduced probability of pregnancy in about 10% of couples. It should be stressed that a majority of these abnormal test results are obtained in women who are in the older age group. By having an abnormal test, these women will have their chances of becoming pregnant further diminished only to a level that may not be greatly different from the overall probability in this age group. If the post-test probability was, indeed, zero, the test would support the decision to refrain from the indicated treatment.

Table 1 Prognostic value of basal FSH for the probability of pregnancy in IVF treatment in five studies where, in unselected cases, only one cycle per couple is analyzed and pregnancy rates are expressed per started cycle

	Study group				
	Ebrahim et al.[14]	*Evers et al.*[15]	*Huyser et al.*[16]	*Bancsi et al.*[17]	*Sharif et al.*[18]
No. of cycles	111	231	139	435	344
Abnormal tests (%)	11	8	14	5	9
Positive likelihood ratio	2.8	3.3	3.7	3.8	4.1
Pretest probability (%)	21	14	17	14	30
Post-test probability (%)	8	5	6	4	10
FSH cut-off level (IU/l)	11.5	17	11.7	15.0	10.8

With the cut-off levels used, the identification of couples with zero chance does not seem possible. Therefore, the application of basal FSH may only be useful to inform the couple on the perspectives of the IVF treatment.

The predictive capacity of basal FSH towards the risk of cancellation due to bad ovarian response has been summarized in Table 2. One study had to be further eliminated because cross-tabulations could not be constructed from the data presented. It seems that here FSH has a slightly better performance in comparison with its predictive ability towards pregnancy. In case of elevated FSH, the post-test probability of having a cancellation due to a bad response may be clearly increased. Still, the majority of these couples will respond adequately to hyperstimulation and obtain some four or more oocytes at the moment of retrieval.

The first conclusion that can be drawn is that the performance of FSH in IVF populations may never lead to FSH being used as a screening device in patients during the initial infertility work-up. It becomes increasingly clear that FSH levels measured during the infertility work-up may have a different meaning than FSH levels measured in a population that is already indicated for IVF[19]. Moreover, raised basal FSH levels in young women may well be a physiological finding or indicate a genetic predisposition to dizygotic twinning[20,21]. On the basis of the results shown above, one may wonder in what sense the basal FSH value prior to IVF treatment would change the management offered to the couple. In case of clearly elevated FSH levels, couples can be informed on the reduced prospects of their IVF treatment. It remains unclear how many couples would actually refrain from proceeding to the first attempt. If abandoning further treatment by the physician is not included as a consequence, then one could decide just to perform IVF and see what happens in couples indicated for IVF, without knowing the basal FSH level. The ovarian response to adequate ovarian stimulation will then provide definite clues as to whether further attempts should be undertaken. This stresses the

Table 2 Prognostic value of basal FSH for cancellation due to a bad response in IVF treatment in four studies where, in unselected cases, only one cycle per couple is analyzed and pregnancy rates are expressed per started cycle

	Author			
	Ebrahim et al.[14]	*Evers et al.*[15]	*Bancsi et al.*[17]	*Sharif et al.*[18]
No. of cycles	111	231	435	344
Abnormal tests (%)	11	7	5	9
Positive likelihood ratio	10.1	8.6	4.0	5.1
Pretest probability (%)	5	20	7	8
Post-test probability (%)	28	40	23	31
FSH cut-off level (IU/l)	11.5	17	15	10.8

need for ovarian reserve tests that are able to correctly predict the ovarian response to hyperstimulation in order to optimize the stimulation regime in the first IVF cycle.

QUANTITATIVE OVARIAN ULTRASONOGRAPHY

The number of remaining follicles in the ovary would obviously be an adequate measure for a woman's fertility potential, as the number of primordial follicles will exponentially decline with advancing age[3]. It is already known from the histological studies performed by Gougeon that small antral follicles with a size between 2 and 10 mm are related to age and probably to the number of primordial follicles present in the ovary[4]. The number of these antral follicles in the ovaries, as visualized by transvaginal ultrasound, may therefore give a representation of the total remaining primordial follicle pool. Moreover, both in the study by Reuss and colleagues[22] and that by Scheffer and co-workers[5], it was shown that the number of small antral follicles decreases gradually with age.

Ultrasound-based antral follicle counts have been found to be correlated very well with the number of oocytes obtained at follicle aspiration in IVF treatment[13,23]. Moreover, antral follicle counts (2–5 mm diameter) were used to evaluate the predictive ability towards pregnancy in a group of patients undergoing IVF, gamete intra-Fallopian transfer or intra-Fallopian embryo transfer[23]. Although the study design does not meet the criteria formulated above, the test results shown in Table 3 indicate that the ability of the test to predict pregnancy bears the same limitations as basal FSH. With regard to cancellations because of bad response, the antral follicle count seems to perform much better and the probability of cancellation due to bad response will rise from 10 to almost 70% in cases with an abnormal test result. This may imply that the finding of a low number of antral follicles in patients indicated for IVF may form the basis of adjustment in the treatment schedule, for instance by raising the dosage of gonadotropin used.

In a study performed on 120 regularly cycling patients undergoing IVF, irrespective of age or basal FSH level, ultrasound and endocrine testing were

Table 3 Prognostic value of ultrasound-based follicle counts (2–5 mm) for two types of outcome (pregnancy probability and cancellation due to bad response) in IVF treatment. Adapted from the study by Chang and colleagues[23]

	Outcome	
	Pregnancy	*Cancellation*
No. of cycles	149	149
Cut-off level	< 4 follicles	< 4 follicles
Abnormal tests (%)	11	11
Positive likelihood ratio	3.6	18.2
Pretest probability (%)	17	10
Post-test probability (%)	5	67

performed in the early follicular phase of the cycle. After a standard long midluteal suppression and ovarian hyperstimulation protocol with a fixed dose of two ampules of Gonal-F®(Serono Benelux, The Hague, The Netherlands), ovarian response was monitored. Ongoing pregnancy was defined as the occurrence of a vital pregnancy carried beyond the 12th week. Low ovarian response was defined as the collection of fewer than four oocytes or the cancellation of aspiration due to insufficient follicle growth. Data were analyzed using logistic regression. With regard to pregnancy probability, neither single nor combined parameters were able to exert any predictive ability. In contrast, in the univariate analysis, three factors (antral follicle count, basal inhibin B and basal FSH) were selected as markers of ovarian response, as indicated from the odds ratios depicted in Table 4. In the multivariate analysis, the antral follicle count was selected first, while basal inhibin B and FSH appeared to contribute independently to the prediction of ovarian response (Table 4). If we compare the test performance of basal FSH and antral follicle count in a receiver operator characteristics curve, the optimal cut-off levels are found in the lower left corner (Figure 1). At these levels of 14 IU/l and four follicles, respectively, the specificity of both tests is high at the expense of the sensitivity, which prevents informing the wrong women to expect a bad response. This implies that the test still will fail to predict some 55% of bad responders. If FSH, antral follicle count and inhibin B are combined in a logistic model, it appears that, with a cut-off of a predicted 50% probability of a bad response as an abnormal test result, over 90% of the patients with a bad response are predicted correctly by the model. By using the model, the sensitivity of the test system has been clearly improved (Figure 1). At the same time, the false-positive rate remains at the same low level as in the single tests (Table 5). From these findings, it may be concluded that, with the use of quantitative ultrasound in combination with endocrine parameters, the ability to predict a bad response in ovarian hyperstimulation becomes largely improved. The prediction of a bad response in the first IVF treatment cycle may lead to adjustments in the gonadotropin dosage schedule in order to ensure maximal ovarian stimulation. Doubt

Table 4 Odds ratios for poor response regarding several potential predictors of ovarian reserve from univariate and multivariate logistic analyses in IVF patients ($n = 120$)

Ovarian response marker	*Univariate logistic regression analysis*		*Multivariate logistic regression analysis*	
	Odds ratio	*p Value*	*Odds ratio*	*p Value*
Antral follicle count 2–5 mm (per follicle)	1.57	0.000	1.31*	0.000
Basal inhibin B (per pg/ml)	1.03	0.000	1.02†	0.002
Basal FSH (per IU/l)	0.71	0.000	0.79‡	0.002
Basal estradiol (per pmol/l)	0.9968	0.049	not selected	0.627
Age (per year)	0.93	0.074	not selected	0.660

*Step 1 (antral follicle count 2–5 mm selected); †step 2 (basal inhibin B selected); ‡step 3 (FSH selected)

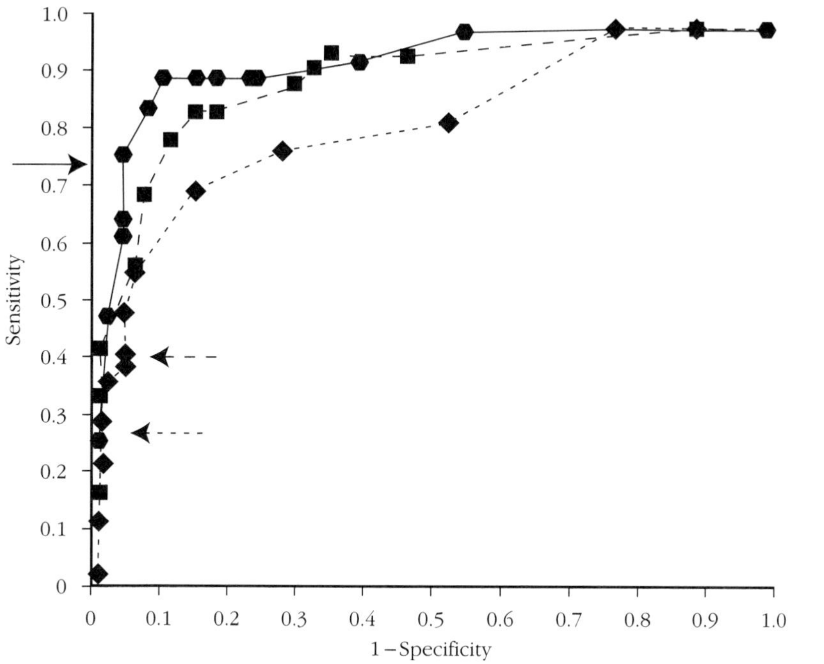

Figure 1 Receiver operator characteristics diagram showing the predictive performance of both the single parameters, FSH (---◆---) and antral follicle count (AFC), (– –■– –) as well as the model (—⬢—) containing the AFC, FSH and inhibin B. Arrows indicate the cut-off points chosen for the comparisons depicted in Table 5

Table 5 Predictive ability for low ovarian response to hyperstimulation in IVF (fewer than four oocytes or cancellation of aspiration due to insufficient follicle growth) by single tests and by a multivariate model containing the antral follicle count (AFC), FSH and inhibin B

	Multivariate model	*AFC*	*FSH*
Cut-off level	50%	< 4 follicles	> 14 IU/l
Abnormal tests (%)	26	15	11
Number of cycles	120	120	120
Sensitivity	0.75	0.47	0.30
Specificity	0.95	0.93	0.98
Positive likelihood ratio	16	8	15
Pretest probability (%)	30	30	30
Post-test probability (%)	87	94	92

exists with regard to the usefulness of raising the dosage of gonadotropins[24] in the management of low ovarian response. However, if adequate stimulation in the first cycle is ensured, the occurrence of a low response will provide final information indicating that ovarian reserve is diminished to such an extent that further treatment is not to be advised.

CONCLUSION

From the data presented and taking into account the criteria for a good test, as mentioned earlier, measuring basal FSH seems to have no significant potential in predicting the outcome of IVF treatment, either with regard to the probability of pregnancy or the occurrence of a bad response. The combined use of the ultrasound-based antral follicle count with early follicular levels of FSH and inhibin B provides us with a potential prognostic system for the response to ovarian hyperstimulation in IVF patients. Validated dose adjustments on the basis of this predictive system may optimize the first treatment cycle and allow definite decisions on further treatment on the basis of the performance of this first cycle. As the predictive capacity towards pregnancy with the use of the combined system is not better than with a single test, outcome prediction in terms of pregnancy probability seems not to be feasible in IVF patients.

REFERENCES

1. Battaglia DE, Goodwin P, Klein NA, Soules MR. Influence of maternal age on meiotic spindle assembly in oocytes from naturally cycling women. *Hum Reprod* 1996;11:2217–22
2. Sauer MV, Paulson RJ, Lobo RA. Pregnancy after age 50: application of oocyte donation to women after natural menopause [see comments]. *Lancet* 1993;341:321–3
3. Faddy MJ, Gosden RG, Gougeon A, Richardson SJ, Nelson JF. Accelerated disappearance of ovarian follicles in mid-life: implications for forecasting menopause. *Hum Reprod* 1992;7:1342–6
4. Gougeon A. Caracteres qualitatifs et quantitatifs de la population folliculaire dans l'ovaire humaine adulte. *Contracept Fertil Sex* 1984;12:527–35
5. Scheffer GJ, Broekmans FJ, Dorland M, *et al.* Antral follicle counts by transvaginal ultrasonography are related to age in women with proven natural fertility. *Fertil Steril* 1999;72:845–51
6. Klein NA, Illingworth PJ, Groome NP, *et al.* Decreased inhibin B secretion is associated with the monotropic FSH rise in older, ovulatory women: a study of serum and follicular fluid levels of dimeric inhibin A and B in spontaneous menstrual cycles. *J Clin Endocrinol Metab* 1996;81:2742–5
7. Scott RT, Toner JP, Muasher SJ, *et al.* Follicle-stimulating hormone levels on cycle day 3 are predictive of *in vitro* fertilization outcome. *Fertil Steril* 1989;51:651–4
8. Seifer DB, Lambert-Messerlian G, Hogan J, *et al.* Day 3 serum inhibin-B is predictive of assisted reproductive technologies outcome. *Fertil Steril* 1997;67:110–14
9. Scott RT, Leonardi MR, Hofmann GE, *et al.* A prospective evaluation of clomiphene citrate challenge test screening of the general infertility population. *Obstet Gynecol* 1993;82:539–44
10. Winslow KL, Toner JP, Brzyski RG, *et al.* The gonadotropin-releasing hormone agonist stimulation test – a sensitive predictor of performance in the flare-up *in vitro* fertilization cycle. *Fertil Steril* 1991;56:711–17
11. Fanchin R, de Ziegler P, Olivennes F, *et al.* Exogenous follicle stimulating hormone ovarian reserve test (EFORT): a simple and reliable screening test for detecting 'poor responders' in *in vitro* fertilization. *Hum Reprod* 1994;9:1607–11

12. Lass A, Skull J, McVeigh E, *et al.* Measurement of ovarian volume by transvaginal sonography before ovulation induction with human menopausal gonadotrophin for *in vitro* fertilization can predict poor response. *Hum Reprod* 1997;12:294–7
13. Tomas C, Nuojua-Huttunen S, Martikainen H. Pretreatment transvaginal ultrasound examination predicts ovarian responsiveness to gonadotrophins in *in vitro* fertilization. *Hum Reprod* 1997;12:220–3
14. Ebrahim A, Rienhardt G, Morris S, *et al.* Follicle stimulating hormone levels on cycle day 3 predict ovulation stimulation response. *J Assist Reprod Genet* 1993;10:130–6
15. Evers JL, Slaats P, Land JA, *et al.* Elevated levels of basal estradiol-17β predict poor response in patients with normal basal levels of follicle-stimulating hormone undergoing *in vitro* fertilization. *Fertil Steril* 1998;69:1010–14
16. Huyser C, Fourie FL, Pentz J, *et al.* The predictive value of basal stimulating and growth hormone levels as determined by immunofluorometry during assisted reproduction. *J Assist Reprod Genet* 1995;12:244–51
17. Bancsi LFJMM, Looman CW, Huijs AM, *et al.* Basal follicle stimulating hormone is of limited value in predicting ongoing pregnancy rates after IVF. *Fertil Steril* 2000; in press
18. Sharif K, Elgendy M, Lashen H, *et al.* Age and basal follicle stimulating hormone as predictors of *in vitro* fertilization outcome. *Hum Reprod* 1998;105:107–12
19. van Montfrans JM, Hoek A, van Hooff M, *et al.* Predictive value of basal FSH in a general subfertility population. Poster presented at *10th Reinier de Graaf Symposium*, 9–11 September 1999, Zeist, The Netherlands
20. Schipper I, de Jong FH, Fauser BC. Lack of correlation between maximum early follicular follicle stimulating hormone concentrations and menstrual cycle characteristics in women under 35 years. *Hum Reprod* 1998;13:1442–8
21. Lambalk CB, Boomsma DI, de Boer L, *et al.* Increased levels and pulsatility of follicle stimulating hormone in mothers of hereditary dizygotic twins. *J Clin Endocrinol Metab* 1998;83:481–6
22. Reuss ML, Kline J, Santos R, *et al.* Age and the ovarian follicle pool assessed with transvaginal ultrasonography. *Am J Obstet Gynecol* 1996;174:624–7
23. Chang MY, Chiang CH, Hsieh TT, *et al.* Use of the antral follicle count to predict the outcome of assisted reproductive technologies. *Fertil Steril* 1998;69:505–10
24. Land JA, Yarmolinskaya MI, Dumoulin JC, *et al.* High dose human menopausal gonadotropin stimulation in poor responders does not improve *in vitro* fertilization outcome. *Fertil Steril* 1996;65:961–5

8

Follicle development before and during the menstrual cycle

N.S. Macklon and B.C.J.M. Fauser

INTRODUCTION

During the 4th month of fetal life, human follicles begin their development and, by the 5th month of intrauterine life, a maximum of approximately 7 million germ cells are present[1]. Thereafter, the pool of immature follicles diminishes so that at birth, each human ovary contains from 266 000 to 472 000 follicles[2]. Each follicle contains an oocyte arrested in prophase of the first meiotic division. Depletion in the number of these primordial follicles, already begun prior to birth, continues throughout childhood, so that by the menarche approximately 500 000 remain[3] (Figure 1). During reproductive life, follicle depletion occurs at a rate of approximately 1000/month. This process occurs either by atresia or by entry into the growth phase. The rate may increase after the age of 35 years[4] until the menopause, when the stock of follicles falls to less than 100[5,6]. The vast majority of follicles are removed from this stock by an atretic process of programmed cell death termed apoptosis[5]. During fetal life and childhood, follicle development occurs up to the early antral stage[6]. From puberty until the menopause, full maturation and ovulation occurs, but only approximately 400 follicles are destined to achieve full maturation.

CHILDHOOD

The hypothalamic–pituitary axis becomes functionally active during the second trimester of pregnancy, enabling fetal gonadotropin secretion under the control of gonadotropin releasing hormone (GnRH). However, steroid negative feedback at the hypothalamus becomes operative towards term, causing a decrease in gonadotropin secretion. After delivery the suppressive effect of placental steroids is removed, and gonadotropin secretion is again activated. In the first 4 months of life, serum luteinizing hormone (LH) concentrations of up to 1 IU/l are present, but follicle stimulating hormone

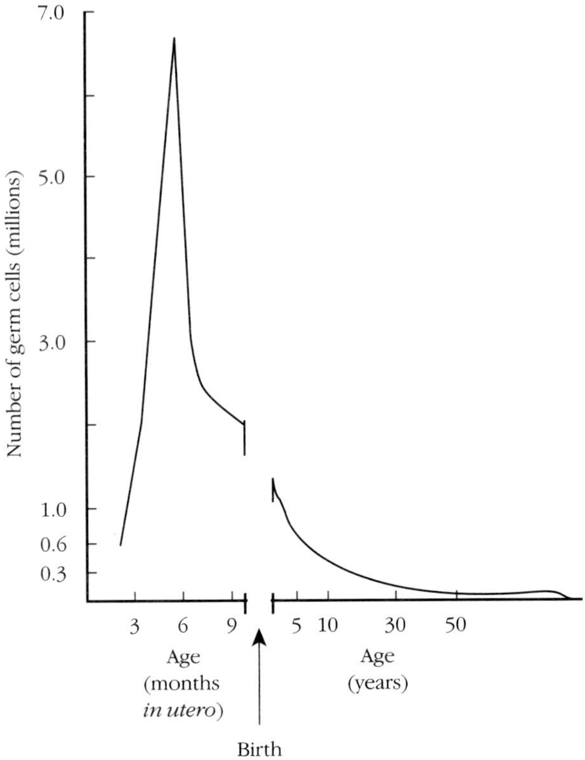

Figure 1 Changes in the total population of germ cells within the human ovary with increasing age. Data from reference 47

(FSH) levels are far higher, exceeding those observed in adult females of reproductive age[7]. These high gonadotropin serum concentrations cause gonadal activation and a rise in sex steroid secretion. However, this situation is short-lived; after 4 months of age gonadotropin and steroid concentrations fall dramatically, reaching basal levels at 1–2 years of age. Between 2 and 9 years of age, mean serum LH concentrations measure just 0.04 IU/l[7]. In the presence of these extremely low gonadotropin levels, estradiol secretion is suppressed. Despite this, ovarian steroid synthesis remains residually active, producing higher estradiol concentrations (2.2 pmol/l) in the mid-childhood female than observed in the mid-childhood male (0.3 pmol/l)[8].

Follicular growth and atresia occur in the ovaries during childhood[9–11]. Very early follicular development to the antral stage (0.25 mm) is independent of gonadotropin secretion[12]. Development beyond the antral stage to the stage at which follicles become potentially able to begin preovulatory development (2–5 mm in diameter) requires the presence of gonadotropins. Despite low gonadotropin levels, follicles measuring up to 5 mm are observed in young children, and the number of follicles exceeding this increases significantly beyond 7 years of age[11]. Although nocturnal, low-amplitude, low-frequency pulsatile gonadotropin secretion occurs in mid-childhood, serum FSH concentrations are not sufficient to sustain development beyond this stage and these follicles are doomed to undergo atresia.

ADOLESCENCE

At puberty, the removal of an as yet undefined central nervous system restraint enables full reactivation of the GnRH pulse generator. On ultrasound, the ovaries appear full of follicles measuring between 5 and 12 mm, with scanty stroma[13]. As puberty progresses, the amplitude of pulsatile gonadotropin and sex steroid secretion increases, resulting in extended follicular maturation[14]. Before ovulation can occur, however, the pituitary must develop the ability to respond with an LH surge in response to estradiol stimulation. This requires a decrease in the sensitivity of the negative feedback system to enable GnRH and gonadotropin levels to rise rather than fall in response to increasing estradiol levels. The development of this positive feedback response marks the maturation of the pituitary–hypothalmic–ovarian axis. Regular ovulatory cycles may take years to become established, however. In the first year following the menarche, cycle length is long and variable. Serial serum progesterone measurements in adolescent girls have indicated that only 15% of cycles are ovulatory in the first postmenarchal year, rising to 41% in the third. By the sixth postmenarchal year 25% of cycles are still anovulatory[15–17]. Metcalf and colleagues[18] found one-third of 209 females between 11 and 24 years of age remaining anovulatory 5 years after the menarche. Anovulation in adolescence appears to be a self-limiting phenomenon in most cases, and by 9–12 years following the menarche over 80% displayed regular ovulatory cycles.

Obesity and insulin resistance have been shown to be associated with prolonged anovulation in adolescence[19]. When compared to age-matched, ovulatory females of similar body mass index, obese anovulatory females were found to have increased fasting insulin levels in the presence of normal serum glucose concentrations, and an increased insulin response to a glucose challenge. This indicates a degree of insulin resistance greater than that associated with obesity; indeed, it is commeasurate with that observed in women with polycystic ovary syndrome (PCOS)[20]. These girls also frequently demonstrate enlarged ovaries on ultrasound, ovarian hyperandrogenism and increased serum LH concentrations[19]. Since these are features also associated with PCOS, the most commonly described cause of anovulatory infertility in adult women, it is likely that obese, anovulatory, hyperinsulinemic adolescent girls are showing early manifestations of this condition[21,22]. In some adolescent females these endocrine abnormalities disappear spontaneously, while in others they are sustained. It would be of interest to undertake further study of potential markers involved in the early detection of children at risk of adult reproductive failure.

FOLLICULAR DEVELOPMENT AND THE NORMAL MENSTRUAL CYCLE DURING ADULTHOOD

Complete maturation of the primordial follicle takes at least 85 days[23]. Initiation of growth of the primordial follicle occurs continuously and in a random fashion. However, the factors that determine when a primordial follicle will enter the growth phase that ultimately leads to atresia or ovulation remain uncertain. The first stage of the growth phase involves enlargement in the size of the oocyte and proliferation of the surrounding layers of granulosa cells to form the primary follicle. After developing its own blood supply the follicular stroma undergoes differentiation into a theca interna and theca externa layer. This stage of development, termed the secondary follicle, is further characterized by the expression in the theca interna of LH receptors[24]. The granulosa cells, in contrast, begin to express FSH receptors as the antral cavity appears[25,26]. The duration of this period of development from the primordial to the preantral follicle takes several months, and the subsequent period of follicular development from the early antral to the preovulatory follicle takes approximately 3 months[27] (Figure 2). Although the initiation of follicle growth appears to be regulated independently of

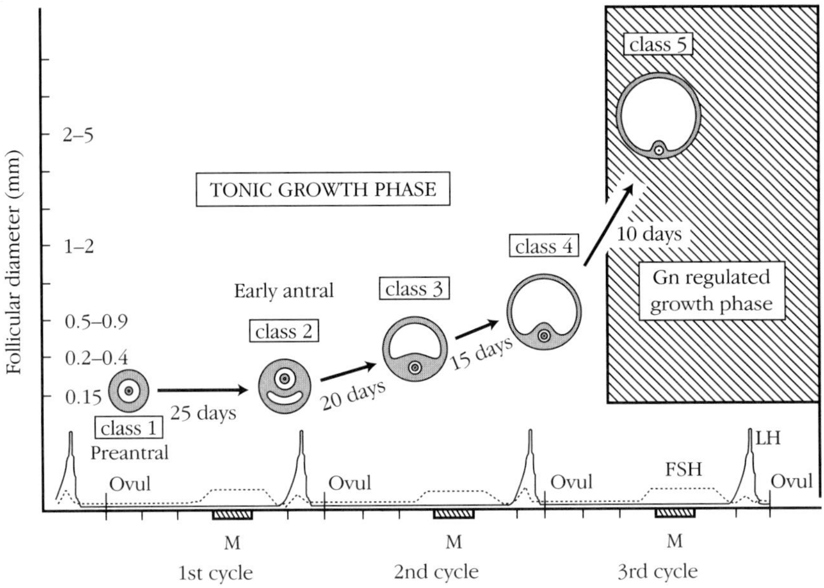

Figure 2 Principal stages of human follicular development. Primordial follicles entering the growth phase form primary follicles. This is followed by gonadotropin-independent (tonic) growth (classes 1–4) and eventually gonadotropin-dependent growth. The overall development takes three cycles. From reference 27. Gn, gonadotropin; Ovul, ovulation; FSH, follicle stimulating hormone; LH, luteinizing hormone; M, menses. Figure reproduced with permission from Fauser BCJM, van Heusden AM. Manipulation of human ovarian function: physiological concepts and clinical consequences. *Endocr Rev* 1997;18:71–106

stimulation by gonadotropins[28], the final stage of follicular development to the preovulatory stage is known to be FSH dependent[29]. The number of follicles that will undergo development to the preovulatory stage is determined by the duration and magnitude of FSH stimulation.

Following the involution of the corpus luteum and the subsequent fall in estrogen production[30], FSH levels rise during the luteal–follicular transition of the normal menstrual cycle. This gives rise to the continued development of a limited cohort of follicles. Subsequent development of this cohort during the follicular phase becomes dependent on continued stimulation by gonadotropins. Only at more advanced stages of development do granulosa cells become responsive to FSH and become capable of converting the theca cell-derived substrate androstenedione to estradiol by induction of the aromatase enzyme. The involvement of two cell types (granulosa and theca cells) and two hormones (LH and FSH) to produce estrogens from cholesterol has led to the concept of the 'two cell, two gonadotropin' theory. In addition to stimulating aromatase activity, FSH also induces LH and further increases FSH receptor formation while stimulating DNA and protein synthesis by the cell[31].

The concept of the FSH 'threshold' proposed by Brown[32] postulated that FSH concentration must exceed a certain level before follicular development will proceed. Once this level is reached, normal follicular growth requires only a minor further increase above this threshold. When the FSH threshold is surpassed in the normal cycle, this stimulates the growth of a cohort of small antral follicles[33] and ensures ongoing preovulatory follicular development[34]. The duration of this period in which the threshold is exceeded is limited in the normal cycle by a decrease in FSH, which occurs in the early to mid-follicular phase[30]. This decrease in FSH concentrations may be the result of negative feedback by increasing estradiol concentrations. Inhibin B, produced by antral follicles in the early follicular phase, may also be involved in initiating decremental serum concentrations by exerting negative feedback at the hypothalamic–pituitary level[35]. Should this period be extended, more follicles will continue development. In the normal cycle, one follicle continues developing despite falling FSH levels because of an increased sensitivity to FSH[36]. The remaining follicles respond to falling FSH levels by undergoing atresia. The duration of elevation of FSH may play a crucial role in determining the number of follicles that will undergo further development. The concept of the FSH 'window' has been proposed[29,37], stressing the significance of the duration of FSH elevation above the threshold level, rather than the level of elevation of FSH, for single dominant selection (Figure 3). This concept has recently been substantiated by the demonstration that elevating FSH levels high above the threshold level for a short period of time in the early follicular phase does not increase the number of dominant follicles[38]. Conversely, when the physiological decrease of FSH in a normal cycle is prevented by administration of FSH in the late follicular phase, the augmented sensitivity to FSH allows several follicles to gain dominance[38].

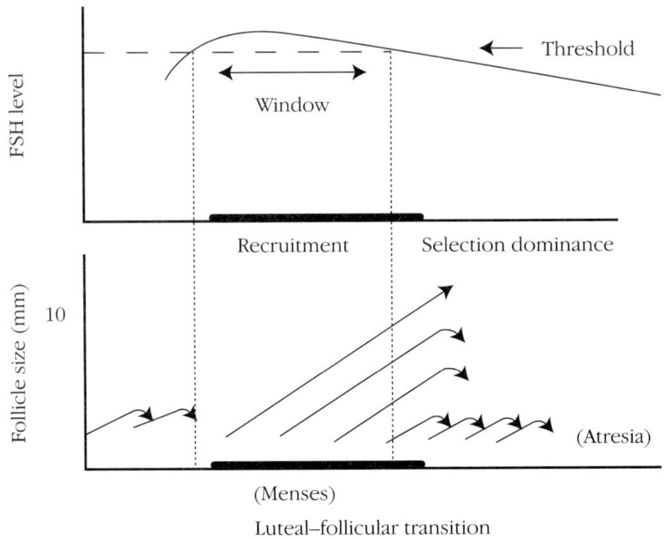

Figure 3 Follicular phase of the normal menstrual cycle. The intercycle rise in serum follicle stimulating hormone (FSH) concentrations exceeds the threshold for recruitment of a cohort of follicles for further development. The number of follicles recruited is determined by the time ('window') in which the serum FSH level is above the threshold at which recruitment occurs. Adapted from reference 29

Figure 4 summarizes the cyclical changes in FSH, LH, estradiol and progesterone, together with the growth of the dominant follicle, as measured in 40 normally cycling volunteers. In the normal ovulatory cycle, a maximum FSH concentration of 6.6 mIU/ml (range 4.4–11.2 mIU/ml) was observed on cycle day 5, followed by a mean linear decrease of 0.5 mIU/ml (range 0.1–0.9 mIU/ml) per day until cycle day 13, 3 days before the LH peak[39]. Between days 5 and 15 the changes in FSH and estradiol concentrations were negatively correlated[39], indicating that the production of estradiol in the late follicular phase may be greater in women with a slower decrease in endogenous FSH concentration and that aromatase enzyme activity in the dominant follicle is related to the degree of stimulation by FSH. When serum FSH concentrations during the follicular phase were correlated with follicle development in normal ovulatory cycles, a 2.5-fold variation in the maximum FSH concentration was observed between subjects[39]. No correlation existed between maximum FSH concentration, follicular phase length or maximum estradiol concentration[39]. A more recent study[40] demonstrated a similar median maximum follicular phase FSH level of 6.2 mIU/ml with a 2.6-fold difference between maximum and minimum values (4.3–11.2 mIU/ml). These studies demonstrate the large interindividual variation in follicular phase FSH levels that exist in normo-ovulatory women.

Androstenedione and testosterone are present in large quantities in follicles of all sizes[41,42]. In contrast, there is a consistent correlation between

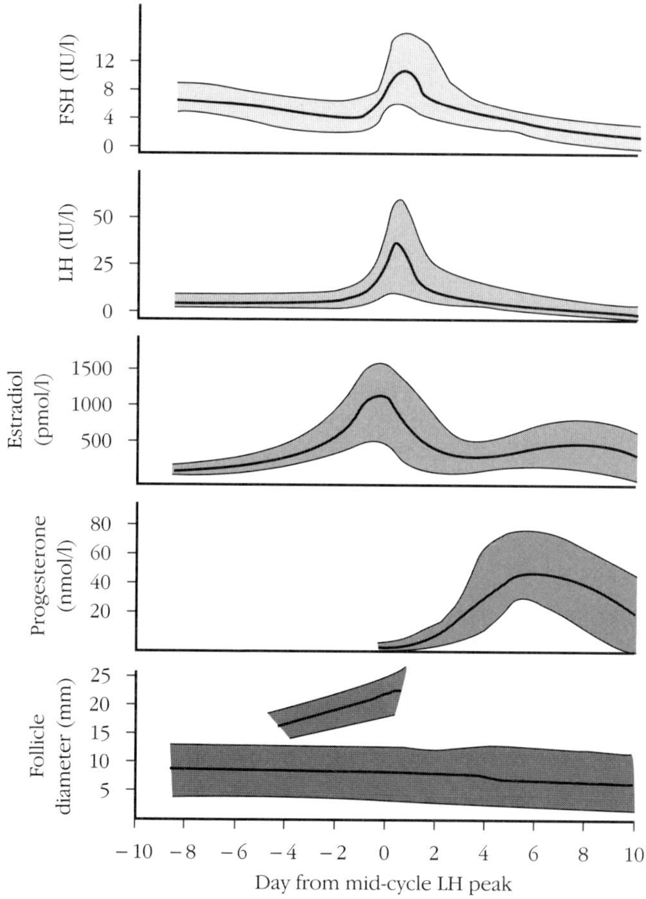

Figure 4 Normal menstrual cycle, examined in 40 regularly cycling women. Mean serum concentrations with 95% centiles are given for luteinizing hormone (LH), follicle stimulating hormone (FSH), estradiol and progesterone from 8 days prior to the mid-cycle LH peak until 10 days after the LH peak. The bottom panel shows the emergence and growth of the dominant follicle in relation to the time of the mid-cycle LH peak

estradiol production and follicular diameter of > 9 mm[39,41,42]. Smaller follicles show no correlation between size and estradiol concentration. These *in vivo* observations are consistent with *in vitro* studies that have demonstrated that the amount of estradiol synthesized by granulosa cells is dependent on the size of the follicle from which cells are obtained, with androstenedione metabolized to estradiol only by granulosa cells from follicles beyond 8–10 mm in diameter[43–45]. Taken together, these observations show that enhanced estradiol biosynthesis is closely linked to preovulatory follicle development and that selection of the dominant follicle occurs relatively late during follicle development, after the recruitment of a pool of follicles. We have observed that the dominant follicle can be identified from median cycle day 7[46] (Figure 5). During the 7 days prior to the LH peak, the diameter of the dominant follicle increased linearly by a mean value of 1.1 mm/day, reaching a median preovulatory size of 20.5 mm[46] (Figure 6). Preovulatory serum estradiol concentrations were correlated with the size of the preovulatory follicle[46] (Figure 7).

In studies of follicular-endocrine dynamics in the normal cycle, our group has also characterized follicular-phase patterns of FSH serum levels and investigated correlations between decremental FSH levels and dominant follicle development[39]. This decrease in FSH levels could be due to negative estrogen feedback on the hypothalamic axis[37]. A profound rise in inhibin B serum levels was recently observed in the follicular phase, suggesting that this is secreted by a recently recruited cohort of follicles in response to FSH. This rapid rise in inhibin B occurs just after the intercycle rise in FSH. It may be proposed that inhibin B limits the duration of the FSH rise (narrowing the FSH window) through negative feedback at the pituitary level and may therefore be crucial for monofollicular development.

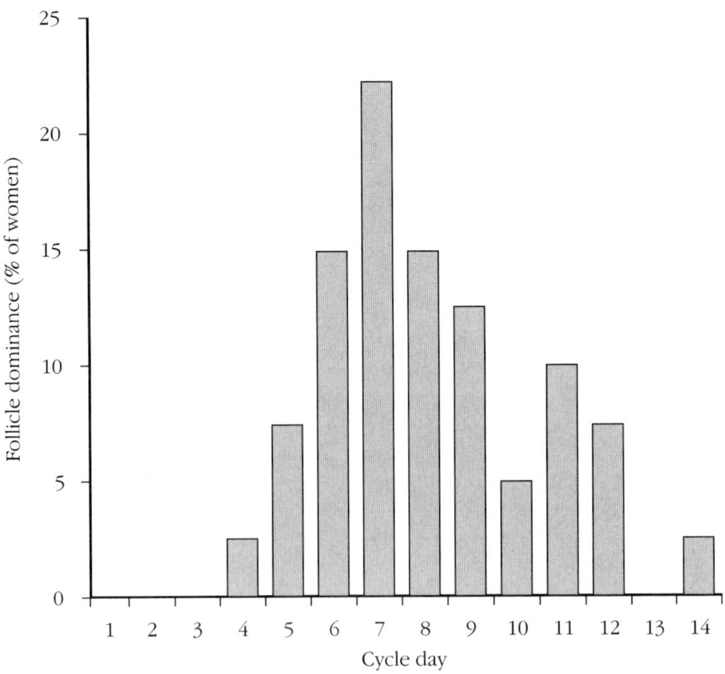

Figure 5 The day on which the dominant follicle was first identified in 40 normally cycling women who underwent daily ultrasound examinations, expressed as a percentage of the study group

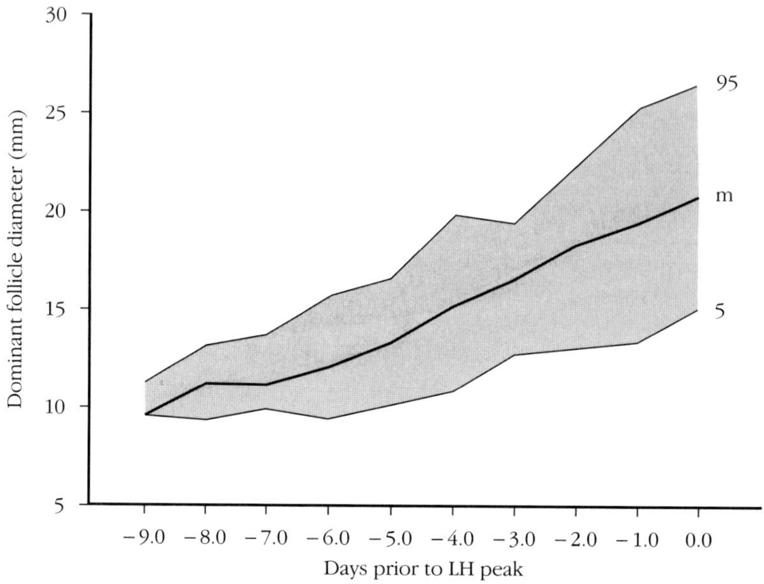

Figure 6 The mean diameter, 5th and 95th percentiles of the dominant follicle measured ultrasonically in 40 normally cycling women on the day of the luteinizing hormone (LH) surge, and the 9 days prior to this

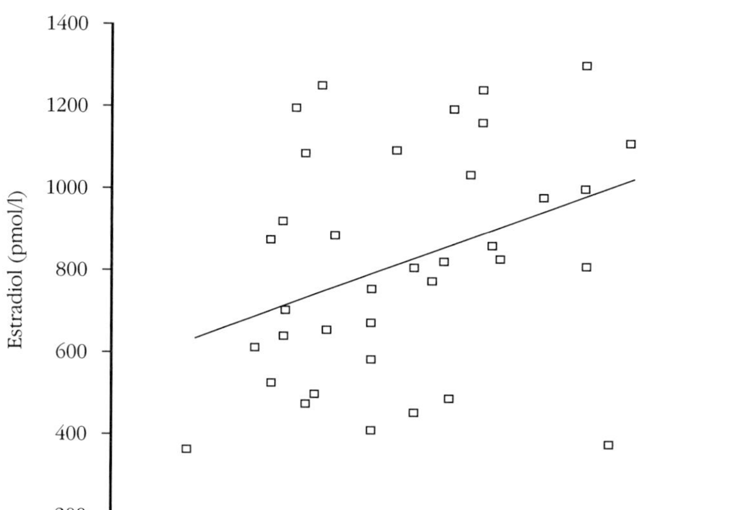

Figure 7 Serum estradiol concentrations on the day on which the maximum diameter of the dominant follicle was measured in 40 normally menstruating women who underwent daily ultrasound examinations and daily estradiol measurements. Pearson correlation 0.338, $p < 0.05$

CONCLUSION

The regulation of ovarian function and follicular development during reproductive life is complex, and many aspects relating to the means by which FSH activity is regulated within the ovary remain to be clarified. Factors influencing early postmenarchal ovarian function and follicular development may subsequently have an important impact on fertility. A greater understanding of the 'physiological' anovulation of adolescence may lead to the development of timely interventions designed to prevent the development of anovulation in an otherwise fertile adult. Many couples in Western society are postponing their wish to conceive to an age where female fertility is already compromised. Since evidence is accumulating that menopausal age (and resulting sterility) is preceeded by a period of reduced fertility related to a decreased follicle pool, a reduced cohort of growing follicles and diminished oocyte quality, efforts should be directed at developing reliable markers for ovarian aging. A better understanding of the control of follicular development from the fetal stage through to the menopause will offer the prospect of developing an effective preventative approach to anovulatory infertility.

REFERENCES

1. Baker TC. A quantitative and cytological study of germ cells in human ovaries. *Proc R Soc B* 1963;158:417–33
2. Forabosco A, Sforza C, De Pol A, *et al*. Morphometric study of the human neonatal ovary. *Anat Rec* 1991;231:201–8
3. Himelstein-Braw R, Byskov AG, Peters H, Faber M. Follicular atresia in the infant human ovary. *J Reprod Fertil* 1976;46:455–9
4. Faddy MJ, Gosden RG, Gougeon A, *et al*. Accelerated disappearance of ovarian follicles in mid-life: implications for forecasting menopause. *Hum Reprod* 1992;7:1342–6
5. Schwartzman RA, Cidlowski J. Apoptosis: the biochemistry and molecular biology of programmed cell death. *Endocr Rev* 1993;14:133–51
6. Lintern-Moore S, Peters H, Moore GP, *et al*. Follicular development in the infant human ovary. *J Reprod Fertil* 1974;39:53–64
7. Neely EK, Hintz RL, Wilson DM, *et al*. Normal ranges for immunochemiluminometric gonadotropin assays. *J Pediatr* 1995;127:40–6
8. Klein K, Baron O, Colli MJ, *et al*. Estrogen levels in childhood determined by an ultrasensitive recombinant cell bioassay. *J Clin Invest* 1994;6:2475–80
9. Sauramo H. Histology and function of the ovary from the embryonic period to the fertile age. *Acta Obstet Gynecol Scand* 1954;33:3–25
10. Winer-Muram H, Emerson D, Muram D, *et al*. The sonographic features of the peripubertal ovaries. *Adolesc Pediatr Gynecol* 1989;2:160–3
11. Cacciatore B, Apter D, Alfthan H, *et al*. Ultrasonic characteristics of the uterus and ovaries in relation to pubertal development and serum LH, FSH and estradiol concentrations. *Adolesc Pediatr Gynecol* 1991;4:15–20
12. Hillier SG. Current concepts of the roles of follicle stimulating hormone and luteinizing hormone in folliculogenesis. *Hum Reprod* 1994;9:188–91

13. Holm K, Mosfeldt Laursen E, Brocks V, *et al*. Pubertal maturation of the internal genitalia: an ultrasound evaluation of 166 healthy girls. *Ultrasound Obstet Gynecol* 1995; 6:175–81
14. Penny R, Parlow F, Olambiwonnu NO, *et al*. Evolution of the menstrual pattern of gonadotropin and sex steroid concentrations in serum. *Acta Endocrinol* 1977;84: 729–37
15. Apter D. Serum steroids and pituitary hormones in female puberty: a partly longitudinal study. *Clin Endocrinol* 1980;12:107–20
16. Apter D, Vihko R. Hormonal patterns of the first menstrual cycles. In Venturoli S, Flamigni C, Givens JR, eds. *Adolescence in Females*. Chicago: Year Book Medical Publishers, 1985:215–38.
17. Apter D, Vihko R. Endocrine determinants of fertility: serum androgen concentrations during follow-up of adolescents into the third decade of life. *J Clin Endocrinol Metab* 1990;71:970–4
18. Metcalf MG, Skidmore DS, Lowry GF, *et al*. Incidence of ovulation in the years after the menarche. *J Endocrinol* 1983;97:213–19
19. Apter D, Bützow T, Laughlin GA, *et al.* Metabolic features of polycystic ovary syndrome are found in adolescent girls with hyperandrogenism. *J Clin Endocrinol Metab* 1995;80:2966–73
20. Poretsky L. Insulin resistance and hyperandrogenism: update. *Endocr Rev* 1994;2:125–9
21. Nestler JE, Clore JN, Blackard WG. The central role of obesity (hyperinsulinemia) in the pathogenesis of the polycystic ovary syndrome. *Am J Obstet Gynecol* 1989;161:1095–7
22. Pasquali R, Casimirri F. The impact of obesity on hyperandrogenism and polycystic ovary syndrome in premenopausal women. *Clin Endocrinol* 1993;39:1–16
23. Gougeon A. Dynamics of follicular growth in the human: a model from preliminary results. *Hum Reprod* 1986;1:81–7
24. Channing CP, Kammerman S. Characteristics of gonadotropin receptors of porcine granulosa cells during follicle maturation. *Endocrinology* 1973;92:531–40
25. Gougeon A. Dynamics of human follicle growth. A morphologic perspective. In Adashi EY, Leung PCK, eds. *The Ovary*. New York: Raven Press, 1993:21–39
26. Oktay K, Briggs D, Gosden RG. Ontogeny of follicle-stimulating hormone receptor gene expression in isolated human ovarian follicles. *J Clin Endocrinol Metab* 1997;82: 3748–51
27. Gougeon A. Regulation of ovarian follicular development in primates: facts and hypothesis. *Endocr Rev* 1996;17:121–55
28. Peters H, Himelstein-Braw R, Faber M. The normal development of the ovary in childhood. *Acta Endocrinol (Copenh)* 1976;82:617–30
29. Fauser BCJM, van Heusden AM. Manipulation of human ovarian function: physiological concepts and clinical consequences. *Endocr Rev* 1997;18:71–106
30. Le Nestour E, Marraoui J, Lahlou N, *et al*. Role of estradiol in the rise in follicle-stimulating hormone levels during the luteal–follicular transition. *J Clin Endocrinol Metab* 1993;77:439–42
31. Hsueh AJ, Bicsak TA, Jia XC, *et al*. Granulosa cells as hormone targets: the role of biologically active follicle-stimulating hormone in reproduction. *Recent Prog Horm Res* 1989;45:209–73
32. Brown JB. Pituitary control of ovarian function – concepts derived from gonadotropin therapy. *Aust NZ J Obstet Gynaecol* 1978;18:47–54
33. Hall JE, Schoen DA, Martin KA, *et al*. Hypothalamic gonadotropin-releasing hormone secretion and follicle-stimulating hormone dynamics during the luteal–follicular transition. *J Clin Endocrinol Metab* 1992;74:600–7

34. Macklon NS, Fauser BC. Follicle development during the normal menstrual cycle. *Maturitas* 1998;30:181–8
35. Groome NP, Illingworth PJ, O'Brien M, *et al*. Measurement of dimeric inhibin B throughout the human menstrual cycle. *J Clin Endocrinol Metab* 1996;81:1401–5
36. Hsueh AJ. Paracrine mechanisms involved in granulosa cell differentiation. *J Clin Endocrinol Metab* 1986;15:117–34
37. Baird DT. A model for follicular selection and ovulation: lessons from superovulation. *J Steroid Biochem* 1987;27:15–23
38. Schipper I, Hop WCJ, Fauser BCJM. The follicle-stimulating hormone (FSH) threshold/window concept examined by differential interventions with exogenous FSH during the follicular phase of the normal menstrual cycle: duration rather than magnitude of FSH increase affects follicle development. *J Clin Endocrinol Med* 1998;83:1292–8
39. Van Santbrink EJP, Hop WC, van Dessel HJHM, *et al*. Decremental follicle-stimulating hormone and dominant follicle development during the normal menstrual cycle. *Fertil Steril* 1995;64:37–43
40. Schipper I, de Jong FH, Fauser BCJM. Lack of correlation between maximum early follicular phase serum follicle-stimulating hormone levels and menstrual cycle characteristics in women under the age of 35. *Hum Reprod* 1998;13:1442–8
41. Pache TD, Hop WC, de Jong FH, *et al*. 17 Beta-oestradiol, androstenedione and inhibin levels in fluid from individual follicles of normal and polycystic ovaries, and in ovaries from androgen treated female to male transsexuals. *Clin Endocrinol (Oxf)* 1992;36:565–71
42. Van Dessel HJHM, Schipper I, Pache TD, *et al*. Normal human follicle development: and evaluation of correlations with estradiol, androstenedione and progesterone levels in individual follicles. *Clin Endocrinol (Oxf)* 1996;44:191–8
43. Hillier SG, van den Boogaard AMJ, Reichert LE, *et al*. Intraovarian sex steroid hormone interactions and the regulation of follicular maturation: aromatization of androgens by human granulosa cells *in vitro*. *J Clin Endocrinol Metab* 1980;50:640–7
44. Erickson GF, Hsueh AJW, Quigley ME, *et al*. Functional studies of aromatase activity in human granulosa cells from normal and polycystic ovaries. *J Clin Endocrinol Metab* 1979;49:514–19
45. Mason HD, Willis DS, Beard RW, *et al*. Estradiol production by granulosa cells of normal and polycystic ovaries: relationship to menstrual cycle history and concentrations of gonadotropins and sex steroids in follicular fluid. *J Clin Endocrinol Metab* 1994;79:1355–60
46. Macklon NS, Fauser BC. Dynamics of ovarian follicle growth throughout life. *Horm Res* 2000;in press
47. Baker TG. Oogenesis and ovulation. In Austin CR, Short RV, eds. *Reproduction in Mammals*, vol 1. *Germ Cells and Fertilization*. London: Cambridge University Press, 1972:14

9

Age-dependent decline of female fecundity is caused by early fetal loss

D.J. Holman, J.W. Wood and K.L. Campbell

INTRODUCTION

Changes in the pace of reproduction over the course of the reproductive lifespan are a complex outcome of physiological, cultural, economic and behavioral changes with age. In many industrialized countries, for example, age-specific fertility rates are largely dominated by the use of contraception for terminating or postponing reproduction as well as for the spacing of births. In these populations, physiological factors play a relatively weak role, except at the beginning and end of the reproductive span. Consequently, it is difficult to study age-related changes in fecundity (the biological capacity to reproduce) under conditions of widespread contraceptive use.

Demographers have addressed this difficulty by turning to populations in which birth control is rarely used. Age-related changes in fecundity can be fruitfully studied in these so-called natural fertility populations, because these strong parity-related controls of fertility are not exercised. A universal finding from decades of demographic research on natural fertility populations is that female fecundity declines with the age of a woman[1]. In examining the causes of this decline, fecundity can be decomposed into two meaningful components. The first component is a true age-related decline in the probability of conception. Demographers measure this component of fecundity as *fecundability*, which is defined as the monthly or cycle-wise probability that a cohabiting couple will experience a conception. The second component of fecundity is *fetal loss*, which is the probability that a pregnancy terminates prior to birth.

The problem with measuring fecundability and fetal loss is that pregnancies are almost impossible to detect non-invasively until well after conception. Sensitive pregnancy assays based on the measurement of human chorionic gonadotropin (hCG) cannot detect a rise in hCG until about 1 week after conception[2,3]. To make matters worse, the risk of pregnancy loss appears to be highest early in pregnancy[4–8], so that, with the best technology available today, some fraction of early pregnancies go unnoticed before terminating.

The difficulty of detecting early pregnancy has led demographers to define several types of fecundability. The term *total fecundability* refers to the probability that fertilization occurs in a single month or cycle for a sexually active woman; this is what we would like to measure, but cannot. The term *apparent fecundability* is the monthly or cycle-wise probability of conception given that the pregnancy survives long enough to be detected using some particular method. In other words, apparent fecundability is a measure that encompasses both the probability of conception and the probability that the conceptus will survive until it can be detected. In the same spirit, we can define *total fetal loss* as the probability of losing a pregnancy between fertilization and birth; *apparent fetal loss* is the probability that a recognized pregnancy does not survive to term.

This confounding of fecundability and fetal loss means that studies of either are sensitive to the technology used to detect pregnancy. A study that uses sensitive endocrine methods to detect pregnancies should yield higher estimates of apparent fecundability and apparent fetal loss than a similar study using mothers' self-reports of pregnancy. The difference arises because many pregnancies that can be biochemically detected terminate before they can be recognized by the mothers. As a consequence, it is difficult to compare values of fecundability and fetal loss among different studies, unless the same method was used to detect pregnancies in each study. Ideally, estimates of apparent fecundability should include a description of the assay for detecting pregnancies along with the gestational age-specific sensitivity of the assay. This information is rarely provided and therefore it is difficult to make direct comparisons of apparent fecundability among studies.

Methodological difficulties aside, the general patterns of age-related changes in fetal loss and fecundability have been examined from studies among natural fertility populations[9]. Figure 1 shows a composite age pattern of apparent fecundability compiled from several natural fertility populations after maximum fecundability was rescaled to one at age 22. Apparent fecundability exhibits a steady decline from the early 20s until it approaches zero in the late 40s. This pattern of age-related changes in fecundability is well accepted, even though it is necessarily based on indirect or incomplete ascertainment of pregnancies.

Figure 1 also shows age-specific apparent fetal loss compiled from several studies after rescaling each study to a common rate of 150 pregnancy losses for 1000 conceptions[10]. Apparent fetal loss shows a steady rise with age, approaching a peak probability of 40% toward the end of the reproductive span. Based on studies of early pregnancy loss, we can conclude that the true overall rate of pregnancy loss is likely to be substantially higher at each maternal age[4,5,7,11], but the overall pattern that shows an increase in the risk of pregnancy loss with age is probably correct.

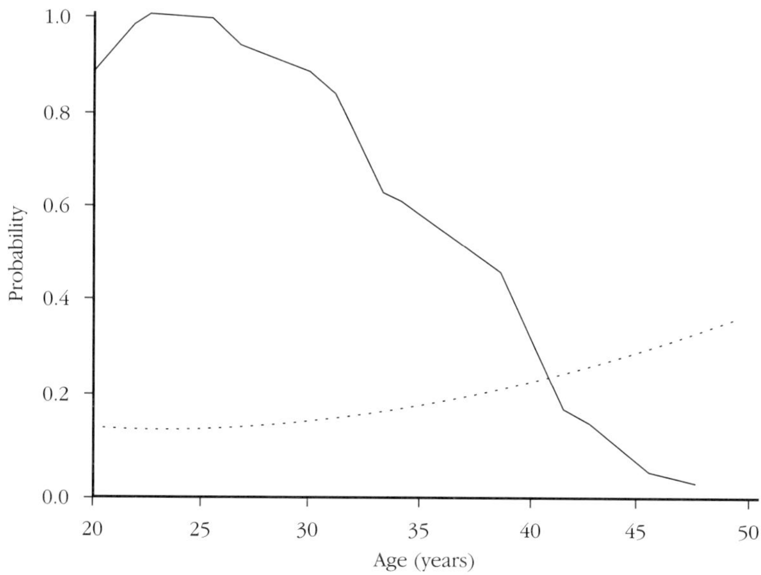

Figure 1 Composite age patterns of apparent fecundability (—) and apparent fetal loss (...) compiled from several natural fertility populations. Apparent fecundability is adjusted so that the maximum value is 1.0 at age 22 (data from reference 9). Apparent fetal loss is from an analysis of nine populations, each adjusted for an overall rate of 150 pregnancy losses per 1000 conceptions (data from reference 10)

Clearly, the increase in apparent fetal loss and decrease in apparent fecundability constitute two important aspects of reproductive aging in women. A fundamental issue for our understanding of human reproductive biology is whether the age-specific decline in fecundability represents a true drop in total fecundability with age or whether it reflects an age-related increase in the probability of early pregnancy losses. Similarly, we would like to ascertain the magnitude of pregnancy loss and the way in which it changes with maternal age.

One way to disentangle total fecundability and fetal loss is to examine the way in which pregnancy losses are distributed across gestation. The top panel of Figure 2 represents a hypothetical study in which a number of menstrual cycles are observed (y-axis) and those that result in a pregnancy are followed to term (x-axis). The horizontal line indicates the number of cycles in which fertilization occurred, and the dashed curve represents the numbers of ongoing pregnancies that survive to each gestational age. After all pregnancies have terminated in this fictitious study, each menstrual cycle can be classified as a non-conception cycle, a cycle that ended in the loss of the pregnancy or a cycle that resulted in a live birth. We could then directly

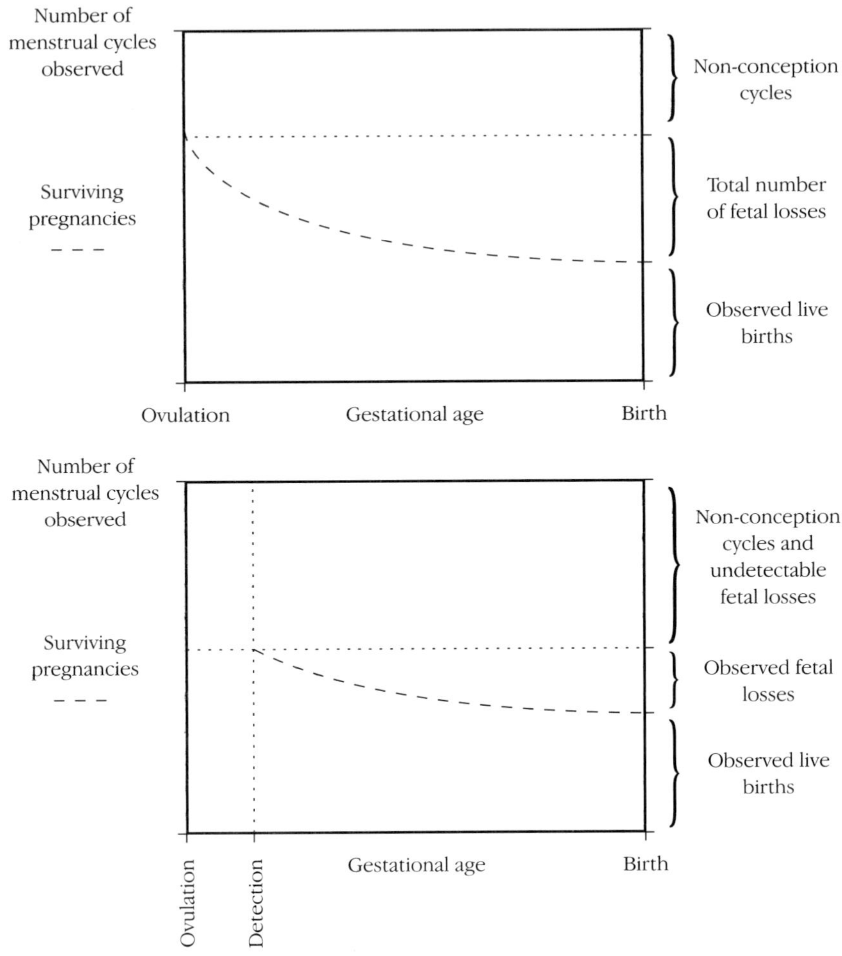

Figure 2 The probability of fetal loss and fecundability are confounded by the incomplete sensitivity of pregnancy assays. The *y*-axis represents the number of menstrual cycles under study and the *x*-axis is time from ovulation to birth. The upper panel shows the classification of each cycle if exact information were known. Fecundability is computed as (fetal losses plus births)/(number of menstrual cycles) and fetal loss is the number of (fetal losses)/(fetal losses plus births). The bottom panel shows what happens when not all pregnancies can be detected. The average gestational age at which the assay can detect pregnancy is shown by the line 'detection'. The earliest fetal losses and the non-conception cycles cannot be differentiated. The correct numerator for fecundability is not known, and the correct numerator and denominator for estimating the total probability of fetal loss are not known[12]

compute total fecundability as the number of pregnancies over the total number of cycles, and the probability of fetal loss as the number of pregnancy losses over the total number of pregnancies. Since we cannot detect pregnancies at fertilization, a more realistic portrayal of what we measured in the fictitious study is shown in the lower panel of Figure 2. The vertical line labelled 'detection' represents the sensitivity limit of the method used to diagnose pregnancies. We cannot detect any pregnancy before this point in gestation. Now, each menstrual cycle must be classified in one of three ways: cycles in which a pregnancy was not detected, cycles that end in the loss of a detected pregnancy and cycles that end in a live birth. Clearly, we do not know the proper denominator for computing either total fecundability or the probability of fetal loss; neither do we know the proper numerator for computing the probability of fetal loss.

One possibility of getting around this problem, as suggested by Figure 2, is to use a parametric mathematical model for the gestational age-specific risk of fetal loss. Given the model, we could, in principle, use observations from the point of detection forward to estimate the entire distribution of pregnancy loss. If so, the resulting estimated distribution could be used to compute total fetal loss, after which estimation of total fecundability is simple. This procedure involves 'back projecting' the distribution of fetal loss to the earliest portion of pregnancy, a method that will be convincing only to the extent that the mathematical model of fetal loss reflects the actual biological mechanisms underlying pregnancy loss. The validity of the fetal loss model will strongly shape our confidence in the resulting estimates of total fecundability and total fetal loss.

THE MODEL

An etiological theory of fetal loss was proposed by Marcus Bishop in 1964[13]. Based on cytogenetic studies of human abortuses and his own work on the cytogenetics of bull sperm, Bishop proposed that most pregnancy losses result from chromosomal abnormalities arising from defects in the gametes and that many of these pregnancies are lost so early in gestation that they are never observed as pregnancies. Furthermore, he postulated that chromosomal abnormalities should increase with parental age.

Many of the basic elements of Bishop's theory were expressed mathematically by Wood[1,9] and independently by Boklage[14]. The underlying logic of the Wood–Boklage model is that, at fertilization, a conceptus can be classified as chromosomally normal or abnormal. The risk of pregnancy loss in the chromosomally abnormal subgroup is modelled as high and constant across gestation. The risk of pregnancy loss in the normal subgroup is modelled as low and constant across gestation. Even though the risk of loss in each subgroup is constant, the combined subgroups show a declining risk of fetal loss with increasing gestational ages (Figure 3). The decline in risk occurs because, on average, abnormal conceptuses are lost earlier in gestation, leaving an increasingly larger fraction of normal conceptuses at later gestational ages.

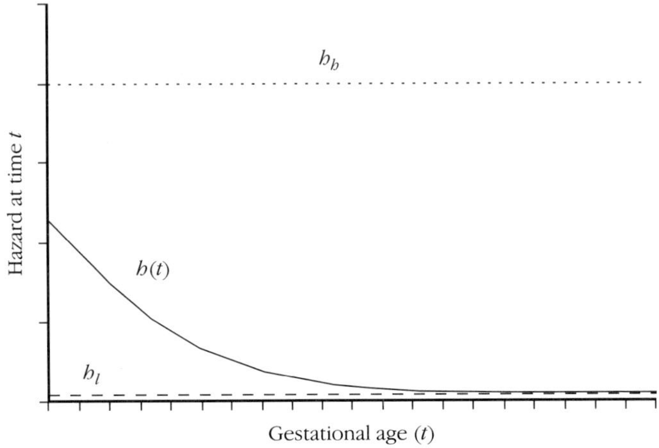

Figure 3 An example of the distribution of fetal loss throughout pregnancy under the Wood–Boklage model. The hazard (or risk) of loss is constant within each subgroup, but the combined hazard declines with age. A third parameter of the model is p, the proportion of abnormal conceptuses at fertilization. (---), Chromosomally normal subgroup; (---), chromosomally abnormal subgroup; (—), combined subgroups. Details of the model can be found in references 1, 9, 12 and 14

Mathematically, we parameterize the model by defining h_h as the hazard for the abnormal (high-risk) subgroup and h_l as the hazard for the normal (low-risk) subgroup. These hazards define a constant risk of fetal loss across gestation. Under these assumptions, the fraction of abnormal conceptuses surviving to gestational age t is $\exp(-h_h t)$. Likewise, the fraction of normal conceptuses surviving to t is $\exp(-h_l t)$.

At fertilization, a certain fraction of conceptuses are chromosomally abnormal. This fraction is denoted p_h. Because the abnormal conceptuses are lost at a greater rate than the normal conceptuses, the surviving proportion of high-risk conceptuses will decline over the course of gestation. The proportion of abnormal conceptuses at gestational age t, denoted $p(t)$, is:

$$p\,(t) = \frac{p_h \exp(-h_h t)}{p_h \exp(-h_h t) + (1 - p_h)\exp(-h_l t)}$$

The hazard for the combined subgroups at some gestational age t is $h(t) = p(t)h_h + [1 - p(t)]h_l$. The distribution of surviving conceptuses at gestational age t is derived directly from $h(t)$ as:

$$S(t) = 1 - \exp\left[-\int_0^t h(u)du\right] = p_h \exp(-p_h t) + (1 - p_h)\exp(-h_l t)$$

This survival distribution is analogous to the conceptus survival curve in Figure 2. Other variables, such as maternal age, can be modelled as affecting one or more of the three parameters of the basic model. Under this model, we are not required to know whether individual pregnancies are normal or abnormal; rather, parameters for the combined-subgroup distribution can be estimated directly from observations.

The Wood–Boklage model of fetal loss was used as the basis of a new model for estimating age-specific total fecundability. The model, which is based on the logic underlying Figure 2, uses pregnancy assay results on a series of menstrual cycles to estimate age-specific total fetal loss and age-specific total fecundability. The mathematical details of the model are given elsewhere[12]; only an overview of the model can be given here. The model incorporates the effects of both assay sensitivity and assay specificity, and incorporates statistically interval-censored and right-censored observations. Additionally, the model statistically controls for a non-susceptible fraction of women (i.e. those who are sterile, sexually inactive or otherwise not at risk of getting pregnant), so that estimates of age-specific fecundability will be one for at least one age, and less than one for all other ages.

The sensitivity of the pregnancy assay refers to the gestational age-specific probability (from fertilization onward) that the hCG assay will detect a true pregnancy. The types of hCG assays used for fetal loss studies have sigmoid-shaped distributions of sensitivity that are zero at fertilization, increase to approximately 0.5 by about 10 days into the pregnancy and approach one by day 25 (see reference 2 for an example). Determination of the sensitivity of a pregnancy assay involves the same difficulties as measuring early pregnancy loss itself. For this reason, our model simultaneously estimates assay sensitivity along with parameters for fetal loss and fecundability.

The specificity of the pregnancy assay is defined as one minus the probability that the assay will falsely diagnose pregnancy in a non-pregnant woman. Pregnancy assays that are more sensitive tend to have a lower specificity. This is because the most sensitive assays are able to detect low levels of background hCG found in non-pregnant women[15,16]. The specificity of a particular assay can be easily determined by quantifying the number of false pregnancies diagnosed in a pool of women who have undergone tubal ligations. For hCG-based pregnancy assays, specificity is likely to be independent of cycle day, so we treat specificity as a constant probability.

In our prospective study, we collected urine samples twice weekly, which were then assayed for the presence of hCG[2]. The start of each 'potential pregnancy cycle' was taken as the estimated day of ovulation. The ending day of the cycle was either the day of the next menses (which includes both non-conception cycles and undetected pregnancies that terminated early), the day on which a detected pregnancy ended or the day of a live birth. Within each type of cycle, one or more pregnancy tests were made. From this collection of observations, the statistical model was used to find parameter estimates of total fecundability (ρ), total fetal loss (p, h_b and h_l), the

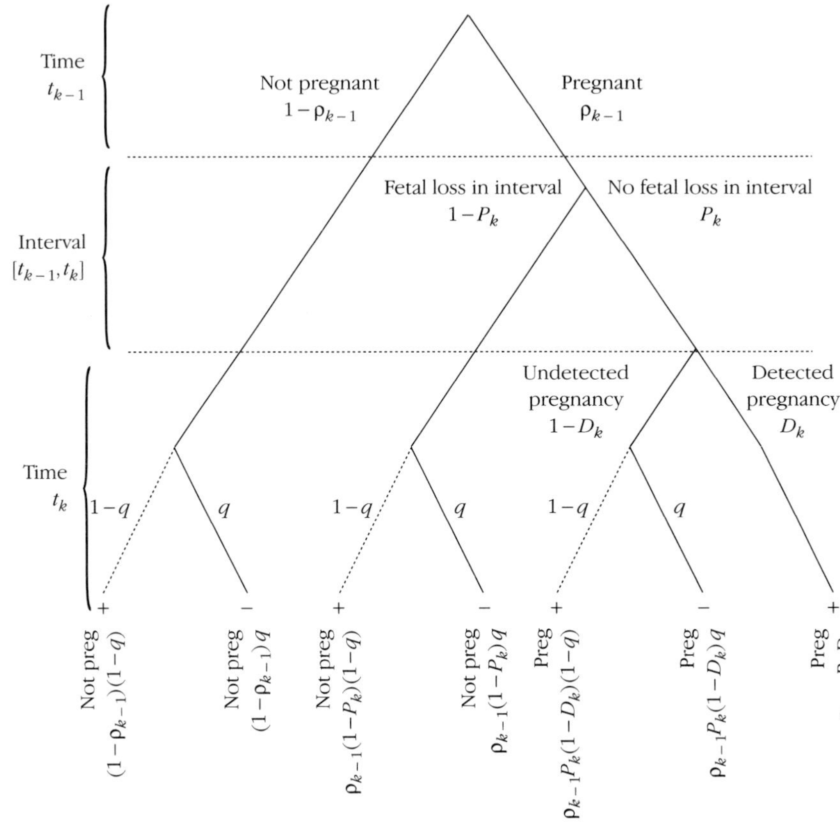

Figure 4 Probability tree showing the relationship among pregnancy assay results, characteristics of the assays and probability of fetal losses across the interval $[t_{k-1}, t_k]$. ρ_k, probability of pregnancy at time k; P_k, probability of no fetal loss occurring in the interval; D_k, sensitivity of the test at time k; q, specificity of the test. At the terminal branches, + and − indicate whether the result of the pregnancy test is positive or negative; 'Preg' and 'Not preg' refer to whether the individual is actually pregnant or not. Below each terminus is an unconditional probability for arriving at that point

gestational-age-specific sensitivity of the pregnancy assay, and maternal age effects on fecundability and fetal loss.

The underlying logic of the method is shown in Figure 4. The basic idea is that events are occurring from one observation (pregnancy assay) to the next. The events occur with probabilities that follow the branches of this tree, yet all we observe are positive or negative assay results at the end of the tree.

At ovulation (time t_0), some fraction of women will be pregnant with probability ρ_0. This parameter will be the estimate of total fecundability. For the sample of women who are not pregnant (probability $1-\rho_0$), the left branch of the tree is traversed. A pregnancy assay given at the first observation after ovulation (time t_1) will give a true negative diagnosis with specificity q, and a false-positive diagnosis with probability $1 - q$. For the women who are pregnant, a fraction $1 - P_1$ will experience a pregnancy loss in the interval $[t_0, t_1]$. The probability P_k arises directly from the Wood–Boklage model as $P_k = S(t_k)/S(t_{k-1})$ and incorporates parameters p, h_b and h_l. Again, specificity q will change the result of the pregnancy assays in terms of probability. For women who do not experience pregnancy losses (with probability P_1), some fraction of their pregnancies will be detected according to the sensitivity, with probability D_1. Likewise, a fraction $1 - D_1$ of pregnancies will not be detected; specificity q changes the result.

As this tree shows, there are four ways of obtaining a positive assay result and three ways of obtaining a negative result for the first pregnancy assay at time t_1. For all women who have positive results, we can compute the probability that they are truly pregnant at time t_1 as the sum of the two pregnant branches that yield positive results divided by the sum of all four positive branches, which simplifies to $\rho_1 = \rho_0 P_1\ [1 - q(1 - D_1)]/[1 - q(1 - \rho_0 D_1 P_1)]$. The probability that these women are not pregnant given a positive assay is $1 - \rho_1$. For women who have negative assay results, the probability that they are pregnant (but the assay could not detect it) is $\rho_1 = \rho_0 P_1 (1 - D_1)/(1 - \rho_0 D_1 P_1)$.

Probability ρ_1 now weights the left and right branches of the tree between the first pregnancy assay and the second pregnancy assay. The tree is traversed again in terms of probability and, given ρ_1, an assay result is used to compute ρ_2. Likewise, we recursively traverse the tree for each assay, always computing the value of ρ_k from ρ_{k-1}.

The preceding description sounds as though values for p, h_b, h_l, ρ_0, D and q are known when, in fact, the goal is to estimate these quantities from observations. Because the model was specified using only probabilities, maximum likelihood could be used to estimate the parameters of the model from observations. Parameter confidence intervals were calculated as the central 95% of bootstrapped parameter estimates. Details of the model, estimation methods, statistical validations and complete results are described elsewhere[12].

SUBJECTS

To estimate the fecundability and fetal loss model, we collected new data from a near-natural fertility population in rural Bangladesh[12] and used a highly sensitive and specific assay to detect pregnancies at early gestational ages[2]. The field study was conducted from February to December 1993 in the rural sub-district of Matlab thana, about 50 km south-east of Dhaka. At the start of the study, female field workers conducted one-time interviews of nearly all married women ($n = 3290$) aged 18–48 years, who permanently resided with their husbands in 28 villages in the region. The 17 villages with the lowest contraceptive prevalence were selected for the 9-month prospective study. The sample included married women of all reproductive statuses, including those who were pregnant or breastfeeding at the start of the study. In this way, we did not select for subfecundity by eliminating those of proven fecundity. Women who were using any form of contraception were excluded from the pool of potential participants. At the start of the study, 320 subjects were randomly drawn from the pool of eligible subjects. The subjects were interviewed twice each week and at the same time a urine sample was collected. The interviews included questions on menses, breastfeeding, contraception and pregnancy. When a subject dropped out of the study or became ineligible (e.g. because of divorce), she was replaced by a new subject randomly selected from the subject pool in the same village.

By the end of the field study, about 19 000 paired interview and urine specimens were collected. A total of 494 subjects had provided urine samples for 1 month or more. After each complete menstrual cycle for a subject, urine samples from the last one-third of the cycle were assayed for hCG[2].

RESULTS

The final set of observations consisted of about 4400 pregnancy assays in 1561 menstrual cycles. A total of 329 pregnancies were followed. Of these, 81 pregnancies were ongoing at the end of the study (statistically right-censored), 151 ended in live births, 84 biochemically detected pregnancies ended early in the pregnancy, ten were later pregnancy losses and three were induced abortions[12].

Effects of age were modelled on the risk of fetal loss in three ways: as affecting the initial fraction of abnormal conceptuses, as changing the risk of loss for abnormal conceptuses and as changing the risk of loss for normal conceptuses. The only significant effect of age, as assessed by likelihood ratio tests, was to increase the fraction of abnormal conceptuses. In other words, maternal age did not significantly influence the risk with which pregnancies of either normal or abnormal conceptuses would terminate. Instead, the effect of age was to increase the probability that a conceptus was abnormal, corresponding to Bishop's prediction[13].

Maternal age significantly affected both fecundability and fetal loss simultaneously. These age effects are summarized in Figure 5. The probability of pregnancy loss steadily increases with maternal age, beginning at about 0.55 for a 20-year-old woman and increasing to 0.96 by the age of 40 years. The age-related increase in the risk of fetal loss closely parallels the increasing proportion of abnormal conceptuses with maternal age.

Total fecundability was remarkably constant across most of the reproductive lifespan. Fecundability was at its maximum of one at the age of

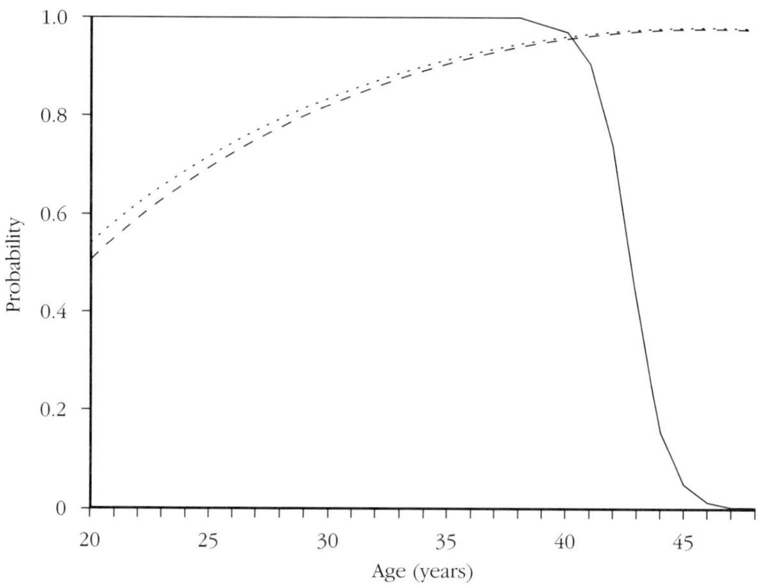

Figure 5 Maternal age-specific total fecundability and fetal loss in Bangladeshi women[12]. (—), Total fecundability; (...), pregnancy loss; (---), abnormal conceptuses

20 years and declined very slowly until the late 30s. From the late 30s onward, fecundability declined rapidly and reached zero by the age of 48 years (Figure 5).

DISCUSSION

The probability of pregnancy loss was surprisingly high: a 20-year-old woman would be expected to lose about half of all her pregnancies. Most of the lost pregnancies would never be detectable, so that they would appear to be non-conception cycles. Boklage[14] previously used the same mathematical model along with results from hCG-based studies of natural conceptions, *in vitro* fertilization studies and twin studies. He estimated an overall probability of pregnancy loss of 0.73. Our results confirm and refine those of Boklage by providing for maternal age-related effects. The best-fitting model of pregnancy loss was one in which maternal age acted by increasing the fraction of conceptuses in the high-risk subgroup. This finding strengthens Bishop's theory of fetal loss and supports his idea that the primary mechanism acting over the reproductive life course is an age-related increase in the proportion of chromosomally abnormal conceptuses. It has long been recognized that many later pregnancy losses result from lethal chromosomal aberrations[17]. More recent investigations have

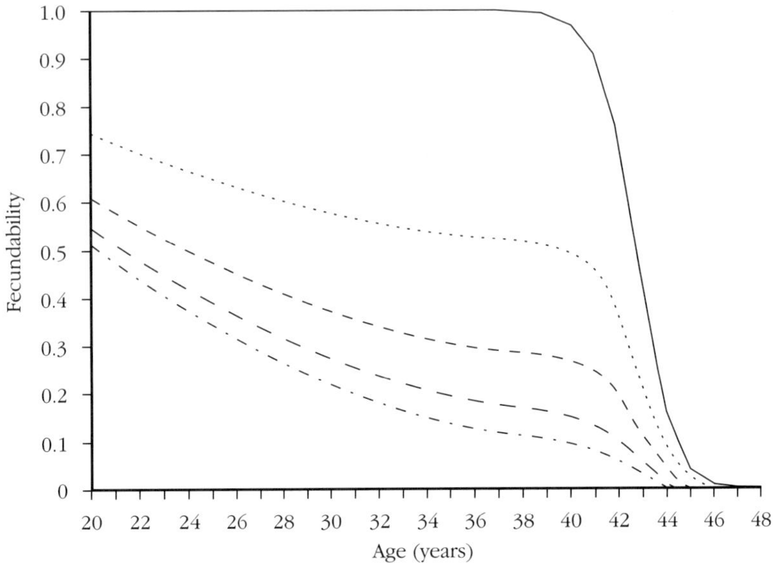

Figure 6 Total fecundability and early fetal loss were mathematically confounded using parameter estimates from the fecundability–fetal loss model. Age-specific apparent fecundabilities were computed given pregnancy detection on days 0, 7, 14, 21 and 28[12]. (—), Total; (...), apparent, day 7; (---), apparent, day 14; (– –), apparent, day 21; (– · – ·), apparent, day 28

begun to uncover the mechanisms by which maternal age increases the probability of non-disjunction during the resumption of meiosis in the oocyte[18–20].

The most surprising result from this work is the age pattern of fecundability, which was high and unaffected by age over much of the reproductive lifespan. This finding is consistent with the modelling results of Wood and Weinstein[10], in which the known biological components of fecundability predicted a total fecundability that is high and constant over much of the reproductive lifespan. We mathematically re-confounded the total fecundability and fetal loss results by generating expected age-related apparent fecundability curves for five different assay sensitivities from 0 to 28 days (Figure 6). Clearly, *apparent* fecundability takes on a strong age-related decline, even when pregnancy can be detected as early as day 7. From 20 to 40 years of age, the decline in fecundability is an artefact of fetal loss and incomplete sensitivity of the pregnancy assay.

Taken together, our results suggest that the observed age-related decline in apparent fecundability over most of the reproductive span is not caused by an age-related decline in total fecundability. Rather, it results from an age-related increase in early fetal loss that is masked by our inability to detect early pregnancies.

ACKNOWLEDGEMENTS

We gratefully acknowledge support from the National Institute on Aging (NIA RO1 AG15141-01), the National Institute of Child Health and Human Development (NICHD F32 HD 07994-02), the National Science Foundation (DBS-9218734) and the Population Council. Research in Bangladesh was supported by a Dissertation Research Grant on International Demographic Issues made on behalf of the Andrew W. Mellon Foundation to the Population Research Institute, the Hill Foundation, the American Institute of Bangladesh Studies, the Centre for Development Research, Bangladesh, and the International Centre for Diarrhoeal Disease Research, Bangladesh. We thank Robert Jones, Kathleen O'Connor, Matthew Steele and Michael Strong for comments and assistance.

REFERENCES

1. Wood JW. *Dynamics of Human Reproduction: Biology, Biometry, Demography*. Hawthorne, NY: Aldine de Gruyter, 1994
2. Holman DJ, Rasheed FN, Stroud CM, *et al*. A commercial pregnancy test modified for field studies of fetal loss. *Clin Chim Acta* 1998;271:25–44
3. Lenton EA. Pituitary and ovarian hormones in implantation and early pregnancy. In Chapman M, Grudzinskas G, Chard T, eds. *Implantation Biological and Clinical Aspects*. London: Springer-Verlag, 1988:17–29
4. Edmonds DK, Lindsay KS, Miller JF, *et al*. Early embryonic mortality in women. *Fertil Steril* 1982;38:447–53
5. Hakim RB, Gray RH, Zacur H. Infertility and early pregnancy loss. *Am J Obstet Gynecol* 1995;172:1510–17
6. Kline J, Stein Z, Susser M. *Conception to Birth: Epidemiology of Prenatal Development*. Oxford: Oxford University Press, 1989
7. Wilcox AJ, Weinberg CR, O'Connor JF, *et al*. Incidence of early loss of pregnancy. *N Engl J Med* 1988;319:189–94
8. Whittaker PG, Taylor A, Lind T. Unsuspected pregnancy loss in healthy women. *Lancet* 1983;1:1126–7
9. Wood JW. Fecundity and natural fertility in humans. *Oxford Rev Reprod Biol* 1989;11:61–109
10. Wood JW, Weinstein M. A model of age-specific fecundability. *Pop Stud* 1988;42: 85–113
11. Miller JF, Williamson E, Glue J, *et al*. Fetal loss after implantation. *Lancet* 1980;2: 554–6
12. Holman DJ. *Total Fecundability and Fetal Loss in Bangladesh*. PhD dissertation. Department of Anthropology, Pennsylvania State University, University Park, PA, 1996
13. Bishop MWH. Paternal contribution to embryonic death. *J Reprod Fertil* 1964;7:383–96
14. Boklage CE. Survival probability of human conceptions from fertilization to term. *Int J Fertil* 1990;35:75–94
15. Alfthan H, Haglund C, Dabek J, *et al*. Concentrations of human choriogonadotropin, its β-subunit, and the core fragment of the β-subunit in serum and urine of men and nonpregnant women. *Clin Chem* 1987;38:1981–7

16. Stenman U-H, Alfthan H, Ranta T, *et al*. Serum levels of human chorionic gonadotropin in nonpregnant women and men are modulated by gonadotropin-releasing hormone and sex steroids. *J Clin Endocrinol Metab* 1987;64:730–6
17. Boué A, Boué J, Gropp A. Cytogenetics of pregnancy wastage. *Adv Hum Genet* 1985;14:1–57
18. Battaglia DE, Goodwin P, Klein NA, *et al*. Influence of maternal age on meiotic spindle assembly in oocytes from naturally cycling women. *Hum Reprod* 1996;11:2217–22
19. Eichenlaub-Ritter U. Genetics of oocyte ageing. *Maturitas* 1998;30:143–69
20. Hassold T, Merrill M, Adkins K, *et al*. Recombination and maternal age-dependent non-disjunction: molecular studies of trisomy 16. *Am J Hum Genet* 1995;57:867–74

10

Genetic parameters of oocyte aging

P.L. Pearson

BACKGROUND

There are compelling social and economic reasons for attempting to understand the process of ovarian aging in humans. The last four decades of the twentieth century have witnessed the widespread use of birth control in economically advanced societies, leading to a greater freedom of choice in family planning. In the Netherlands this trend has resulted in an increase in the average maternal age, from 24.4 years to 29.0 years, in the period 1970–1997. Moreover, the same trends apply to the majority of Western European countries, albeit with some regional and ethnic differences. One consequence of delaying starting a family is a progressively increased inability to conceive because of infertility associated with raised maternal age[1]. Various studies indicate that average female fertility, expressed as the likelihood of conception in each cycle, decreases from a maximum at age 30, is halved by 35 and is essentially zero by the age of 41. However, it must be emphasized that these are average values, and it has long been realized that there is a wide variation between individual women; some women will become infertile in their early 30s and others may extend fertility into their late 40s. There are no reliable studies providing firm information on the distribution of variation in fertility within the population for a given chronological age, although for reasons advanced later, it is probably reasonable to assume that the variation approximates a Gaussian distribution. Conventional wisdom states that ovarian aging is a complex derivative of several factors: principally, the initial size of the ovarian pool and its rate of atresia, the regularity of cyclical variations in levels of essential hormones and the efficiency of metabolic maintenance mechanisms. Due to homeostatic regulation, these factors are not entirely independent of each other and the individual contribution of each factor to the aging process is difficult to determine. The chronological changes occurring in these interacting factors are what constitute the process of ovarian aging.

OVARIAN AGING MARKERS

Many attempts have been made to identify biological markers that reliably predict the ovarian aging characteristics of individual women. Changes in follicle stimulating hormone (FSH) levels have been shown to be a poor predictor of future ovarian functionality; ironically, the exception is a long-term and stable increase in FSH, denoting that infertility has already been reached. Determining the frequency of antral follicles using sophisticated three-dimensional analysis of ultrasound images of the ovary appears to have predictive potential[2]. Attempts have been made to predict the reproductive potential of women on the basis of residual follicle counts at various ages[3]. Recently Broekmans and colleagues (Chapter 7) provided support for the predictive value of antral follicle frequency. However, it is too early to know what the prognostic power of antral follicle frequency will be when applied to individual women. One of the major problems in using an aging parameter such as the number of antral follicles is that the end-point (in this case the number of follicles) has a high measurement error and is extremely variable between women of the same chronological age. For these reasons, it is difficult to link antral follicle frequency to a defined position in the ovarian aging process for a given individual.

Given that atresia plays such an important role, both in determining the size of the ovarian pool at menarche and the subsequent loss of oocytes in addition to those recruited during the estrous cycle, it is not surprising that apoptosis has been proposed as one of the major determinants of ovarian aging[4–7]. It is clear that studies defining oocyte differentiation checkpoints and their associated apoptotic sequelae will show how, when and where oocytes undergo programmed cell death. In particular, checkpoint control and apoptosis genes or even apoptotic antagonists[8] are now being identified. However, such studies will not necessarily reveal why the rate of oocyte atresia differs between women, whether such differences are preprogrammed and what constitutes the nature of the program. Exactly the same reservations apply to all the factors proposed as are involved in the ovarian aging process.

It has been argued that age of menopause is a more suitable parameter for assessing ovarian aging; it can be accurately defined and there is no dubiety over its chronological relationship with ovarian aging[9]. Commencement of menopause implies final exhaustion of the oocyte pool and the establishment of irreversible infertility. On the negative side, as with increased FSH levels, by the time menopause manifests the women concerned are already infertile. Age at menopause cannot be used directly as a biological marker for predicting ovarian aging; its power lies in its use for establishing correlates with alternative markers. Ideally, these will be independent of ovarian aging in their expression and with an ability to predict the future ovarian aging profiles of individual women. DNA markers potentially meet these requirements. They may ultimately prove to be the only markers with the power to adequately discriminate between women with an increased risk of premature ovarian aging and those who can afford to make reasonable delays in completing their families without fear of early infertility.

GENETIC EVIDENCE FOR OVARIAN AGING

Preprogrammed ovarian aging implies a genetic predisposition for a particular ovarian aging profile. This will be inherited and will demonstrate more homogeneity within families than between families or in the population as a whole. The similarities in ovarian aging between individuals with known levels of genetic similarity can be used to quantify the inherited predisposition for ovarian aging. This parameter, referred to as heritability, is normally expressed as a decimal fraction; for example, a value of 0.80 denotes that 80% of the observed variation in ovarian aging is determined genetically and 20% by environmental factors. An assumption made in this calculation is that a relatively large number of genes are involved in determining the genetic trait being studied.

There are cogent arguments supporting the hypothesis that the age at which normal menopause commences mirrors the chronological staging of the preceding phases in ovarian aging. te Velde (Chapter 3) has reasoned that the distributions within the population for age-related decreases in the size of the ovarian pool, decreases in fertility, loss of regularity of menses, and commencement of menopause are parallel and equidistant for all ages. Whether this is coincidence, or whether it reflects a general underlying mechanism regulating the rate of ovarian aging at all phases, remains to be explored. However, as advanced below, determining whether the same genetic variants are involved in determining the aging profiles of different stages in the ovarian aging process would be an important confirmation of the hypothesis. The hypothesis predicts that a woman who enters menopause at an early age will have previously become infertile at an early age and vice versa. Surprisingly, and regrettably, there are no data available to test whether a positive correlation exists between the age of last childbirth and the age at which women enter menopause, which would also be expected from the hypothesis. The age range for commencement of normal menopause varies between 40 and 60 years with an average of approximately 51 years in the Netherlands. Although the distribution is almost Gaussian, there is evidence of skewness with a mild excess of women on the left (young) side of the distribution. The age at which women become infertile can only be inferred from the age at last childbirth in natural populations that do not practice anti-conception. In other studies in natural populations, the average age of last childbirth was 41 years[25], which agrees with estimates for the Dutch population and suggests that this is a constant feature for most human populations.

It has been previously proposed that the absence of any clear single causative environmental factor to account for variation in the age of menopause suggested the involvement of genetic factors[10]. Several studies have confirmed this[11]. Torgerson and colleagues[12] noted a positive association between the age of menopause in mothers and that of daughters, but made no estimate of the extent of heritability. Twin studies performed in Australia and England estimated the heritability to be between 0.4 and 0.63 respectively[13,14]. More recently, our own group has confirmed this familial similarity and determined the heritability of age of menopause to be 0.85 (0.61–0.92, 90% confidence interval) in 243 pairs of sisters taken from a large randomly selected group of women assembled some 25 years previously for epidemiological purposes[26]. Furthermore, this analysis also demonstrated the absence of any measurable environmental contribution to the variation. The much-discussed relationship between smoking and reduction in the age of menopause is small, and owes its high statistical significance to the large number of observations made, rather than to the size of the contribution of smoking to total variation, which is less than 2%[15–17]. We conclude that variation in the age of menopause is largely, if not entirely, genetically determined.

GENETIC MODELS

There are several reasons for believing that the genetic model that best fits the type of variation and inheritance pattern observed in normal age of menopause is multifactorial. These include the following: that the normal age at menopause is clearly not inherited as a single-gene trait such that there is a clear division of children within a given sibship into just two phenotypic categories; and the daughters of mothers, who themselves have had either a very late or very early menopause, will tend to have a less extreme age of menopause shifting towards the population mean. Such a regression towards the mean is routinely observed for many other complex genetic traits including height, weight, IQ and blood pressure in the children of parents demonstrating extremes on one or the other side of the population distribution. This implies that the age of menopause, as for many other complex traits, is determined by a combination of several genes, and perhaps environmental factors. Just how many genes, which genes and what the relative contribution of each gene is to the total variation in age of menopause are the crucial questions to be answered. However, given that the variation is largely genetically determined, then the observed Gaussian distribution is explicable by the combined expression of multiple genes and their alleles.

Let us for the sake of argument and simplicity assume the following: that there are three different genes involved; that each gene can occur as two types of allele in the parents, one of which predisposes to early menopause and the other to late menopause; that the frequencies of both types are equal; that the interaction between genes and alleles to produce a phenotype is purely additive; that the genes are carried on different chromosomes and segregate independently relative to each other. Given that each gene is represented by two alleles, and that each allele has an equal chance of coding for either early or late menopause, this produces a total of six alleles and 2^6 (64) possible allelic combinations when both maternal and paternal contributions are taken into account. In a population exhibiting random mating, this results in seven different types of phenotype combinations in the next generation. These range from all six alleles coding for early menopause at one extreme, three alleles coding for early and three for late menopause in the middle of the distribution and all six alleles coding for late menopause at the other extreme. Despite there being only three genes involved, there is already a good approximation to a Gaussian distribution. Using the same assumptions for five genes results in ten alleles, 1024 allelic combinations and eleven phenotype combinations respectively, and provides a smoother fit to a Gaussian distribution. In these simplified examples with just two types of phenotypic class (early and late menopause) in equal frequency, the frequency distribution of phenotype combinations corresponds to the simple binomial expansion of $(q+p)^{2n}$, where n represents the number of genes, $2n$ the number of alleles and q and p the frequency of alleles contributing to early and late menopause, respectively.

The modelling rapidly becomes more complex when other variables are taken into account, including differences in the number of alleles per gene, the frequency of alleles and the relative contribution of different alleles to the total variation. This contribution may not be purely additive, as in our simplified model, but multiplicative, which would suggest a synergy between different alleles in their contribution to the total phenotypic variation. When more than two phenotypic classes are taken into account, the contribution of individual genes and alleles to the total variation can now best be described by a multinomial expansion of the form $(p_1q_ix_1+p_2q_ix_2 \ldots + p_iq_ix_i)^n$ where n now represents the number of phenotypic classes contributing to the total variation, p is the number of genes, q is the frequency of a given allele, i is the total number of alleles for a given gene, and x the contribution of a given allele to the total phenotypic variation. This latter term also incorporates whether or not the given allele has an additive or a multiplicative interaction with other defined alleles. It is entirely plausible that the number of phenotypic classes required to model this much more complex situation is still relatively low. Five evenly distributed classes may be sufficient to describe the phenotypic contribution of various types of allele, with the original two extreme phenotypic classes of early and late menopause from our simple model now being separated by three intermediate ones. However, as in our simple model, it is not only the number of phenotypic classes which provides the close approximation to a Gaussian distribution, but mainly the large number of allelic combinations, which rises exponentially as the number of genes increases. Moreover, despite the fact that the overall distribution of phenotypic variation comprises a complex admixture of individual genetic components, deviations towards the two extremes on average will be evenly divided and the distribution will remain approximately Gaussian. This model permits us to study the role of selected parameters, including complexities such as multiplicative allelic interaction, and enables us to define more critically the specific contribution of individual genes to the total variation under various conditions.

GENETIC MAPPING

The availability of high-resolution genetic maps of highly polymorphic markers has made it feasible to map genes involved in the etiology of complex human traits. To date, the locations of genes predisposing to complex traits have been determined by whole genome screens using highly polymorphic markers in several types of segregation or association analysis[18–20]. In principle, this general approach can be applied to all traits with a complex genetic inheritance pattern, including traits such as ovarian aging, given that the trait has a high heritability.

Since there is presumably a large amount of genetic variation contributing to total variation in age of menopause, a strategy for reducing the genetic heterogeneity and maximizing the chance of detecting the contribution of individual genes is to compare the allelic variation of individual genes between and within the two extremes of variation and to ignore the rest[21]. A convenient definition of extreme variation might be between the ages of 40–45 years for early menopause and 55–60 years for late menopause, which corresponds more or less to the fifth and 95th percentile limits, respectively. The comparison could be carried out as a case-controlled study in which allele frequencies for selected candidate genes are compared between individuals within and between the two groups. However, the choice of genes and the determination of whether the allelic variation being used is causal to differences in age of menopause is extremely problematic. Furthermore, fluctuations in allelic frequencies between populations and/or ethnic groups can easily result in spurious associations with the trait under study. An alternative and much more powerful strategy is to carry out identity by descent linkage studies (IBD) using many small families and polymorphic markers randomly distributed over the whole genome. Essentially, this is a quantitative trait locus extension (QTL) of the affected sib-pair analysis in which many pairs of sisters exhibiting either early or late menopause and two additional first-degree relatives are investigated. Since in many cases the parents of menopausal women will be already dead at the time of analysis, the inclusion of two other sibs, in addition to the menopausal sisters, means that four chromosomes of each parent will be sampled. This permits determination of the parental genotypes with 88% accuracy even when the parents are dead. Another large bonus in determining the parental genotypes is that it makes it possible to construct haplotypes of the alleles of adjacent polymorphic markers. For example, consider two polymorphic markers A and B, which are adjacent to each other on a particular chromosome, and carry the alleles A1 and A2, and B1 and B2, on the respective homologous chromosomes. The information which can be obtained on the possible involvement of this particular chromosome region in the inheritance of a genetic trait is much more specific when we know which A marker allele associates with which B marker allele on the same chromosome – in other words whether the chromosome haplotypes are of the form A1,B1/A2,B2 or A1,B2/A2,B1. When the gene determining a given genetic trait is located between two markers forming a haplotype, then the probability of defining the map location of the gene is much higher. If a particular haplotype or individual allele is significantly linked to a gene determining either early or late menopause, it will be inherited more frequently within the given menopause group than expected by chance alone. Further, it might be expected that association of a particular haplotype or allele with either early or late menopause would result in enrichment of other haplotypes or alleles in the other menopause category. It can be concluded that the sib-pair method provides a powerful method for defining chromosome regions containing genes impacting on the age at which menopause commences. The statistical methods for mapping genetically complex traits have developed rapidly during the last decade and many novel approaches are likely to emerge over the coming years.

We have performed power studies which show that an initial genome screen using approximately 400 highly polymorphic markers on 120 sister-pairs in which at least one member of each pair comes from either the early or late menopause cohort, would result in one or more chromosome regions being detected with a 60% reliability. Positive regions could then be rescreened using a much higher density of markers within the given chromosome region and an independent set of sister-pairs. Once the involvement of particular chromosome regions has been confirmed, suitable candidate genes from the same chromosome region can be selected from public databases, which contain information on the map location of coding sequences, including ESTs (expressed sequence tags). Each candidate gene so defined would then be sequenced using DNA samples taken from selected early and late menopause individuals to determine whether particular sequence variants cosegregate with the alleles of the polymorphic marker(s) used to identify the particular chromosome region in the first place. Such association depends on linkage disequilibrium existing between the DNA sequence variant and the polymorphic marker variation; this implies that the two types of variation are so close together on the same chromosome that their association (linkage) will never or seldom be interrupted by meiotic crossing-over. Following stringent analysis of such associations and assessment of the possible effect of the discovered sequence variation on gene function, it might be concluded that the discovered sequence variant is indeed part of the genetic variation contributing to differences in the age of menopause. The same procedure would then be followed for all chromosome regions detected in the first genome screen.

CANDIDATE GENES

Various candidate genes have been proposed that may contribute to ovarian aging and age of menopause. In a case-controlled study, Weel and co-workers[24] showed that homozygosity of the wild type allele of an intronic restriction site polymorphism within the estrogen receptor gene was associated with a 1.1-year reduction in the average age of menopause. However, the power of this analysis might have been significantly improved by the use of a much more informative polymorphic marker, namely a $[TA]_n$ repeat polymorphism also carried within the estrogen receptor gene. It has been claimed that this polymorphism associates with the premutation state in females with FRA-X syndrome, resulting in premature ovarian failure (POF)[22]. POF has been arbitrarily defined as the onset of menopause below the age of 40 years. It is important to recognize that important etiological differences exist between POF and the normal process of menopause (above 40 years). Between 12 and 30% of POF individuals exhibit either Mendelian segregation in families or chromosome abnormalities, particularly deletions in the long arm of the X chromosome, indicating involvement of a single major disease-causing mutation. This is in contradistinction to the situation described above in which normal menopause is caused by the interaction of several genes and presumably involves genetic variations within the genes which are much more common than POF mutations and individually make a much smaller contribution to the menopause phenotype. It is likely that POF-inducing mutations disrupt production of the gene product by either gene deletion or premature termination of transcription by frameshift or stop-codon mutations, whilst genetic variants associated with normal menopause will be mild missense mutations. Although any genes believed to be involved in POF are also potential candidate genes for determining the process of normal menopause, the spectrum of genetic changes involved in the two phenomena will be entirely different. It has been recently argued that there is an overlap both in phenotype and in etiology between idiopathic POF and cases of early menopause (between 40 and 45 years)[23]. However, for mapping studies based on linkage analysis we should be careful not to mix the two forms since this will seriously degrade the power of the analysis. Accordingly, menopausal sister-pairs within the normal range only should be selected.

Similarly, the genes believed to be involved in either ovarian apoptosis or metabolic maintenance pathways are candidate genes for normal menopause. Whilst it is true that apoptosis studies detail the pathways and genes involved, the nature of the work does not provide insights into how genetic variation in such genes might determine the onset of menopause in particular and ovarian aging in general. One of the major problems in defining whether or not a particular candidate gene contributes to variations in the age of menopause is that there are usually no known genetic polymorphisms that can be used as a marker in IBD investigations to establish such an involvement. This situation can potentially be resolved by first mapping the gene concerned using a PCR detection system on a radiation hybrid mapping panel. Such a mapping system can map genes to an accuracy of less than 1–2 megabases. Subsequently anonymous highly polymorphic markers can be selected which are located in the same region as that containing the candidate gene. Implementation of this strategy should provide a rapid means of establishing the role of candidate genes in the onset of menopause, once the molecular genetic infrastructure to carry out the studies has been established.

THE FUTURE

We are currently engaged in a gene mapping enterprise such as has been discussed above. This requires a close collaboration between a molecular genetics department with the necessary expertise and infrastructure to carry out the molecular investigations (Professor Pearson, Utrecht), a department of gynecology with a research interest in ovarian aging (Professor te Velde, Utrecht) and a department of epidemiology to direct the population analysis (Professor Grobbee, Utrecht). Our goal is to define the range of genotypes that predict where a woman fits into the phenotypes of ovarian aging; as it were, to create a genetic fingerprint for female reproductive capacity. These developments can potentially add important new dimensions to the ways in which clinicians will regard the problem of premature ovarian aging in future. At the least, the investigations will provide further insights into the etiology of the problem and at the best they can provide information on which to base future advisory or therapeutic strategies. The advisory dimension will involve identifying women with an increased risk of premature ovarian aging (on the basis of genotyping analyses of the type described here) and informing them about the possible consequences. The therapeutic dimension may come from our increased knowledge of the genes concerned and insights into how gene function can be modulated to delay the ovarian aging process.

REFERENCES

1. Chandra A, Stephen EH. Impaired fecundity in the United States: 1982–1995. *Fam Plann Perspect* 1998;30:34–42
2. Scheffer GJ, Broekmans FJ, Dorland M, *et al*. Antral follicle counts by transvaginal ultrasonography are related to age in women with proven natural fertility. *Fertil Steril* 1999;72:845–51
3. Faddy MJ, Gosden RG. A model conforming the decline in follicle numbers to the age of menopause in women. *Hum Reprod* 1996;1:1484–6
4. Putowski LT, Skrzypczak M, Zielewicz J, *et al*. The relevance of c-myc to the physiology of the human ovary. *Gynecol Endocrinol* 1997;11:5–10
5. Perez GI, Robles R, Knudson CM, *et al*. Prolongation of ovarian lifespan into advanced chronological age by Bax-deficiency. *Nat Genet* 1999;21:200–3
6. Morita Y, Tilly JL. Oocyte apoptosis: like sand through an hourglass. *Dev Biol* 1999;213: 1–17
7. Hsu SY, Hsueh AJ. Intracellular mechanisms of ovarian cell apoptosis. *Mol Cell Endocrinol* 1998;145:21–5
8. Hsu SY, Lai RJ, Finegold M, Hsueh AJ. Targeted overexpression of Bcl-2 in ovaries of transgenic mice leads to decreased follicle apoptosis, enhanced folliculogenesis, and increased germ cell tumorigenesis. *Endocrinology* 1996;137:4837–43
9. te Velde ER, Dorland M, Broekmans FJ. Age at menopause as a marker of reproductive ageing. *Maturitas* 1998;30:119–25
10. Van Noord PA, Dubas JS, Dorland M, *et al*. Age at natural menopause in a population-based screening cohort: the role of menarche, fecundity, and lifestyle factors. *Fertil Steril* 1997;68:95–102
11. Cramer DW, Xu H, Harlow BL. Family history as a predictor of early menopause. *Fertil Steril* 1995;64:740–5
12. Torgerson DJ, Thomas RE, Reid DM. Mothers and daughters menopausal ages: is there a link? *Eur J Obstet Gynecol Reprod Biol* 1997;74:63–6
13. Treloar SA, Do KA, Martin NG. Genetic influences on the age at menopause. *Lancet* 1998;352:1084–5
14. Snieder H, MacGregor AJ, Spector TD. Genes control the cessation of a woman's reproductive life: a twin study of hysterectomy and age at menopause. *J Clin Endocrinol Metab* 1998;83:1875–80
15. Cooper GS, Sandler DP, Bohlig M. Active and passive smoking and the occurrence of natural menopause. *Epidemiology* 1999;10:771–3
16. Kato I, Toniolo P, Akhmedkhanov A, *et al*. Prospective study of factors influencing the onset of natural menopause. *J Clin Epidemiol* 1998;51:1271–6
17. Cramer DW, Harlow BL, Xu H, *et al*. Cross-sectional and case-controlled analyses of the association between smoking and early menopause. *Maturitas* 1995;22:79–87
18. Lander ES, Green P. Construction of multilocus genetic linkage maps in humans. *Proc Natl Acad Sci USA* 1987;84:2363–7
19. Lander E, Kruglyak L. Genetic dissection of complex traits: guidelines for interpreting and reporting linkage results. *Nat Genet* 1995;11:241–7
20. Todd JA. Genetic analysis of type 1 diabetes using whole genome approaches. *Proc Natl Acad Sci USA* 1995;92:8560–5
21. Risch N, Zhang H. Extreme discordant sib pairs for mapping quantitative trait loci in humans. *Science* 1995;268:1584–9
22. Syrrou M, Georgiou I, Patsalis PC, *et al*. Fragile X premutations and $(TA)_n$ estrogen receptor polymorphism in women with ovarian dysfunction. *Am J Med Genet* 1999;84:306–8

23. Tibiletti MG, Testa G, Vegetti W, *et al*. The idiopathic forms of premature menopause and early menopause show the same genetic pattern. *Hum Reprod* 1999;14:2731–4
24. Weel AE, Vitterlinden AG, *et al*. Estrogen receptor polymorphism predicts the onset of natural and surgical menopause. *J Clin Endocrinol Metab* 1999;84:3146–50
25. Wood JW. Fecundity and natural fertility in humans. In Milligen SR, ed. *Oxford Reviews of Reproductive Biology*. Oxford, UK: Oxford University Press, 1989;2:61–109
26. de Bruin JP, Bovenhuis H, *et al*. The role of genetic factors in age at natural menopause. Submitted for publication

11

The determinants of non-disjunction and their possible relationship to oocyte aging

U. Eichenlaub-Ritter

INTRODUCTION

No species other than the human exhibits such high rates of reproductive wastage associated with errors in chromosome segregation during the reductional and equational division of chromosomes in oogenesis[1]. Maternal age is the main etiological factor associated with numerical chromosomal aberrations in oocytes, trisomy in the embryo and liveborn, and significantly reduced developmental potential of the pre- and postimplantation embryo[1–5]. Postponing childbearing to advanced reproductive ages, as is common in modern societies, has increased dramatically the number of subfertile couples. The reproductive age of most women attending fertility clinics is over 30, but there is no method available to predict the relative risk for non-disjunction in oocytes of patients apart from maternal age. Despite the advances in molecular biology and genetics, the determinants of non-disjunction in female meiosis are still unknown. For detecting the mechanisms responsible for non-disjunction in oogenesis, it is essential to know at which stage (premeiotic, meiosis I, meiosis II or postfertilization) errors in chromosome segregation occur, what chromosome-specific characteristics exist in magnitude and type of non-disjunction events (e.g. meiotic versus mitotic), and what data are available on genetic, physiological or toxicological risk factors[5–7]. Finally, it is imperative to identify the feature(s) unique to mammalian oocytes and, in particular, to human oogenesis that are affected by age and make oocytes more susceptible to errors in chromosome segregation in comparison to spermatocytes or mitotically dividing cells, e.g. the longevity of oocytes and the incontinuous meiotic process, factors associated with chronological or physiological age of the female, the processes associated with selection of aberrant gametes (apoptosis) or of surviving and developing oocytes and follicles, hormonal homeostasis in female meiosis and altered cell populations in depleted ovaries, regulation of cell cycle progression and/or molecular processes specific for governing spindle formation in oocytes. Several recent studies in the human and experimental animals have suggested that there may be more than one contributing factor that may influence the susceptibility to malsegregation of meiotic chromosomes in the oocyte of an aged female. In the following, I will first review data on the analysis of the origin of extra chromosomes in trisomies in the human. I will then represent experimental evidence from studies in a mouse model, showing that there are correlations between (i) the chromosomal constitution, (ii) reduced quality of mammalian oocytes associated with disturbed cell cycle progression, and (iii) loss of fidelity of chromosome distribution. Furthermore, specific risk factors for reduced developmental capacity of oocytes, and oocyte-specific features of cell cycle regulation and spindle formation that relate to susceptibility to errors in chromosome segregation and trisomy formation with advanced maternal age, will be discussed.

NON-DISJUNCTION OF INDIVIDUAL CHROMOSOMES AND MATERNAL AGE

Most, if not all, chromosomes in the human appear to be susceptible to non-disjunction in oogenesis[8–11]. However, the relative increase in trisomy formation within maternal age groups differs between chromosomes[5,11–14]. The long chromosomes of the A and B groups are rarely found in a spontaneous abortus, stillbirth or liveborn, regardless of maternal age. In contrast, trisomy 16 increases early in reproductive life and there is a linear correlation with maternal age. The rate of trisomy 21 and the small acrocentrics increases exponentially from about the mid-30s[13]. Preimplantation diagnosis also suggests that individual chromosomes are differentially susceptible to non-disjunction[9,11,15–18]. However, recent cytogenetic studies of preimplantation embryos revealed that chromosomes found infrequently in trisomies in the postimplantation embryo, which were assumed to be comparatively resistant to non-disjunction, are frequently involved in numerical aberrations of the preimplantation embryo[11]. Imbalance of these chromosomes in the embryo may be incompatible with normal development and could be responsible for arrest or delays in the cell cycle and implantation failures, in this way contributing to the reduced fertility associated with advanced maternal age[11]. Therefore, analysis of trisomic conditions, their origin and association with chromosome-specific features may provide some information on possible etiological factors, but probably will not uncover the whole range of processes leading to the reduced developmental capacity of the 'aged' egg.

Judging from the trisomy data of prenatal diagnosis, there is no general pattern in susceptibility detectable in terms of density of genes, morphological criteria or heterochromatin content explaining the mechanisms leading to aneuploidy and the differences between individual chromosomes to become involved in trisomy formation[10]. However, recent molecular analyses of the origin and recombination of extra chromosomes in trisomies using polymorphic markers have revealed some consistent features of chromosomes associated with non-disjunction. They have shown that most non-disjunction in female meiosis occurs at anaphase I, while some chromosomal configurations may have rather a high chance of causing second meiotic errors and failures in the separation of chromatids at meiosis II. Relationships with the recombinational history of the non-disjoining chromosome suggest that there is a link between predisposition to non-disjunction and the very early events in the development of the mammalian oocyte, when oocytes undergo meiotic prophase, homologous chromosomes pair and crossing over takes place in the embryonal ovary (Figure 1). Since malsegregation of chromosomes actually occurs at a much later time, when

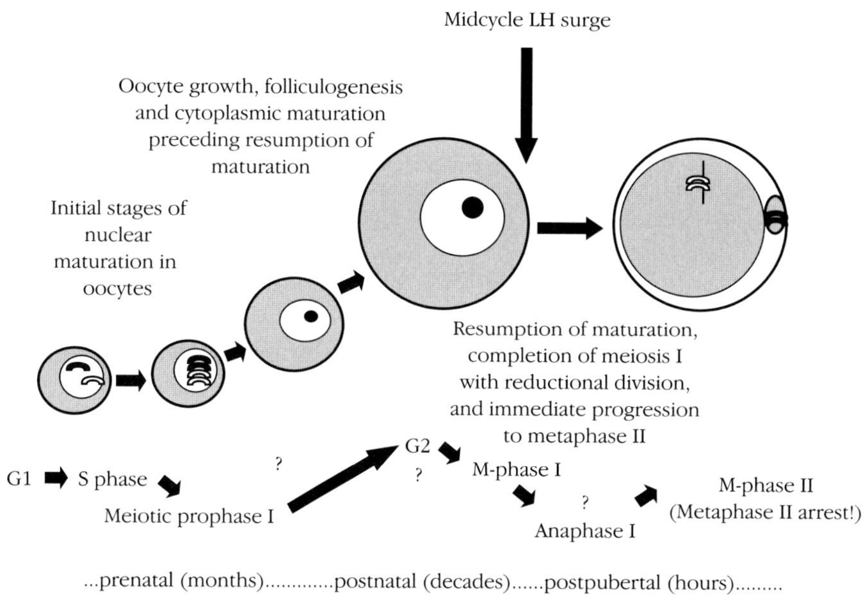

Figure 1 Discontinuous meiosis and the cell cycle in oocytes: question marks designate transitions where checkpoint controls may be present. Replication of parental homologous chromosomes in the S phase of the embryonal ovary is followed by prophase I, during which pairing between homologs and recombination take place. Meiotic arrest in the G2 phase can last decades in the human. Transition from the G2 phase to the meiotic M phase requires folliculogenesis, oocyte growth and cytoplasmic maturation of the oocytes to full meiotic competence. The midcycle luteinizing hormone (LH) surge triggers the resumption of maturation in the meiotically competent oocytes inside of mature Graafian follicles. Cell cycle progression from the G2 phase through meiosis I, with the reductional separation of homologous chromosomes, and progression to metaphase II requires only hours. M-phase arrest at metaphase II is dependent on active cytostatic factor in the presence of a functional spindle and well-aligned chromosomes. For further explanation, see text

the oocyte resumes maturation (Figure 1), the concept of a correlation between the recombinational history of an oocyte and its chromosomes would predict that early, as well as late, events may predispose to aneuploidy[4,19,20]. The observations in oocytes of aged rodents have suggested that a pool of oocytes exists in the embryonal ovary that is destined to remain meiotically arrested in the ovary for long periods. The latter may resume the growth phase inside their follicle and mature to metaphase II only at an advanced maternal age, close to the end of the reproductive phase[21–25]. From morphological criteria, there is no evidence for the existence of distinct cohorts of oocytes or follicles in the human embryonal ovary. However, in rodents, experiments involving pulse-labelling of DNA during the S phase have suggested that, in this species, oocytes resume maturation in the sexually mature animal according to the 'first in, first out' pattern[7,26], in agreement with the concept of a production line[21] (see also discussion below).

IS THERE A CORRELATION BETWEEN EARLY EVENTS IN OOGENESIS AND NON-DISJUNCTION WITH AGE?

It is beyond the scope of this article to review in detail the literature on the incidence of meiotic non-disjunction, its relation to maternal age and the association with recombination in individual chromosomes, and readers are referred to recent reviews. However, a brief summary of data from retrospective studies on the origin and recombination of extra chromosomes in trisomies is provided in Table 1, including recent reports and observations on cases of uniparental disomy 15, where the embryo contains two maternal copies of a chromosome while the paternal chromosome was probably lost due to secondary non-disjunction early in embryogenesis.

Molecular analysis generally confirms the observations made by conventional cytogenetic and molecular cytogenetic analyses in spare or donated human oocytes and sperm, showing that the aneuploidy rate is extremely high in oocytes compared to sperm or mitotically dividing cells. The average hyperploidy rate after meiosis I in human oocytes is 8.6% and the conservative estimate of aneuploidy is accordingly over 15%[5]. In contrast, on average, 1% to maximally 4% of all sperm from healthy men carry numerical chromosomal aberrations after completion of both meiotic divisions[5,27–29]. Extra chromosomes in the embryo appear to be predominantly of maternal meiotic orgin. This is only different for the sex chromosomes. The extra X chromosome in XXY and triple X cases seems to be paternally derived in about 50% of all cases studied[30]. Paternal gonosomal non-disjunction appears to be caused by failures in recombination between sex chromosomes in male meiosis[31,32].

Trisomies 13, 15, 18 and 21 are similar in that about 90% of them are derived from meiotic errors in oogenesis[33] (Table 1). Trisomy 8 is a rare condition that is mostly mosaic in the embryo or offspring and appears to be incompatible with a continuing pregnancy. It differs from the other trisomies in that one-third of all cases studied by molecular analysis so far had an extra paternal chromosome of postmeiotic orgin. In addition, one-third of all studied cases were due to a mitotic error involving a maternal chromosome and only in one-third of cases was the extra chromosome 8 of maternal meiotic orgin (for references and discussion see reference 33). Trisomy 16 appears to be exclusively of maternal meiotic origin[34], in contrast to trisomy 8 and different from trisomies 13, 15, 18 and 21 (Table 1).

About three-quarters of all maternal meiotic errors giving rise to trisomy 15 and maternal uniparental disomy 15 (mUPD 15) or trisomy 21 involve errors in segregation of the homologous chromosomes and non-disjunction at meiosis I of oogenesis. Trisomy 16 is exceptional, with 100% meiosis I errors. Trisomy 18 of maternal meiotic origin predominantly (65.8%) appears to be derived by failures in segregation of sister chromatids at anaphase II (Table 1).

Correlations between altered recombination and age-related non-disjunction have been detected by now for trisomy/mUPD 15, trisomy 16, trisomy 18 and trisomy 21 (Table 1), but the type of alteration differs again for each chromosome.

In trisomy 16, recombination of the non-disjoined chromosomes is associated with a 25% reduction in recombination. However, this does not lead to a proportional shortening of the recombination map at all studied intervals. Instead, there is a markedly reduced recombination in the vicinity of the centromeres, in the proximal short and long arms of chromosome 16, with nearly normal recombination at other sites. All non-disjoined chromosomes 16 still appear to possess at least one chiasma and there is no evidence for total absence of recombination and, accordingly, the presence of univalents, which might explain the loss in fidelity of segregation of this chromosome[34].

Similar to trisomy 16, recombination in trisomy 21 of maternal meiosis I origin also appears to be reduced. However, the overall length of the recombination map is reduced much more in trisomy 21 as compared to trisomy 16, from 72 cM in the control to 33 cM in the maternal meiosis I errors (a reduction of 54%). Again, recombination is altered non-randomly: it is reduced in proximal, but increased in distal, parts of non-disjoined chromosomes 21. Nearly half (42%) of all errors in segregation of chromosome 21 at anaphase I are consistent with the total absence of recombination[35]. This means that still more than half of all errors in disjunction of this chromosome occur at maternal meiosis I, in spite of the presence of a crossing-over event[19]. Strikingly, non-disjunction of sister chromatids at meiosis II is also associated with altered recombination frequencies, although one would expect that the presence and positioning of a chiasma influences only meiosis I where the homologous chromosomes disjoin. In contrast to meiosis I errors, extra maternal chromosomes of trisomy 21 with unseparated chromatids (meiosis II errors) have increased recombination in the intervals close to the centromere. This suggests that the initial event causing second

Table 1 Origin of extra chromosome in trisomies or additional maternal chromosome in maternal uniparental disomy, as determined by DNA polymorphism analysis (modified from reference 33)

Chromosome (no informative cases)	*Paternal (%)*	*Maternal (%)*	*Association with meiotic recombination*
Trisomy 8[123–126]			
Total ($n = 15$)	33.3	66.7	
Mitotic	33.3	33.3	
Meiotic		33.3	?
Trisomy 13[127,128]			
Total ($n = 42$)	11.9	88.1	?
Trisomy 15[127–129]			
Total ($n = 17$)			
Meiotic	11.8	88.2	
Maternal trisomy 15 plus maternal UPD 15[36]			
Total ($n = 127$)		100	
Mitotic		9.4	
Meiotic		90.6	
Of the meiotics ($n = 116$): meiosis I		83.6	Overall reduced recombination all along chromosome; approximately 21% achiasmate; maternal age group < 30 years: 100% with 0–1 crossover; age > 40 years: approximately 40% with 3–4 crossovers
meiosis II		16.4	Probably no association
Trisomy 16[34]			
Total ($n = 62$)		100	
Meiosis I ($n = 56$)		100	Reduced recombination in proximal short and long arms, but all chiasmate
Trisomy 18[130–132]			
Total ($n = 176$)	8.5	91.5	
Informative for stage ($n = 7$ paternal plus 86 maternal = 93)			
Mitotic	5.4	7.5	
Meiotic	2.1	84.9	
Of the meiotics:			
meiosis I		34.2	Reduced recombination
meiosis II		65.8	

Table 1 *Continued*

Table 1 *Continued*

Chromosome (no informative cases)	*Paternal (%)*	*Maternal (%)*	*Association with meiotic recombination*
Trisomy 21[19,133]			
Total (n = 880)	8.5	91.5	
Informative for stage (n = 807)			
Mitotic	1.7	2.1	
Meiotic	5.4	90.7	
Of the meiotics:			
meiosis I	38.6	76	Maternal: reduced recombination with reductions in proximal and increases in distal regions: about 45% achiasmate
meiosis II	61.4	24	Maternal: increased recombination and excess recombination in proximal parts

UPD, uniparental disomy

meiotic non-disjunction may be initiated at meiosis I and that this then predisposes oocytes to failures in chromatid segregation.

The overall length of the recombination map is also reduced in mUPD 15 and trisomy 15, from 137.5 cM in the controls to 100.6 cM in the non-disjunction cases. Unlike in trisomies 21 and 16, the recombination is reduced to about the same extent at all intervals and there is no evidence for an overproportional shortening in proximal parts, as in trisomies 16 and 21. Twenty-one per cent of all errors in chromosome segregation are compatible with an absence of recombination, explaining most of the reduction in the recombination map. However, unexpectedly, the involvement of achiasmatic chromosomes 15 in aneuploidy appears to differ between different maternal age groups. Robinson and colleagues[36] reported that two-thirds of mUPD 15 and trisomy 15 cases from a meiotic I origin showed no evidence of crossing over in the group of women under 30 years of age. In contrast, the relative frequency of achiasmatic chromosomes in mUPD 15 and trisomy 15 cases was decreased to only around 10% in the oldest age group (> 40 years). At the same time, there appeared to be a positive correlation between the involvement of chromosomes with three to four crossovers in aneuploidy and increased maternal age. Extra, non-disjoined, chromosomes from women under 30 years did not possess more than two chiasmata, while over 40% of all non-disjoined chromosomes in the age group over 40 years had three to four chiasmata. These observations suggest that recombinant tetrads of chromosome 15 may be more susceptible to maternal age than the achiasmatic ones, and achiasmatic ones might have a high risk for malsegregation at all ages.

Taken together, the currently available data from retrospective molecular analyses of extra chromosomes from prenatal and postnatal diagnosis suggest that a correlation exists between the relative risk of a chromosome to malsegregate at meiosis I or II and its recombinational history; in particular, the distribution and number of chiasmata appear to be important. Those bivalents with one distal chiasma appear to be particularly susceptible to first meiotic errors, while those with excess proximal recombination in the vicinity of the centromere may have increased chances of failing to segregate chromatids at meiosis II. This is similar to findings in yeast or higher eukaryotes, such as *Drosophila,* which are amenable to genetic analysis[37–39]. There are no published studies which suggest that recombination is globally altered in the chromosomes of human oocytes and children of aged women, in contrast to the expected situation when a cohort of oocytes with insufficient recombination exists and resumes maturation at the end of the reproductive period, according to the hypothesis of a production line. However, detailed studies on the distribution of recombination at different intervals of individual chromosomes in relation to maternal age are still sparse in the human, such that it is unknown whether subtle or substantial changes in recombination involving some or all chromosomes exist. One recent study on the overall recombination rates in trisomy 21 cases originating from achiasmatic maternal meiosis of this chromosome suggested that, in fact, the crossing-over frequency between markers on other chromosomes was also reduced[35]. Therefore, in these cases, the cohort of oocytes undergoing nondisjunction might have suffered from a global reduction in recombination, strengthening the hypothesis of the existence of a production line. However, numbers of these thoroughly studied cases are still too small to reveal distinct etiological factors.

EVIDENCE FOR THE EXISTENCE OF A PRODUCTION LINE IN THE MOUSE AND ITS CONSEQUENCES FOR CHROMOSOME SEGREGATION IN OOGENESIS

Curious end-to-end associations of chromosomes were previously found in aged oocytes of some mammals[21,24]. It was suggested that they comprise functional or true univalents. In the absence of recombination, univalents may segregate randomly at meiosis I due to failures in proper alignment on the spindle[21]. The presence of only one distal chiasma may likewise represent a risk factor for proper segregation of the homologs in meiosis I, as has been indicated by studies in yeast as well as *Drosophila* and mammals[37–39]. Angell and colleagues[40,41] suggested that certain chiasmatic chromosomes in oocytes of aged women might segregate untimely at meiosis I (termed predivision), thus forming functional univalents which then either randomly segregate or undergo an equational division of chromatids at meiosis I instead of meiosis II. In fact, some univalents of a trisomic cell line from a human ovary segregated equationally at meiosis I of oogenesis[42], and the single X chromosome in oocytes of the X0 mouse may also either segregate randomly as a univalent at anaphase I or undergo predivision with one or both chromatids migrating to one spindle pole[43]. This is different for univalents in oocytes of a mouse lacking proteins for recombination (knockouts for the *Mlh1* mismatch repair gene), which remain in a metaphase I stage for extended lengths of time and do not appear to segregate precociously into chromatids prior to anaphase I[44].

Initial observations in our group have shown that aneuploidy is increased in oocytes of aged female mice of the CBA/Ca strain after maturation *in vitro*[5,45]. This strain of mice is characterized by possessing a limited follicle pool which is depleted by the end of the reproductive period, similar to the human, but unlike other strains of mice where cessation of ovulation appears to be determined mainly by aging of the hormonal axis[46,47]. The CBA strain is therefore marked by premature reproductive decline, maternal age-related fetal aneuploidy and high levels of pre- and postimplantation mortality[48,49].

The aim of a new cytogenetic study was to determine whether the number of univalents or bivalents with only one distal chiasma was different between age groups in oocytes of the CBA mouse, and whether there was any evidence for a precocious disjoining of homologs during the spontaneous resumption of maturation of oocytes, e.g. such involving bivalents with telomeric associations or very distal chiasmata. For this study, the chromosomal constitution of mouse oocytes was analyzed after defined times of maturation in culture, following their isolation from large antral follicles, to determine whether non-disjunction was based on the presence of increased numbers of true univalents in aged oocytes in accordance with the concept of a production line. Sequential analysis was performed *in vitro* at two time intervals (at 3 h and 6 h of maturation) to detect also precocious segregation of homologous chromosomes/univalents, due to an untimely resolution of chiasmata, prior to anaphase I, once chromosomes were under tension from spindle fibers. Oocytes of young and aged mice (3–4 months or ≥ 9 months) were spread shortly after germinal vesicle breakdown (GVBD) (designated the 3 h group) or after 6 h of maturation *in vitro*. In a third group, spreading and fixation were performed under identical conditions after 16 h of culture and maturation of the oocytes of both age groups, when the oocytes had progressed through first anaphase and had reached metaphase II.

Shortly after GVBD (3 h group), the oocytes were still in the circular bivalent stage, with numerous asters of microtubules in the vicinity of the chromosomes, but these oocytes had not established a bipolar spindle (Figure 2A and C). Under these conditions, homologs in bivalents should not be exposed to strong pulling or pushing forces into opposite directions, as evident from their highly contracted state and more or less random orientation. After spreading under these conditions, one would expect to be able to identify true univalents that failed to recombine during early prophase I in the fetal ovary. At 6 h of maturation *in vitro*, a bipolar spindle was assembled in most oocytes (Figure 2B and D). Oocytes were usually in an advanced prometaphase I stage by this time, and chromosomes were in the process of congression at the spindle equator. Centromeres of most homologs pointed to opposite spindle poles, and appeared stretched and bipolarly oriented at 6 h of culture. The arms of homologs between the centromeres and the first chiasma of bivalents were nearly all aligned parallel to the long axis of the spindle (Figure 2B′ and D′), suggesting that homologs were subjected to pushing and/or pulling forces on their kinetochores or on the chromatin in the chromosome arms at this time of maturation. Under these conditions, untimely segregation might become visible after spreading, when labile associations between homologs were lost and functional or true univalents had formed precociously prior to anaphase I.

Unexpectedly, chromosomal analysis of spread oocytes revealed that only one oocyte of a young mouse contained two chromosomes presenting possibly true univalents without any chiasma or physical attachment. In this single case, the two homologs were located away from each other after spreading over a distance exceeding the length of the whole chromosome, although they were still bipolarly aligned. Neither at 3 h of culture nor at 6 h were any other univalent chromosomes found in another oocyte.

In contrast, we frequently observed bivalents with only one distal chiasma in oocytes of young as well as aged mice (Figure 3A and B). In many of the oocytes, the Giemsa-stained telomeres of homologs visibly touched each other, indicative of the presence of a true chiasma in the very distal part of the homologous chromosomes attached to each other. However, an unstainted 'gap' of 0.8–2.5 μm was also frequently observed between the distal chromosome tips of homologs in bivalents. Telomeres of the homologs were still facing each other and chromosomes were oriented away from each other, similar to those bivalents with a distal chiasma. On morphological criteria, the bivalents with distal chiasmata and/or telomeric associations with or without a gap could clearly be distinguished from those possessing a subtelomeric chiasma. In the latter case, telomeres of homologs extended away from the distal chiasma and were located perpendicularly to the long axis of the arms of the homologous chromosomes in the bivalent (Figure 3A and B).

For quantitative analysis of the relative abundance of bivalents with one distal chiasma with or without a gap, only those oocytes were evaluated which had 20 well-spread and recognizable bivalents. Scoring the number of bivalents with distal chiasma (excluding the subtelomeric ones, but including those configurations with a gap) showed that the relative numbers and the percentage of such distally placed physical attachments of homologs were significantly different between the two age groups after 3 h of maturation (Figure 4). A larger percentage of bivalents of aged as compared to young oocytes possessed a distal chiasma or a telomeric association.

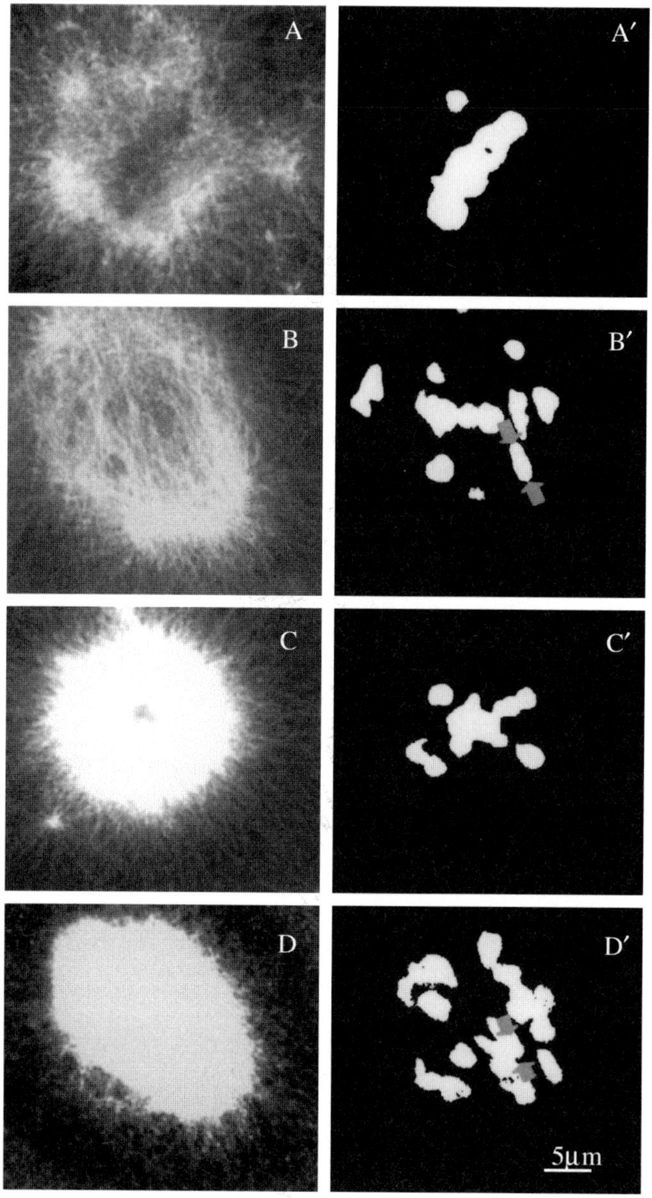

Figure 2 Spindles and chromosomes in oocytes of young (A, A′, B and B′) or aged (C, C′, D and D′) CBA mice, matured for 3 h *in vitro*, shortly after germinal vesicle breakdown (A, A′, C and C′), or cultured for 6 h (B, B′, D and D′), when a bipolar spindle has formed (B and D). Centromeres of homologs of some bipolarly oriented chromosomes in oocytes of young (B′) or aged (D′) mice matured for 6 h are marked by arrows. For further explanation see text. A, B, C, D: confocal images of spindles after antitubulin staining; A′, B′, C′, D′: Dapi-stained chromosomes in respective oocytes

There was no increase in the relative numbers or in the percentage of bivalents with one distal chiasma (including those with and those without a gap) when oocytes matured for 3 more hours during culture *in vitro* (6 h group). No univalents were found at the later prometaphase I stage (6 h of maturation), showing that there was no predivision at this time. The age-related significant difference in numbers of bivalents with distal chiasmata was retained and the relative frequency of such configurations was similarly higher in oocytes of the aged as compared to the young group, irrespective of culture time.

Counting only those bivalents with one distal chiasma visibly touching another, excluding those with a gap, showed that the percentage of such

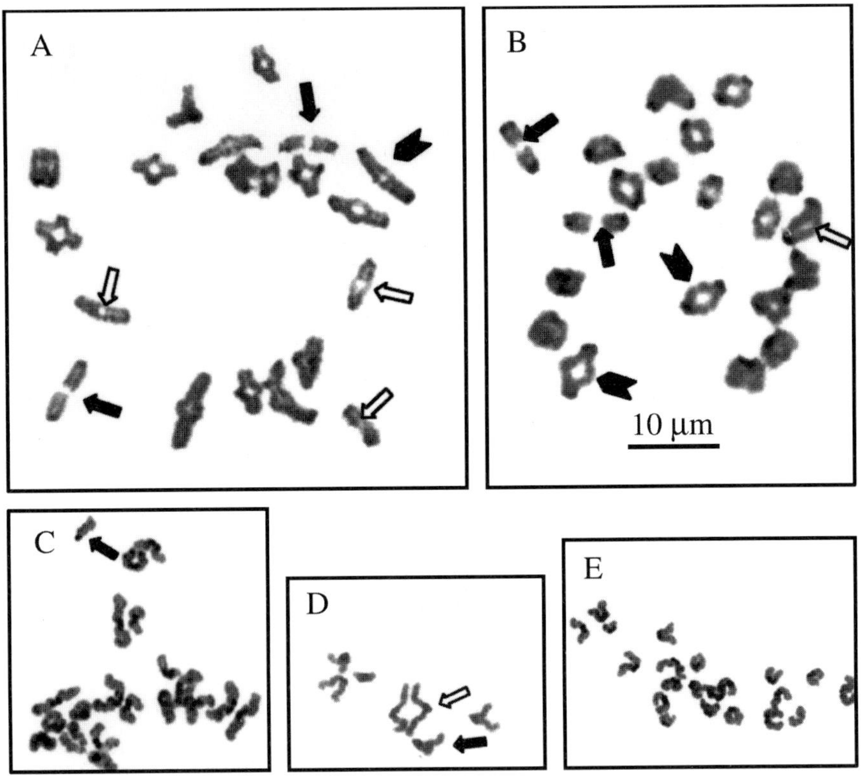

Figure 3 C-banded chromosomes of oocytes of young (A) or aged (B–E) mice matured for 3 h (A and B) or 16 h (C–E) *in vitro*. Oocytes of young (A) and aged (B) mice may possess bivalents with only one distal chiasma without a gap (open arrow) or with an unstained region between the telomeres of homologs (designated 'with gap') (solid arrows). Bivalents with a subterminal chiasma can clearly be identified (solid arrowheads in B). Metaphase-II oocytes of aged mice often contain single chromatids (predivision, solid arrow in C and D), seldom bivalent-like chromosomes (open arrow in D), and increased numbers are hyperploid with more than 20 metaphase-II chromosomes (E)

bivalents was not statistically different between age groups. Accordingly, the percentage of bivalents with chromosomes with telomeric associations with an unstained gap between 0.8 μm and 2.5 μm was much higher in aged oocytes[50] (Figure 4). Still, bivalents with distal associations were not restricted to aged oocytes. Such bivalents with homologs separated by an unstained gap were also commonly found in young oocytes.

Overall, 90% of all oocytes from the young, as well as the old, age group contained one or several bivalents with a distal chiasma with or without a gap. Comparable to the analysis of the total number of bivalents possessing a distal chiasma, when the numbers of oocytes possessing such bivalents with distal chiasmata without a gap were compared between age groups, there was no significant difference. Therefore, the average numbers of such configurations per oocyte appear similar in the young and aged groups. However, significantly more aged than young oocytes had at least one or several bivalents with a telomeric association and an unstained gap between homologous chromosomes (Figure 5). The relative number of oocytes with a gap remained more or less constant and was always higher in aged oocytes, irrespective of the period of culture/maturation and the time when spreading was performed (3 h or 6 h; Figure 5).

These observations support the notion that there seems to exist a production line with a cohort of oocytes from aged females possessing one or several bivalents with only one extremely distal chiasma or a mere telomeric

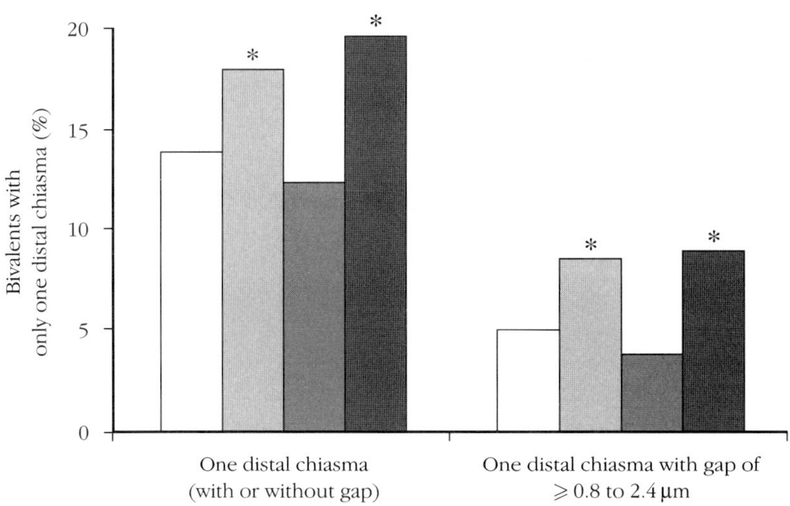

Figure 4 Percentage of bivalents from oocytes of young (y) or aged (a) mice, matured for 3 h or 6 h, with a single distal chiasma (total: with or without a gap) or with an unstained gap of more than 0.8 μm (⩾ 0.8–2.4 μm). For further explanation, see text. $^*p < 0.001$ (significantly different to young group. □ y, 3 h (n = 2680); ▨ a, 3 h (n = 1760); ▩ y, 6h (n = 2020); ■ a, 6 h (n = 2260)

association. The maximal number of bivalents with distal chiasmata was 11 in oocytes of both groups. Plotting the number of oocytes with one to 11 bivalents with one distal chiasma, including those with a gap and an unstained region between the homologs, revealed that the overall numbers of such configurations shifted to higher rates in aged oocytes as compared to young ones. There was no second peak in numbers of such bivalents per oocyte in the old age group. Therefore, the aged oocytes do not appear to consist of two cohorts, one with normal numbers of distal chiasmata/telomeric associations and one with an unusual increase in numbers of such configurations (Michels *et al.*, in preparation). Oocytes of young mice contained, on average, 3.4 bivalents with a telomeric association with a gap, while oocytes of aged mice had, on average, 4.2 such chromosomal configurations[50]. These data show that both young, as well as aged, oocytes possess bivalents in which homologs are connected physically at the very distal portion of the chromosome. Provided that these configurations are generally at high risk for errors in orientation at prometaphase I and segregation at first anaphase, one would expect to find aneuploidy in metaphase II in oocytes of both age groups.

However, the relative rate of both aneuploidy and predivision was low in the young age group when oocytes from hormonally unstimulated mice were spread after 16 h of *in vitro* maturation. Thus, the oocytes of the old age group had higher rates of hyperploidy and chromatids at metaphase II,

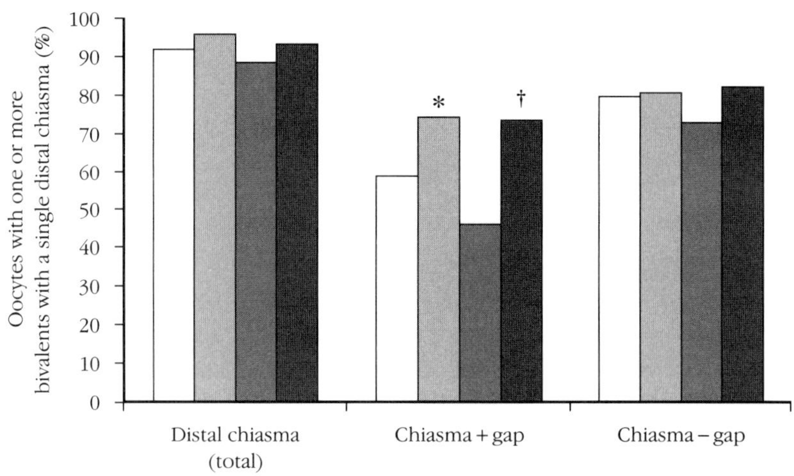

Figure 5 Percentage of oocytes of young (y) or aged (a) mice that contain one or several bivalents with a distal chiasma (total), those containing one or several bivalents with a chiasma with a gap (chiasma + gap) or those with bivalents with a single distal chiasma without a gap (chiasma – gap) after 3 h or 6 h of maturation *in vitro*. *$p < 0.05$; †$p < 0.001$ (significantly different to young group). ☐ y, 3 h ($n = 134$); ▨ a, 3 h ($n = 88$); ▨ y, 6 h ($n = 101$); ■ a, 6 h ($n = 113$)

and the overall rate of oocytes with numerical chromosomal aberrations and single or multiple chromatids was significantly higher in aged as compared to young mice (Figure 6).

Age-related differences in hyperploidy were retained, but did not reach any more statistically significant levels when oocytes were isolated from mice primed with pregnant mare serum (PMS) prior to oocyte retrieval (reference 5 and Michel *et al*., in preparation). The overall rate of hyperploidy was slightly increased in the stimulated as compared to the unstimulated cycles, suggesting that age and hormonal status may both contribute to a predisposition to non-disjunction. Since oocytes from follicles of young and aged mice from stimulated cycles matured under identical conditions *in vitro*, predisposition to non-disjunction appears to depend on the one hand on maternal age and follicular depletion of the ovaries, but on the other hand on those periods of oocyte development comprising folliculogenesis, oocyte growth and acquisition of meiotic competence prior to the resumption of maturation. The latter respond to hormonal status.

Significantly more oocytes of aged mice from hormonally unstimulated, PMS-primed cycles still had single or multiple chromatids (Figure 3C; Figure 6). Oocytes and their polar bodies could both be analyzed in some cases and each contained a single chromatid. Therefore, predivision of homologs, and precocious, equational separation of chromatids, must have occurred at anaphase I instead of at anaphase II in these oocytes and have given rise to the aneuploid constitution. Instead of the separation of the arms of chromatids, which is believed to induce chiasma resolution, the centromeres of sister chromatids also apparently separated during the progression to second metaphase.

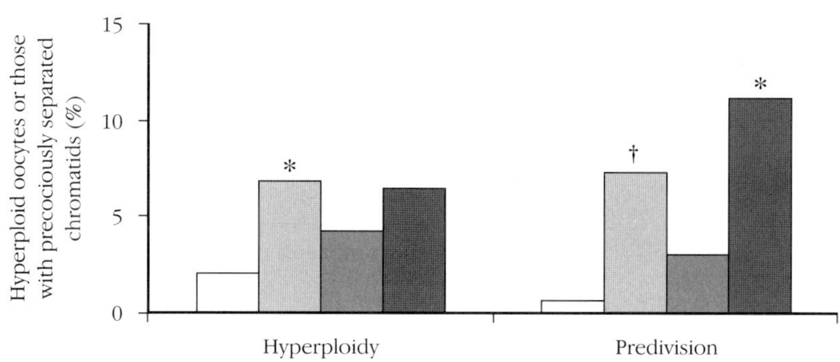

Figure 6 Aneuploidy in oocytes of young and aged mice, from unstimulated or pregnant mare serum-primed cycles, matured under identical conditions *in vitro* for 16 h. Hyperploidy is significantly different between age groups in oocytes from unstimulated cycles. Predivision (presence of single or multiple chromatids) is significantly elevated in aged oocytes from unstimulated as well as PMS-primed cycles. For further explanation, see text. *$p < 0.02$; †$p < 0.01$ (significantly different to young group). □ Unstimulated, young ($n = 162$); ▨ Unstimulated, aged ($n = 192$); ▨ PMS-primed, young ($n = 166$); ■ PMS-primed, aged ($n = 125$)

This suggests that the timing of chromosome segregation and the resolution of chiasmata or labile telomeric associations is perturbed in oocytes of aged females. The failures in cell cycle control are predetermined by oocyte age/depletion of the follicle pool and by the constitution of the oocytes prior to the resumption of maturation. Although hormonal status modifies and possibly increases the risk for untimely segregation, the perturbation in chromatid segregation appears to be primarily predetermined by the age of the female and less so by the hormonal status of the follicle prior to the resumption of maturation. Occasionally, true bivalents with unseparated chiasmata were also found in metaphase II oocytes (Figure 3D). However, their number was very small.

In conclusion, the observations on prometaphase I stages of mouse oocytes suggest that certain chromosomal constitutions, those comprising homologs with distal associations exhibiting an unstained gap after spreading, are enriched but not exclusively present in aged oocytes. There is no evidence that these physical connections are so unstable that presegregation occurs when a spindle is formed. Considering that failures in the recombination of homologs in mutant mice result in the presence of true univalents that behave independently and do not appear physically connected[44], we believe that the distal chiasma with a gap results from a recombination event in the prophase stage of meiosis and does not comprise merely a proteinaceous association between telomeres of homologs. However, chiasma formation at such distal sites may not necessarily be accompanied by a true genetic exchange when repetitive telomeric sequences are involved, as suggested by the observations of Imai and co-workers[51] in male meiosis. However, the frequent observation of chromatids in metaphase-II oocytes of aged mice suggests that the timing of segregation of chromatids, possibly related to the enrichment in bivalents with an extremely telomeric, distal chiasma, is disturbed frequently in aged oocytes. The loss of control of timing for homolog and chromatid separation relative to anaphase I progression appears to contribute to the age effect, and this appears to be related to, but possibly not exclusively caused by, an increased number of potentially susceptible chiasmate configurations.

IS THE PRESENCE OF A SUSCEPTIBLE CHIASMATE CONFIGURATION SUFFICIENT TO PREDISPOSE TO ANEUPLOIDY: EVIDENCE FOR A 'SECOND HIT' AND LOSS OF CONTROL OF CELL CYCLE-REGULATED EVENTS

The percentage of aged oocytes possessing one or more chromosomes with a gap and telomeric association was increased by about 15–25% in the old relative to the young age group. However, at least each second oocyte of the young group also had at least one bivalent with such a peculiar chromosomal configuration. Provided homologs of such bivaleonts are at high risk to undergo non-disjunction or presegregation, one would expect to find frequently numerical aberrations and chromatids in young as well as aged metaphase-II oocytes, but the relative rate of hyperploidy and predivision was low in the young age group. This suggests that oocytes are generally able to deal with a certain number of such critical chromosomal configurations, and only when there is a further, critical increase in their numbers, as found in aged oocytes, does faithful chromosome segregation become compromised. Likewise, critical chromosomal configurations may be rather safe in the cytoplasm and spindle of a young oocyte, while back-up controls and mechanisms controlling the orientation, congression and separation of homologs with only one distal chiasma or a telomeric association, including a gap, are predominantly compromised in the cytoplasm of an aged oocyte.

We have previously reported that the kinetics of cell cycle progression differ between oocytes from young and aged mice[5,45,52]. Previous studies had indicated that there are also differences in gene expression and in the status of post-translational modifications/phosphorylation of proteins between GV-stage oocytes of the two age groups, which might be responsible for the differences in meiotic progression[52]. To test for differential activity of major cell cycle-driving and cell cycle-controlling kinases in correlation with maternal age, we performed an *in vitro* assay to analyze the relative activities of maturation promoting factor (MPF) and mitogen-activated protein (MAP) kinases in the cytoplasm of oocytes. Under appropriate conditions, the phosphorylation of H1-histone, a substrate of MPF, provides a marker for MPF activity in assays with oocyte cell extracts[53,54]. The initial activation of MPF activity appears to be independent of *de novo* protein synthesis at the resumption of maturation in the mouse[55] (see also discussion below); MPF activity increases steeply around the time of GVBD in mouse oocytes[53–55]. Later, at prometaphase I and metaphase I, a plateau in activity is reached, which requires constant and new cyclin B synthesis. At anaphase I progression, MPF becomes inactivated in oocytes. At meiosis II, activity is again high and decreases after fertilization, when oocytes progress into anaphase II[53,54].

MAP kinases are components of the cytostatic factor. They become activated in a signalling cascade downstream from the activity of the c-mos kinase[56]. C-mos protein synthesis is highly regulated in oogenesis and is initiated only at the resumption of maturation (for review see reference 57). MAP kinases increase in their activity shortly after the activation of MPF in mammalian oocytes[54]. In contrast to MPF, MAP kinases do not become inactivated at first anaphase, but their activity is retained until some hours after fertilization[56]. Inactivation of MAP kinase is not triggered by degradation, but rather by dephosphorylation after the rapid inactivation of MPF at anaphase II. MAP kinase activity ceases upon the formation of the male and female pronucleus and the progression of eggs to first mitotic interphase, some hours after fertilization[56]. The activity of the MAP kinases can be monitored semi-quantitatively by analyzing the phosphorylation of one of their substrates, myelin basic protein (MBP), in assays involving oocyte cytoplasm[56].

We examined the relative activities of MPF and MAP kinases in cell extracts of oocytes from hormonally unstimulated young and aged mice after isolation from follicles (in the GV stage), and at 3 h and 6 h or at 16 h of maturation. Assays always involved individual samples of three oocytes each. To detect alterations in MPF activity at anaphase I, the first three oocytes of the young or aged group that had emitted a first polar body were isolated and used in the assay. For the GV stages and oocytes matured for 3 h or 6 h *in vitro*, the phosphorylation of substrate was determined in triplicate samples of three oocytes each, of young or aged mice. Phosphorylation of substrate (H1 histone or MBP) in assays with cell extracts of oocytes matured for 3 h (t3) was designated as 100 arbitrary units and compared to that at the GV stage (time zero, t0) and that at 6 h (t6) of maturation in each age group (each with triplicate samples).

Consistently, there was little MPF or MAP kinase activity in cell extracts of oocytes from both groups immediately after isolation (Figure 7). There was no significant difference between the age groups at this time. However, reproducibly, there was a significant difference in the kinase activities of cell extracts between oocytes obtained from young and aged mice that were matured for 3 h *in vitro*. Later, at 6 h of maturation, the relative activity of both kinases was slightly, but not significantly, different between the age groups (Figure 7). This indicates that the activation profiles of the two cell cycle-driving kinases differ between oocytes of young and aged mice, and the relative increase in activity of both kinases is slower in aged as compared to young oocytes at the resumption of maturation.

In previous studies, we found that oocytes of aged mice progress more synchronously and earlier into anaphase I than young oocytes[45,58]. Accordingly, MPF activity also decreased dramatically and early in oocytes of aged mice when they progressed to anaphase I (Michel *et al.*, in preparation). Usually, the first oocytes from the young group emitted a first polar body slightly later than those from the aged group. Progression into anaphase I was always accompanied by a characteristic drop in H1-histone kinase (MPF) activity in the young as well as the aged oocytes. In spite of the relative asynchrony in anaphase I progression in both oocyte populations from hormonally unstimulated cycles, the decrease in MPF activity was usually first seen in samples from the old-age group. At 16 h of maturation, when the oocytes of both groups had reached metaphase II, there was no consistent difference between kinase activities in the two age groups (data not shown).

In summary, the observations suggest that the kinetics of cell cycle progression differ in the oocytes of young and aged mice. The pattern of increases in kinase activities at 3 h of maturation implies that cytoplasmic maturation is delayed in aged as compared to young oocytes at the early

(a)

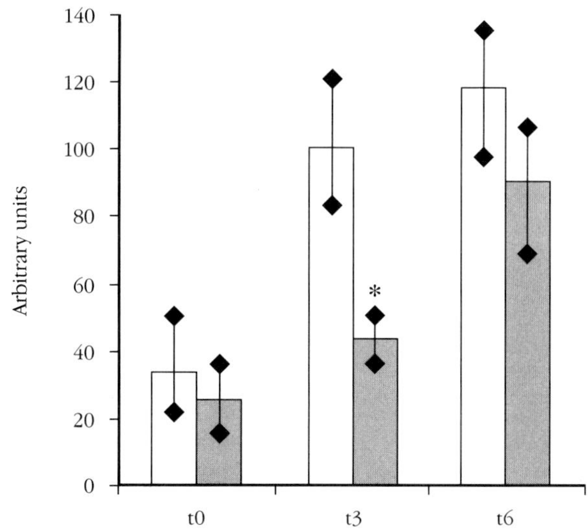

(b)

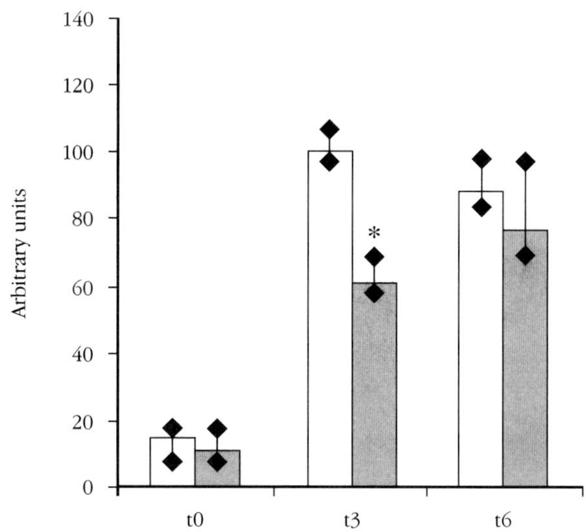

Figure 7 Activity of maturation promoting factor (MPF) measured as relative phosphorylation of H1-histone in (a) that of mitogen-activated protein (MAP) kinases as phosphorylation of myelin basic protein (MBP) in (b) in cell extracts of oocytes of young or aged mice after isolation from follicles at the GV stage (t0), or after 3 h (t3) or 6 h (t6) of maturation *in vitro*. $^{*}p < 0.001$ (significantly different to young group). □, young; ■, aged

meiotic phases. In spite of this, there is a tendency to trigger anaphase I earlier in the oocytes of aged mice as compared to those from young mice. Concomitantly, the relative duration of prometaphase I and metaphase I is shortened in aged oocytes. Precocious anaphase I progression may relate to the presence and presegregation of homologs in bivalents with an extremely distal chiasma (characterized in the spreads by an unstained gap). It might also present a risk for bivalents with proximal and more than one chiasma to fail to segregate in time and therefore undergo non-disjunction[5].

One can speculate that the slow increase in MPF and MAP kinase activities affects the synchrony between chromatin condensation and spindle formation and all the events associated with the phosphorylation of substrates of the kinases that are necessary for timed expression of meiotic genes[59,60] and for proper congression, alignment and separation of homologous chromosomes. In concert with an early progression into anaphase I, the relative shortening of the period between GVBD and anaphase I might therefore predispose chromosomes to errors in distribution. Provided that chromosomes with distal chiasmata or achiasmatic chromosomes with telomeric associations are always especially susceptible to misalignment or presegregation, both the positioning and relative abundance of chiasmata, as well as an altered cell cycle, may synergistically lead to the high risk for errors in segregation. The observations therefore support the 'two-hit' hypothesis, suggesting that susceptible chiasmate configurations, as well as characteristic disturbances in cytoplasmic maturation due to damage or immaturity of aged oocytes, which affect the timing of homolog or chromatid separation, critically contribute to aneuploidy and predispose to trisomy after fertilization.

CYTOPLASMIC QUALITY, RECOMBINATION AND CELL CYCLE REGULATION, AND PECULIARITIES OF SPINDLE FORMATION IN MAMMALIAN OOCYTES: TARGETS FOR THE FIRST AND THE SECOND HIT

It is not known which intrinsic factors or signalling pathways are responsible for the preprogrammed cell cycle block during the long period of meiotic quiescence until the growth phase of the follicle and oocyte has been completed and the oocyte has stockpiled all those molecules necessary to support early embryogenesis. It appears that control over arrest in the G2 phase is mainly dependent on hormonal homeostasis, growth factors and inhibitory activities in the follicular fluid (for recent review see reference 61). Oocytes that have not reached full meiotic competence can thus spontaneously develop to metaphase I and only arrest there when isolated from larger, but still immature, follicles[62]. Since metaphase-I blocked immature oocytes can be triggered to go into anaphase I and to emit a polar body by exposure to calcium ionophores[62], maturation of the processes governing calcium homeostasis appears to be a prerequisite for the successful resumption of oogenesis. Oocytes themselves play a major role in promoting dynamic changes in gene expression by granulosa cells that are appropriate to the stage of follicular development prior to meiotic resumption[63,64]. For instance, the synthesis of meiosis activating sterol (MAS) in follicle cells, which contributes to the resumption of maturation in oocytes in the presence of inhibitory molecules in follicular fluid, appears to be initiated by signalling between the oocyte and the follicle cells[65]. We recently obtained evidence that MAS may also have a function in modulating cell cycle progression in oocytes[66]. Compromized folliculogenesis in depleted ovaries of aged females[67], in concert with altered hormonal feedback, oxidative damage, impaired mitochondrial function and other disturbances in the aged oocyte, may therefore influence the quality of the oocyte prior to the resumption of maturation and thereby reduce its capacity to separate chromosomes faithfully, to mature to metaphase II and to support early embryogenesis. We have previously argued that an oocyte 'remembers' its past. Disturbances in follicles and oocytes by follicle depletion, altered hormonal homeostasis and a number of noxae may thereby affect the quality of the oocyte during meiotic dormancy and the growth phase, especially in the human, where oocytes rest for decades before resuming maturation[4,5]. In support of this, there now exists evidence that trisomy formation may be related to elevated follicle stimulating hormone (see other chapters). Reduced oxygen supply and mitochondrial dysfunction are other parameters that may critically influence the quality of 'aged' oocytes prior to or during maturation (for discussion see references 68–70), contributing to the second hit. Delayed activation of major cell cycle-driving kinases, as observed in our mouse model, can serve as an indicator that the quality of aged oocytes is, in fact, reduced and that this has consequences for the fidelity of chromosome segregation. The relative significance of the reduced cytoplasmic quality of the oocyte versus its genetic constitution, as predetermined by processes including recombination at prophase I in embryogenesis and DNA damage during meiotic arrest, can hopefully be elucidated by studies in which nuclei of aged oocytes are transferred to the cytoplasm of enucleated young oocytes, or cytoplasm is injected into recipient oocytes, to evaluate meiotic competence and the fidelity of chromosome segregation under these conditions[71].

To understand the implications of altered activities of cell cycle-regulating kinases in oocytes, it is important to understand the processes involved in the resumption of maturation and cell cycle control during oogenesis, since they may reveal why oocytes are so much more susceptible to non-disjunction and aneuploidy compared to somatic or male meiotic cells. The cell cycle in mitotic, as well as all meiotic, cells is driven by the activity of MPF (maturation promoting factor or cyclin-dependent kinases, Cdk2). In fact, the regulatory subunit of MPF, cyclin B, as well as its catalytic subunit, $p34^{cdc2}$ (cdc2), are already synthesized during the growth phase of oogenesis, prior to the acquisition of meiotic competence[55,72]. In the meiotically competent oocyte, the inactive complex, pre-MPF, is present, in which cdc2 is already associated with cyclin B, but still phosphorylated at inhibitory threonine

14 and tyrosine 15 residues. The resumption of maturation and the activation of the pre-MPF to active MPF is regulated by the relative activity of the Wee1/Mik1 kinases, which maintain the inhibitory tyrosine and threonine phosphorylation on cdc2 and the distribution and activity of the Cdc25 phosphatase, which removes the critical tyrosine and threonine phosphorylation and, in this way, activates pre-MFP (Figure 8).

The relative activities of Mik1 and Cdc25 are themselves dependent on post-translational modifications by the phosphorylation of specific residues. Phosphatases of the PP2A family can positively and negatively influence the activity of Wee1 kinases and Cdc25 phosphatase, respectively[73]; they are also involved in anaphase progression[74], and PP2A phosphatase activity is tightly regulated in mammalian oogenesis[75]. Cdc25 appears to be sequestered in a complex with 14-3-3 protein in meiotically competent oocytes when phosphorylated by the Chk1 kinase in the vertebrate's ooplasm[76–78]. The sequestration may remove free Cdc25 from the pool and in this way prevent Cdc25 from interacting with and activating pre-MPF. Therefore, oocytes remain in the GV stage. It is unknown in which way the luteinizing hormone surge ultimately causes the resumption of maturation in meiotically competent, mature oocytes and induces the activation of pre-MPF downstream. In *Xenopus*, new proteins were identified that induce meiotic progression[79,80]. It is debated whether MAS has a similar role in mammalian oocytes[65]. The reduction in cyclic adenosine monophosphate (cAMP) and the transient inactivation of cAMP-dependent protein kinase are intimately involved in meiotic progression. Other signalling events involved in the early steps of the commitment to the resumption of maturation that interact with cell cycle-regulating kinases and phosphatase activities still have to be identified. However, it is noteworthy to mention that the Chk1 kinase is a highly conserved kinase involved in checkpoint control at the G2-phase to M-phase transition of mitotic cells[77]. It is involved in a pathway that induces arrest at the G2 phase in the presence of damaged or unreplicated DNA (Figure 8). Oocytes do not appear to possess a sensor for unreplicated or damaged DNA. When unreplicated DNA is transferred to the cytoplasm of an oocyte, cell cycle progression is not inhibited[81], and when oocytes are exposed to ultraviolet radiation, they still resume maturation[82]. As pointed out by several recent studies, there is evidence that the regulation of mitotic and meiotic division differs in important aspects. Oocytes have a unique pre-programmed meiotic arrest at the dictyate stage (see Figure 1), which is essential for growth and the acquisition of meiotic competence. Therefore, oogenesis may miss certain checkpoints, or the role of conserved components in cell cycle control, such as Chk1, may be different in oogenesis as compared to male meiosis and mitosis. So far, the role and importance of Chk1 in mammalian oogenesis remains an enigma.

Once the levels and activity of Cdc25 reach a critical threshold upon the resumption of maturation in meiotically competent oocytes, MPF becomes activated by the dephosphorylation of the inhibitory tyrosine and threonine residues (Figure 8). The phosphorylation of Cdc25 by MPF triggers a further rapid increase in kinase activity, and MPF activity rises steeply at around the time of GVBD and in the first hours thereafter. Polo-like kinases (Plx1 kinase, Figure 8) represent further regulatory molecules present in mammalian oocytes that are associated with the spindle and support the activity of Cdc25 and thereby that of MPF[83–85].

While the initial rise in MPF activity is independent of *de novo* protein synthesis, synthesis of cyclin B is required for the following prometaphase I and metaphase I stages. There is evidence from the mouse suggesting that the relative length of the cell cycle and the period between GVBD and anaphase

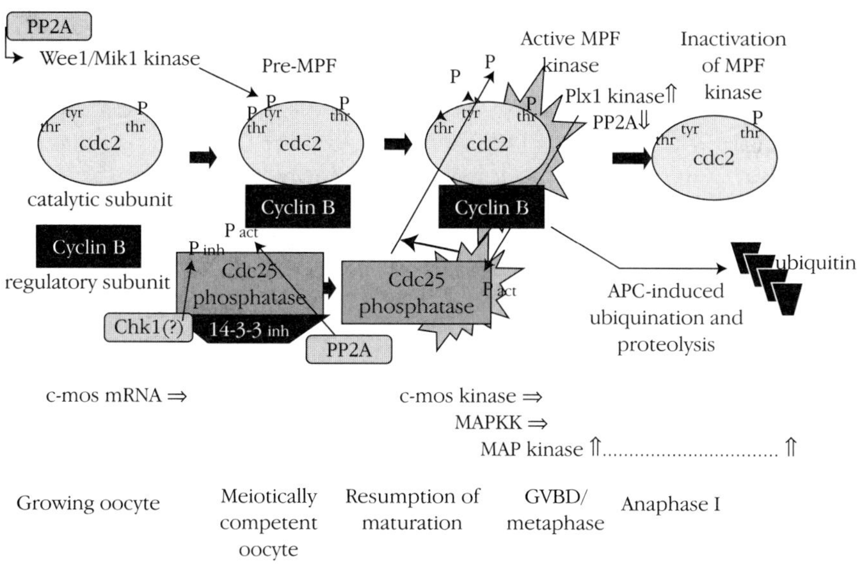

Figure 8 Activation and inactivation of maturation promoting factor (MPF) in oocytes. Catalytic (p34 cdc2) and regulatory (cyclin B) subunits of MPF are present in a complex of inactive pre-MPF in fully grown oocytes with phosphorylated threonine 14, tyrosine 15 and threonine 161 residues. Phosphorylation is mediated by Wee1/Mik1 kinases and influenced by phosphatase PP2A. Upon the resumption of maturation, Chk1 kinase appears to cease to phosphorylate Cdc25 phosphatase, thus releasing it from 14-3-3 protein[134]. Cdc25 phosphatase induces initial tyrosine/threonine dephosphorylation, thus activating MPF. In an autophosphorylation loop, further phosphorylation by MPF and increased activity of Plx kinase[85,135] and reduced activity of PP2A phosphatase then support further phosphorylation and activation of Cdc25 phosphatase, thus boosting MPF activity[83]. The anaphase I transition is triggered by anaphase-promoting complex (APC); a ubiquitin ligase which induces proteolysis of cyclin B and other proteins, thus inactivating MPF[109]. C-mos RNA is accumulated in the growing oocyte and, after translation at the resumption of maturation, c-mos kinase induces mitogen-activated protein kinase kinase (MAPKK or MEK), which in turn phosphorylates and activates MAP kinases. For further explanation and references, see text

I transition appears to depend mainly on the rate of synthesis of cyclin B[54,86]. Judging from the fast progression of oocytes of aged mice into anaphase I, it can be speculated that protein synthesis is less efficient in aged as compared to young oocytes, once the aged oocytes have undergone GVBD, such that the length of prometaphase I in the aged CBA mouse oocyte may become shortened in the presence of reduced levels of cyclin B. Human oocytes are actively synthesizing proteins throughout maturation, and hence reduced efficiency of synthesis may cause a delay in meiotic progression during this stage, as previously reported[67].

The progression into anaphase in mitosis and meiosis is triggered by the ubiquination of cyclin B through the anaphase-promoting complex (APC), an ubiquitin ligase that triggers ubiquitin-dependent proteolysis of cyclin B, the regulatory subunit of MPF, and thereby causes the inactivation of MPF (for recent reviews see references 87–89). Molecular dissection of anaphase progression and cell biological studies have shown that, besides cyclin B, other molecules that are involved in sister chromatid cohesion at centromeres, microtubule motor molecules and other proteins become degraded via the ubiquitin pathway at the beginning of anaphase[90] (Figure 8). For instance, in yeast, chromatid separation is initiated by APC-mediated proteolysis of the Pds1 protein (its mutation causes **p**remature **d**issociation of **s**ister chromatids[91]). The latter exists in a complex with another separating protein, Esp1 (a separin), which, when liberated from the complex, induces the dissociation of a cohesion protein, Scc1[91,92]. Scc1 itself becomes cleaved by proteolysis, and this is believed to induce the separation of sister chromatids, a prerequisite for chromosome segregation[92,93]. The Scc1 cleavage site is conserved in Scc1-like proteins, required also for meiotic chromosome segregation in yeasts[93]. One of these Scc1-like proteins, Rec8, is a cohesin protein that persists throughout meiosis I and disappears only from the centromeres of chromosomes at meiosis II[94,95]. Deletion of Rec8 causes equational, instead of reductional, separation of chromosomes at meiosis I in yeast[94], reminiscent of what we find for meiotic chromosomes in the oocytes of aged females. Krawchuk and colleagues[96,97] reported recently that mutations in *rec8*, *rec10* and *rec11* in fission yeast also compromised recombination, but only in the central regions of chromosomes, while recombination near telomeres was almost normal. These observations demonstrate that there is a link between recombination and the positioning of chiasmata and molecules involved in chromatid cohesion at anaphase I and II. In contrast to *rec8*, mutations in the *rec10* and *rec11* genes affected mainly the fidelity of chromosome segregation at meiosis II. Similarly, judging from our findings in mouse oocytes, there may be correlations between the relative decrease in bivalents with interstitial chiasmata and the increase in those with one extremely distal chiasma in aged oocytes, and the relative risk for premature segregation and errors in chromosome distribution at meiosis I. Genes and proteins with functions like *rec8* are therefore possible targets of age-related

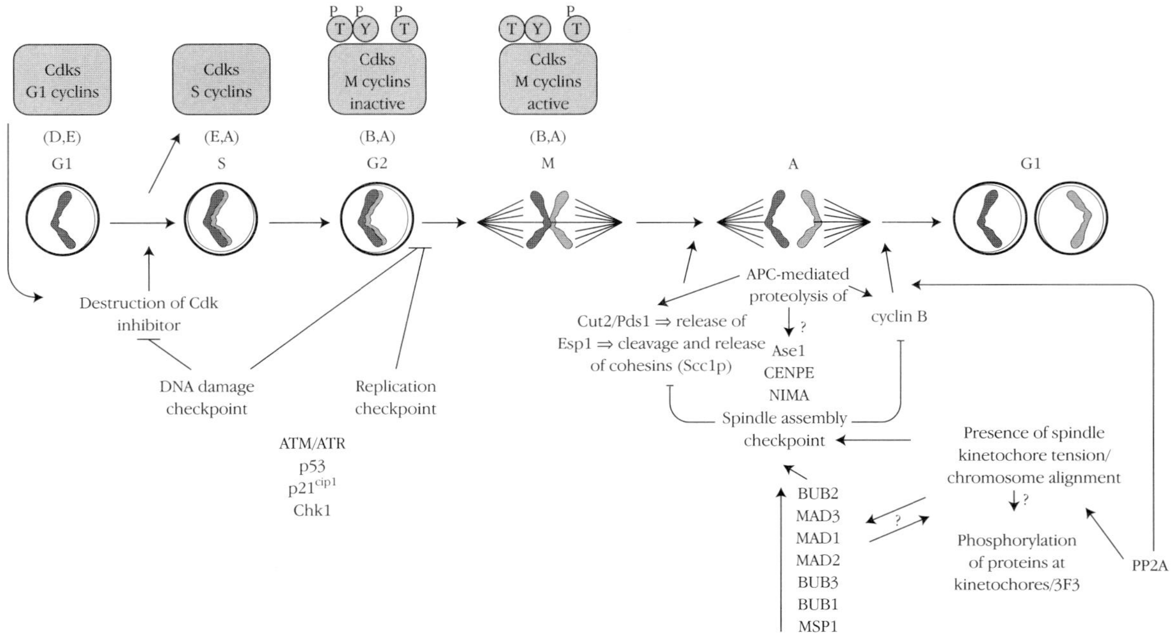

Figure 9 Overview of the checkpoints in cell cycle control. The cell cycle is driven by the activity of specific Cdk–cyclin complexes (as schematically depicted in the upper part of Figure 9; cyclins involved in the individual complexes are indicated underneath: cyclin D, cyclin E, etc.). G2-phase to M-phase progression involves the dephosphorylation of tyrosine and threonine residues. G1-phase to S-phase transition involves the destruction of Cdk inhibitor. Checkpoints in response to DNA damage and unreplicated DNA are indicated and involve genes/proteins ATM/ATR, p53, p21^{cip1} and Chk1. Transition from the M phase (M) to anaphase (A) involves anaphase-promoting complex (APC)-mediated proteolysis of Cut2/Pds1, cyclin B and other proteins. The spindle assembly checkpoint arrests cells in the M phase and prevents APC-mediated proteolysis when spindle integrity, kinetochore attachment/tension and/or chromosome alignment are compromised. A number of proteins (MSP1 to BUB2)[136] and the reversible phosphorylation of proteins at kinetochores and those recognized by an antibody against phosphorylated epitopes (3F3) are involved in checkpoint control. For references and further explanation, see text

disturbances, in the context of a production line, which may be responsible for maternal age-related aneuploidy, linking early meiotic events (recombination) with cell cycle disturbances at the resumption of maturation. A Rec8p homolog was recently discovered in human germ cells[98]. Still, it is too early for any direct comparisons between species, since there are distinct differences in the components and mechanisms mediating chromosome cohesion and anaphase progression between unicellular and multicellular organisms, and between mitosis and meiosis (for discussion see reference 99); for example, the cleavage site of yeast Scc1 protein is not conserved in vertebrate cells[93]. The products of the *mei-s332* and *ord* genes have been implicated in centromere cohesion in *Drosophila*. The Mei-s332 protein remains located at the centromeres of meiotic chromosomes until anaphase II[100] and *ord* mutants prematurely separate chromosomes after anaphase I and prior to meiosis II[101].

Other targets for APC-mediated proteolysis include the Ase1 protein[102], the centromere protein E (CENPE), which belongs to the family of the kinesis-like microtubule motor proteins, and the products of the *PIMPLES* and *NIMA* genes[88].

Many studies on cell cycle progression in mitotic cells have revealed that there are several checkpoints and back-up mechanisms that may arrest mitotic progression until lesions are repaired and a normal constitution has been achieved in a proliferating cell[103] (Figure 9). Studies on anaphase progression in unicellular organisms such as yeast, as well as in mitotic and meiotic cells of multicellular organisms, have shown that targeting of substrates and the activity of APC are tightly regulated[87,88]. Checkpoints exist to ensure that ubiquination of cyclin B and other molecules is only initiated when a spindle is present, kinetochores of all chromosomes are saturated with microtubules and are under tension, and chromosomes are properly aligned at the spindle equator (for recent discussion and references see references 104–106). Cascades of phosphorylation events and differential interactions between proteins (MSP1, BUB1, BUB3, MAD2, MAD1, MAD3, BUB2) may cause association with or dissociation of proteins from kinetochores of individual chromosomes, depending on the state of microtubule attachment and tension, and phosphorylation of proteins at the kinetochores[104–110]. The cell cycle usually becomes arrested when chromosomes are not attached and aligned or a spindle is missing. We and others showed that mammalian oocytes possess a spindle checkpoint and that homologs do not disjoin in oocytes in which the spindle was depolymerized by an antimicrotubular agent[45,111–113]. However, a recent study by Brunet and co-workers[114] revealed that a delay in anaphase-I progression is predominantly caused by a disturbance in spindle integrity in the final hours prior to anaphase-I progression and not at the earlier prometaphase-I stage. Exposure of oocytes to nocodazole during the period from GVBD to late prometaphase I hardly affected the time when oocytes triggered anaphase I; only the transient depolymerization of the spindle close to anaphase I significantly affected the progression into second meiosis after the removal of the drugs[114]. Therefore, any disturbance in chromosome congression during the initial stages of prometaphase I, as was noticed in aged oocytes of the mouse, has the potential to cause errors in chromosome segregation, since there is no additional time provided to correct for misalignment or other deficiencies.

We recently showed that oocytes exposed to the pesticide trichlorfon may progress into anaphase I in spite of the presence of unaligned chromosomes[115]. From the observation of chromosomes in trichlorfon-exposed oocytes, it appeared that each bivalent segregated its homologs on its own spindle fibers. Mice that do not possess the functional DNA mismatch repair gene *Mlh1* are sterile. Females do still possess oocytes, but meiotic recombination is dramatically reduced and most chromosomes in oocytes are thus univalents without physical attachment to their homolog. Spindle formation is aberrant and chromosomes do not align in these oocytes, but some oocytes are still able to progress into anaphase and emit a polar body, provided they can establish a bipolar spindle[44]. This indicates that checkpoint controls sensing chromosome displacement may be rather permissive in mammalian oocytes and this may present a sex-specific risk factor for aneuploidy in oogenesis. In spite of the ability of mammalian oocytes to form bipolar spindles in the absence of chromosomes or chromatin[116], the observations of Woods and associates in the *Mlh1* knockout mouse suggest that, in the presence of chromosomes, bivalent configurations are indispensible for bipolar spindle formation[44]. This implies that the chromosomal constitution of the oocyte is of importance and is one factor that determines the risk for spindle aberrations and aneuploidy. Fusion experiments with insect spermatocytes imply that the chromosomes themselves, and not the cytoplasm, direct chiasma resolution and the loss of cohesion between sister chromatid arms, as in reductional meiosis I, or, instead, cause the loss of cohesion at centromeres of sister chromatids, as is characteristic of second meiosis and mitosis[117]. In accordance with this, spermatocyte chromosomes can segregate reductionally when introduced into metaphase-II oocytes that are activated, while oocytes segregate their chromatids at anaphase II[118]. The constraints to the loss of cohesion of sister chromatids, especially in the presence of a single extremely distal physical attachment, appear to be reduced at anaphase I in aged oocytes. It will be of major importance to determine whether this untimely segregation is due to a decay of cohesion proteins, alterations in chromosome condensation and structure at kinetochores, spindle disturbances or global asynchrony in cellular signalling and cell cycle events. At the same time, the sensing of misplaced bivalents appears to be relaxed in mammalian oocytes. Under normal conditions, a healthy oocyte may not be at high risk to trigger anaphase I with unaligned chromosomes, since prometaphase I is a comparatively long period in mammalian oogenesis, providing time for kinetochore maturation and the formation of a stable bipolar attachment of chromosomes to spindle fibers. Only when cytoplasmic maturation is significantly affected and oocyte quality reduced, as may be the case in aged oocytes, or when chromosome alignment is delayed while the spindle checkpoint sensing spindle aberrations is compromised, e.g. due to exposures to chemicals in the environment[115], may oocytes have a high risk of going into anaphase I and failing to segregate homologs in time. Observations in somatic cells have shown that the signal to progress into anaphase once chromosomes start to segregate can spread from one spindle to another in a common cytoplasm[119] and that chromosome segregation is usually instantaneous and synchronous at anaphase progression. We previously found evidence that the separation of homologs may be rather more gradual in mammalian oocytes[45]. The targeting of APC and proteolytic processes, as well as the post-translational modification of proteins involved in cell cycle control may be frequently compromised, e.g. due to reduced oxygen supply[68,69,120,121], to mitochondrial dysfunction[70] and to reduced availability of high-energy substrates[122]. As a consequence this can lead to a situation where cell cycle progression is altered and once oocytes initiate anaphase I the segregation of homologs is delayed and asynchronous, in this way predisposing to non-disjunction and errors in chromosome distribution.

SUMMARY AND PERSPECTIVES

In conclusion, our observations in the mouse and those of retrospective studies on the origin of extra chromosomes in trisomies in the human all support the concept that the chromosomal constitution of any individual chromosome and the distribution and efficiency of recombination differentially predispose to aneuploidy in a specific, age-dependent fashion. Follicle pool size and the history of each oocyte and its follicle ultimately determine oocyte quality and the risk for errors in chromosome segregation. While it is not possible to influence the chromosomal constitution of an oocyte once it has developed past prophase I in the embryonal ovary and has accumulated critical chiasmate configurations, it is of greatest importance to identify parameters predicting oocyte quality and to perform further studies to elucidate parameters that are unique to oocyte maturation and are additionally affected by age, according to the concept of a second predisposing lesion, leading to aneuploidy and trisomy. In continuation of the research on human reproductive health that has been undertaken by one of the most prominent and innovative scientists in reproductive medicine, Reinier de Graaf, it is imperative to pursue his work on the regulation of oogenesis in mammals in order to identify and reduce the risks of environmental exposures and of behavioral patterns that cause depletion of the follicle pool or adversely affect follicular and hormonal status and the integrity of oocytes. Future research should be aimed at developing methods that improve the capacity of aged oocytes to mature normally and to support the development of a genetically normal embryo and a healthy child. It has never been more obvious that this research requires interdisciplinary and combined clinical, medical, cell and developmental biological, molecular and genetic approaches.

REFERENCES

1. Bond DJ, Chandley AC. *Aneuploidy*. Oxford Monographs on Medical Genetics No. 11. Oxford: Oxford University Press, 1983
2. Abruzzo MA, Hassold TJ. Etiology of non-disjunction in humans. *Environ Mol Mutagen* 1995;26:38–47
3. Eichenlaub-Ritter U. Mechanisms of non-disjunction in mammalian meiosis. In Pederson RA, ed. *Current Topics in Developmental Biology*, vol 29. New York: Academic Press, 1994:281–324
4. Eichenlaub-Ritter U. Parental age-related aneuploidy in human germ cells and offspring: a story of past and present. *Environ Mol Mutagen* 1996;28:211–36
5. Eichenlaub-Ritter U. Genetics of oocyte ageing. *Maturitas* 1998;30:143–69
6. Wyrobek AJ, Aardema M, Eichenlaub-Ritter U, *et al*. Mechanisms and targets involved in maternal and paternal age effects on numerical aneuploidy. *Environ Mol Mutagen* 1996;28:254–64
7. Hirshfield AN. Heterogeneity of cell populations that contribute to the formation of primordial follicles in rats. *Biol Reprod* 1992;47:466–72
8. Hassold TJ, Abruzzo M, Adkins K, *et al*. Human aneuploidy: incidence, origin, and etiology. *Environ Mol Mutagen* 1996;28:167–75
9. Jamieson ME, Coutts JRT, Connor JM. The chromosome constitution of human preimplantation embryos fertilized *in vitro*. *Hum Reprod* 1994;9:709–15
10. Warburton D, Kinney A. Chromosomal differences in suceptibility to meiotic aneuploidy. *Environ Mol Mutagen* 1996;28:237–47
11. Bahce M, Cohen J, Munne S. Preimplantation genetic diagnosis of aneuploidy: were we looking at the wrong chromosomes? *Assist Reprod Genet* 1999;16:176–81
12. Hassold TJ, Chiu D. Maternal age-specific rates of numerical chromosome abnormalities with special reference to trisomy. *Hum Genet* 1985;70:11–17
13. Griffin DK. The incidence, origin, and etiology of aneuploidy. *Int Rev Cytol* 1996;167:263–96
14. Dailey T, Dale B, Cohen J, Munné S. Association between non-disjunction and maternal age in meiosis II human oocytes. *Am J Hum Genet* 1996;59:176–84
15. Benadiva C, Kligman I, Munné S. Aneuploidy 16 in human embryo increases significantly with maternal age. *Fertil Steril* 1996;66:248–55
16. Kuo HC, Ogilvie CM, Handyside AH. Chromosomal mosaicism in cleavage-stage human embryos and the accuracy of single-cell genetic analysis. *J Assist Reprod Genet* 1998;15:276–80
17. Verlinsky Y, Cieslak J, Ivakhnenko V, *et al*. Prevention of age-related aneuploidies by polar body testing of oocytes. *Assist Reprod Genet* 1999;16:165–9
18. Handyside AH, Ogilvie CM. Screening oocytes and preimplantation embryos for aneuploidy. *Curr Opin Obstet Gynecol* 1999;11:301–5
19. Lamb NE, Freeman SB, Savage-Austin A, *et al*. Suceptible chiasmate configurations of chromosome 21 predispose to non-disjunction in both maternal meiosis I and meiosis II. *Nature Genet* 1996;14:400–5

20. Koehler KE, Hawley RS, Sherman S, *et al.* Recombination and non-disjunction in humans and flies. *Hum Mol Genet* 1996;5:1495–504
21. Henderson SA, Edwards RG. Chiasma frequency and maternal age in mammals. *Nature (London)* 1968;217:22–8
22. Luthardt FW, Palmer CG, Yu BL. Chiasma and univalent frequencies in ageing female mice. *Cytogenet Cell Genet* 1973;12:68–79
23. Polani PE, Jagiello G. Chiasmata, meiotic univalents, and age in relation to aneuploid imbalance in mice. *Cytogenet Cell Genet* 1976;16:505–29
24. Speed RM. The effects of ageing on the meiotic chromosomes of male and female mice. *Chromosoma* 1977;64:241–54
25. Sugawara S, Mikamo K. Absence of correlation between univalent formation and meiotic non-disjunction in aged female Chinese hamster. *Cytogenet Cell Genet* 1983;35:34–40
26. Polani PE, Crolla JA. A test of the production line hypothesis of mammalian oogenesis. *Hum Genet* 1991;88:64–70
27. Jacobs PA. The chromosome complement of human gametes. In Milligan SR, ed. *Oxford Reviews of Reproductive Biology*, vol 14. Oxford: Oxford University Press, 1992:47–72
28. Martin RH, Ko E, Rademaker A. Distribution of aneuploidy in human gametes: comparison between human sperm and oocytes. *Am J Med Genet* 1991;39:321–31
29. Hassold TJ. Non-disjunction in the human male. *Curr Top Dev Biol* 1998;37:383–406
30. MacDonald M, Hassold TJ, Harvey J, *et al.* The origin of 47,XXY and 47,XXX aneuploidy: heterogeneous mechanisms and role of aberrant recombination. *Hum Mol Genet* 1994;3:1365–71
31. Hassold TJ, Sherman SL, Pettay D, *et al.* XY chromosome non-disjunction in man is associated with diminished recombination in the pseudoautosomal region. *Am J Hum Genet* 1991;49:253–60
32. Lorda-Sanchez I, Binkert F, Maechler M, *et al.* Reduced recombination and paternal age effect in Klinefelter syndrome. *Hum Genet* 1992;89:524–30
33. Nicolaidis P, Petersen MB. Origin and mechanisms of non-disjunction in human autosomal trisomies. *Hum Reprod* 1998;13:313–19
34. Hassold TJ, Merrill M, Adkins K, *et al.* Recombination and maternal age-related non-disjunction: molecular studies of trisomy 16. *Am J Hum Genet* 1995;57:867–74
35. Shen JJ, Sherman SL, Hassold TJ. Centromeric genotyping and direct analysis of non-disjunction in humans: Down syndrome. *Chromosoma* 1998;107:166–72
36. Robinson WP, Kuchinka B, Bernasconi F, *et al.* Maternal meiosis I non-disjunction of chromosome 15: dependence of the maternal age effect on level of recombination. *Hum Mol Genet* 1998;7:1011–19
37. Ross L, Maxfield R, Dawson D. Exchanges are not able to enhance meiotic chromosome segregation in yeast. *Proc Natl Acad Sci USA* 1996;93:4979–83
38. Ross L, Rankin S, Flatters M, *et al.* The effects of morphology, size and exchange on the meiotic segregation in chromosomes in *Saccaromyces cerevisae*. *Genetics* 1996;142:79–89
39. Koehler KE, Boulton CL, Collins HE, *et al.* Spontaneous X chromosome MI and MII disjunction events in *Drosophila melanogaster* have different recombination histories. *Nature Genet* 1996;14:406–14
40. Angell RR, Xian J, Keith J, *et al.* First meiotic abnormalities in human oocytes: mechanism of trisomy formation. *Cytogenet Cell Genet* 1994;65:194–202
41. Angell R. First-meiotic-division non-disjunction in human oocytes. *Am J Hum Genet* 1997;61:23–32

42. Cozzi J, Conn CM, Harper J, *et al.* A trisomic germ cell line and precocious chromatid segregation leads to recurrent trisomy 21 conception. *Hum Genet* 1999;104:23–8
43. LeMaire-Adkins E, Radke K, Hunt PA. Lack of checkpoint control at the metaphase–anaphase transition: a mechanism of meiotic non-disjunction in mammalian females. *J Cell Biol* 1997;139:1611–19
44. Woods LM, Hodges CA, Baart E, *et al.* Chromosomal influence on meiotic spindle assembly: abnormal meiosis I in female *Mlh1* mutant mice. *J Cell Biol* 1999;145: 1395–406
45. Eichenlaub-Ritter U, Boll I. Nocodazole sensitivity, age-related aneuploidy, and alterations in the cell cycle during maturation of mouse oocytes. *Cytogenet Cell Genet* 1989;52:170–6
46. Fabricant JD, Schneider E. Studies on the genetic and immunologic components of the maternal age effect. *Dev Biol* 1978;66:41–5
47. Gosden RG, Faddy MJ. Biological bases of premature ovarian failure. *Reprod Fertil Dev* 1998;10:73–8
48. Fabricant JD, Dunn G, Schneider EL. Maternal age related pre- and post-implantation fetal mortality: a strain survey. *Mech Ageing Dev* 1978;8:227–31
49. Brook JD, Gosden RG, Chandley AC. Maternal ageing and aneuploid embryos – evidence from the mouse that biological and not chronological age is the important influence. *Hum Genet* 1984;66:41–5
50. Betzendahl I, Cukurcam S, Michel G, *et al.* Cell cycle control and chemically or age-related predisposition to nondisjunction in mammalian oocytes. *Cytogenet Cell Genet* 1999;85:33
51. Imai HAT, Wada MY, Hirami H, *et al.* Cytological, genetic and evolutionary functions of chiasmata based on chiasma graph analysis. *J Theor Biol* 1999;198:239–57
52. Eichenlaub-Ritter U, Sobek-Klocke I. Implications of cell cycle disturbances for meiotic aneuploidy: studies on a mouse model system. In Vig BK, ed. *Chromosome Segregation and Aneuploidy.* Nato ASI Series 72. Berlin: Springer Verlag, 1993:173–82
53. Fulka J Jr, Jung T, Moor RM. The fall of biological maturation promoting factor (MPF) and histone H1 kinase activity during anaphase and telophase in mouse oocytes. *Mol Reprod Dev* 1992;32:378–82
54. Polanski Z, Ledan E, Brunet S, *et al.* Cyclin synthesis controls the progression of meiotic maturation in mouse oocytes. *Development* 1998;125:4989–97
55. Mitra J, Schultz RM. Regulation of the acquisition of meiotic competence in the mouse: changes in the subcellular localization of cdc2, cyclin B1, cdc25C and wee1, and in the concentration of these proteins and their transcripts. *J Cell Sci* 1996;109:2407–15
56. Verlhac MH, Kubiak JZ, Weber M, *et al.* Mos is required for MAP kinase activation and is involved in microtubule organization during meiotic maturation in the mouse. *Development* 1996;122:815–22
57. Gebauer F, Richter JD. Synthesis and function of Mos: the control switch of vertebrate oocyte meiosis. *Bioessays* 1997;19:23–8
58. Eichenlaub-Ritter U, Michel G, Betzendahl I. Predivision and altered maturation are implicated in maternal age-related errors in chromosome segregation in mammalian oogenesis. *Eur J Hum Genet* 1998;6(suppl 1):83
59. Culp PA, Musci TJ. C-mos and cdc2 cooperate in the translational activation of fibroblast growth factor receptor-1 during *Xenopus* oocyte maturation. *Mol Biol Cell* 1999;10:3567–81
60. Howard EL, Charlesworth A, Welk J, *et al.* The mitogen-activated protein kinase signaling pathway stimulates mos mRNA cytoplasmic polyadenylation during *Xenopus* oocyte maturation. *Mol Cell Biol* 1999;19:1990–9

61. Driancourt MA, Thuel B. Control of oocyte growth and maturation by follicular cells and molecules present in follicular fluid. A review. *Reprod Nutr Dev* 1998; 38:345–62
62. Eppig JJ, Schultz RM, O'Brien M, *et al*. Relationship between the developmental programs controlling nuclear and cytoplasmic maturation of mouse oocytes. *Dev Biol* 1994;164:1–9
63. Picton H, Briggs D, Gosden R. The molecular basis of oocyte growth and development. *Mol Cell Endocrinol* 1998;145:27–37
64. Joyce IM, Pendola FL, Wigglesworth K, *et al*. Oocyte regulation of kit ligand expression in mouse ovarian follicles. *Dev Biol* 1999;214:342–53
65. Byskov AG, Yding Andersen C, Hussaini A, *et al*. Cumulus cells of oocyte–cumulus complexes secrete a meiosis-activating substance when stimulated with FSH. *Mol Reprod Dev* 1997;46:296–305
66. Hegele-Hartung C, Kuhnke J, Lessl M, *et al*. Nuclear and cytoplasmic maturation of mouse oocytes after treatment with synthetic meiosis-activating sterol *in vitro*. *Biol Reprod* 1999;61:1362–72
67. Volarcik K, Sheean L, Goldfarb J, *et al*. The meiotic competence of *in vitro* matured human oocytes is influenced by donor age: evidence that folliculogenesis is compromised in the reproductively aged ovary. *Hum Reprod* 1998;13:154–60
68. Van Blerkom J, Antczak M, Schrader R. The developmental potential of the human oocyte is related to the dissolved oxygen content of follicular fluid: association with vascular endothelial growth factor levels and perifollicular blood flow characteristics. *Hum Reprod* 1997;12:1047–55
69. Van Blerkom J. Epigenetic influences on oocyte developmental competence: perifollicular vascularity and intrafollicular oxygen. *J Assist Reprod Genet* 1998;15: 226–34
70. Yin H, Baart E, Betzendahl I, *et al*. Diazepam induces meiotic delay, aneuploidy and predivision of homologues and chromatids in mammalian oocytes. *Mutagenesis* 1998;13:567 80
71. Liu H, Wang CW, Grifo JA, *et al*. Reconstruction of mouse oocytes by germinal vesicle transfer: maturity of host oocyte cytoplasm determines meiosis. *Hum Reprod* 1999;14:2357–61
72. Choi T, Aoki F, Mori M, *et al*. Activation of p34 cdc2 protein kinase activity in meiotic and mitotic cell cycles in mouse oocytes and embryos. *Development* 1991;113:789–95
73. Millward TA, Zolnierowicz S, Hemmings BA. Regulation of protein kinase cascades by protein phosphatase 2A. *Trends Biochem Sci* 1999;24:186–91
74. Vorlaufer E, Peters JM. Regulation of the cyclin B degradation system by an inhibitor of mitotic proteolysis. *Mol Biol Cell* 1998;9:1817–31
75. Winston NJ, Maro B. Changes in the activity of type 2A protein phosphatases during meiotic maturation and the first mitotic cell cycle in mouse oocytes. *Biol Cell* 1999;91:175–83
76. Sanchez Y, Wong C, Thoma RS, *et al*. Conservation of the Chk1 checkpoint pathway in mammals: linkage of DNA damage to Cdk regulation through Cdc25. *Science* 1997;277:1497–501
77. Russell P. Checkpoints on the road to mitosis. *Trends Biochem Sci* 1998;23:399–402
78. Nakajo N, Oe T, Uto K, Sagata N. Involvement of Chk1 kinase in prophase I arrest of *Xenopus* oocytes. *Dev Biol* 1999;207:432–44
79. Ferby I, Blazquez M, Palmer A, *et al*. A novel p34(cdc2)-binding and activating protein that is necessary and sufficient to trigger G(2)/M progression in *Xenopus* oocytes. *Genes Dev* 1999;13:2177–89

80. Lenormand JL, Dellinger RW, Knudsen KE, *et al*. Speedy: a novel cell cycle regulator of the G2/M transition. *EMBO J* 1999;18:1869–77
81. Fulka J Jr, Kalab P, First NL, *et al*. Damaged chromatin does not prevent the exit from metaphase I in fused mouse oocytes. *Hum Reprod* 1997;12:2473–6
82. Bradshaw J, Jung T, Fulka J Jr, *et al*. UV irradiation of chromosomal DNA and its effect upon MPF and meiosis in mammalian oocytes. *Mol Reprod Dev* 1995;41:503–12
83. Karaiskou A, Jessus C, Brassac T, *et al*. Phosphatase 2A and polo kinase, two antagonistic regulators of Cdc25 activation and MPF auto-amplification. *J Cell Sci* 1999; 112:3747–56
84. Nigg EA. Polo-like kinases: positive regulators of cell division from start to finish. *Curr Opin Cell Biol* 1998;10:776–83
85. Wianny F, Tavares A, Evans MJ, *et al*. Mouse polo-like kinase 1 associates with the acentriolar spindle poles, meiotic chromosomes and spindle midzone during oocyte maturation. *Chromosoma* 1998;107:430–9
86. Kubiak JZ, Weber M, de Pennart H, *et al*. The metaphase II arrest in mouse oocytes is controlled through microtubule-dependent destruction of cyclin B in the presence of CSF. *EMBO J* 1993;12:3773–8
87. Nasmyth K. Separating sister chromatids. *Trends Biochem Sci* 1999;24:98–104
88. Peters JM. Subunits and substrates of the anaphase-promoting complex. *Exp Cell Res* 1999;248:339–49
89. Clute P, Pines J. Temporal and spatial control of cyclin B1 destruction in metaphase. *Nature Cell Biol* 1999;1:82–7
90. Yamamoto A, Guacci V, Koshland D. Pds 1 p, an inhibitor of anaphase in budding yeast, plays a critical role in the APC and checkpoint pathway(s). *J Cell Biol* 1996;133: 99–110
91. Tinker-Kulberg RL, Morgan DO. Pds1 and Esp1 control both anaphase and mitotic exit in normal cells and after DNA damage. *Genes Dev* 1999;13:1936–49
92. Uhlmann F, Lottspeich F, Nasmyth K. Sister-chromatid separation at anaphase onset is promoted by cleavage of the cohesin subunit Scc1. *Nature (London)* 1999; 400:37–42
93. Glotzer M. Samurai separation of Siamese sisters. *Curr Biol* 1999;9:531–4
94. Watanabe Y, Nurse P. Cohesin Rec8 is required for reductional chromosome segregation at meiosis. *Nature (London)* 1999;400:461–4
95. Klein F, Mahr P, Galova M, *et al*. A central role for cohesins in sister chromatid cohesion, formation of axial elements, and recombination during yeast meiosis. *Cell* 1999;98:91–103
96. Krawchuk MD, Wahls WP. Centromere mapping functions for aneuploid meiotic products. Analysis of rec8, rec10 and rec11 mutants of the fission yeast *Schizosaccharomyces pombe*. *Genetics* 1999;153:49–55
97. Krawchuk MD, DeVeaux LC, Wahls WP. Meiotic chromosome dynamics dependent upon the rec8(+), rec10(+) and rec11(+) genes of the fission yeast *Schizosaccharomyces pombe*. *Genetics* 1999;153:57–68
98. Parisi S, McKay MJ, Molnar M, *et al*. Rec8p, a meiotic recombination and sister chromatid cohesion phosphoprotein of the Rad21p family conserved from fission yeast to humans. *Mol Cell Biol* 1999;19:3515–28
99. Rieder CL, Cole R. Chromatid cohesion during mitosis: lessons from meiosis. *Cell Sci* 1999;112:2607–13
100. Moore DP, Page AW, Tang T, *et al*. The cohesion protein MEI-S332 localizes to condensed meiotic and mitotic centromeres until sister chromatids separate. *J Cell Biol* 1998;140:1003–12

101. Bickel SE, Wyman DW, Orr-Weaver TL. Mutational analysis of the *Drosophila* sister-chromatid cohesion protein ORD, and its role in the maintenance of centromere cohesion. *Genetics* 1997;146:1319–31
102. Juang YL, Huang J, Peters JM, *et al*. APC-mediated proteolysis of Ase1 and the morphogenesis of the mitotic spindle. *Science* 1997;275:1311–14
103. Elledge SJ. Cell cycle checkpoints: preventing an identity crisis. *Science* 1996;274:1664–72
104. Gorbsky GJ, Kallio M, Daum JR, *et al*. Protein dynamics at the kinetochore: cell cycle regulation of the metaphase to anaphase transition. *FASEB J* 1999;13(suppl 2): 231–4
105. Waters JC, Chen RH, Murray AW, *et al*. Mad2 binding by phosphorylated kinetochores links error detection and checkpoint action in mitosis. *Curr Biol* 1999; 9:649–52
106. Rieder CL, Schultz A, Cole R, *et al*. Anaphase onset in vertebrate somatic cells is controlled by a checkpoint that monitors sister kinetochore attachment to the spindle. *Cell Biol* 1994;127:1301–10
107. Martinez-Exposito MJ, Kaplan KB, Copeland J, *et al*. Retention of the BUB3 checkpoint protein on lagging chromosomes. *Proc Natl Acad Sci USA* 1999;96:8493–8
108. Chan GK, Jablonski SA, Sudakin V, *et al*. Human BUBR1 is a mitotic checkpoint kinase that monitors CENP-E functions at kinetochores and binds the cyclosome/APC. *J Cell Biol* 1999;146:941–54
109. Kotani S, Tanaka H, Yasuda H, *et al*. Regulation of APC activity by phosphorylation and regulatory factors. *J Cell Biol* 1999;146:791–800
110. Chen RH, Brady DM, Smith D, *et al*. The spindle checkpoint of budding yeast depends on a tight complex between the Mad1 and Mad2 proteins. *Mol Biol Cell* 1999;10:2607–18
111. Can A, Albertini DF. Stage specific effects of carbendazim (MBC) on meiotic cell cycle progression in mouse oocytes. *Mol Reprod Dev* 1997;46:351–62
112. Fulka J Jr, Moor RM, Fulka J. Sister chromatid separation and the metaphase–anaphase transition in mouse oocytes. *Dev Biol* 1994;165:410–17
113. Soewarto D, Schmiady H, Eichenlaub-Ritter U. Consequences of non-extrusion of the first polar body and control of the sequential segregation of homologues and chromatids in mammalian oocytes. *Hum Reprod* 1995;10:2350–60
114. Brunet S, Maria AS, Guillaud P, *et al*. Kinetochore fibers are not involved in the formation of the first meiotic spindle in mouse oocytes, but control the exit from the first meiotic M phase. *J Cell Biol* 1999;146:1–12
115. Yin H, Cukurcam S, Betzendahl I, *et al*. Trichlorfon exposure, spindle aberrations and non-disjunction in mammalian oocytes. *Chromosoma* 1998;107:514–22
116. Brunet S, Polanski Z, Verlhac MH, *et al*. Bipolar meiotic spindle formation without chromatin. *Curr Biol* 1998;8:1231–4
117. Nicklas RB. Chromosome distribution: experiments on cell hybrids and *in vitro*. *Philos Trans R Soc Lond B Biol Sci* 1977;277:267–76
118. Sasagawa I, Kuretake S, Eppig JJ, *et al*. Mouse primary spermatocytes can complete two meiotic divisions within the oocyte cytoplasm. *Biol Reprod* 1998;58:248–54
119. Rieder CL, Khodjakov A, Paliulis LV, *et al*. Mitosis in vertebrate somatic cells with two spindles: implications for the metaphase/anaphase transition checkpoint and cleavage. *Proc Natl Acad Sci USA* 1997;94:5107–12
120. Hu Y, Betzendahl I, Cortvrindt R, *et al*. Spindles and chromosomes in mouse oocytes from pre-antral follicle culture: effects of low O_2 and ageing. *Mol Cell Endocrinol* 2000; in press

121. Gaulden ME. Maternal age-effect: the enigma of Down syndrome and other trisomic conditions. *Mutation Res* 1992;296:69–88
122. Van Blerkom J, Davis PW, Lee J. ATP content of human oocytes and developmental potential and outcome after *in-vitro* fertilization and embryo transfer. *Hum Reprod* 1995;10:415–24
123. DiBrasi D, Genuardi M, Agostino A, *et al*. Double autosomal/gonosomal mosaic aneuploidy: study of non-disjunction in two cases with trisomy of chromosome 8. *Hum Genet* 1995;95:519–25
124. Robinson WP, Binkert F, Bernasconi F, *et al*. Molecular studies of chromosomal mosaicism: relative frequency of chromosome gain or loss and possible role of cell selection. *Am J Hum Genet* 1995;56:444–51
125. James RS, Jacobs PA. Molecular studies of the aetiology of trisomy 8 in spontaneous abortions and the liveborn population. *Hum Genet* 1996;97:283–6
126. Seghezzi L, Maserati E, Minelli A, *et al*. Constitutional trisomy 8 as first mutation in multistage carcinogenesis: clinical, cytogenetic, and molecular data on three cases. *Genes Chromosom Cancer* 1996;17:94–101
127. Zaragoza MV, Jacobs PA, James RS. Non-disjunction of human acrocentric chromosomes: studies of 432 trisomic fetuses and liveborns. *Hum Genet* 1994;94:411–17
128. Robinson WP, Langois S, Schuffenhauer S, *et al*. Cytogenetic and age-dependent risk factors associated with uniparental disomy 15. *Prenat Diagn* 1996;16:837–44
129. Robinson WP, Lorda-Sachez I, Malcolm S, *et al*. Increased parental ages and uniparental disomy 15: a paternal age effect? *Eur J Hum Genet* 1993;1:280–6
130. Ya-gang X, Robinson WP, Spiegel R, *et al*. Parental origin of the supernumary chromosome in trisomy 18. *Clin Genet* 1993;44:57–61
131. Fisher JM, Harvey JF, Morton NE, *et al*. Trisomy 18: studies of the parent and cell division of origin and effect of aberrant recombination on non-disjunction. *Am J Hum Genet* 1995;56:669–75
132. Eggermann T, Nöthen M, Eiben B, *et al*. Trisomy of human chromosome 18: molecular studies on parental origin and cell stage of non-disjunction. *Hum Genet* 1996; 97:218–23
133. Antonarakis SE, Avramopoulos D, Bloin J-L, *et al*. Mitotic errors in somatic cells cause trisomy 21 in about 4.5% of cases and are not associated with advanced maternal age. *Nature Genet* 1993;3:146–50
134. Yang J, Winkler K, Yoshida M, *et al*. Maintenance of G2 arrest in the *Xenopus* oocyte: a role for 14-3-3-mediated inhibition of Cdc25 nuclear import. *EMBO J* 1999; 18:2174–83
135. Matsubara N, Yanagisawa M, Nishimune Y, *et al*. Murine polo like kinase 1 gene is expressed in meiotic testicular germ cells and oocytes. *Mol Reprod Dev* 1995;41:407–15
136. Hardwick KG, Li R, Mistrot C, *et al*. Lesions in many different spindle components activate the spindle checkpoint in the budding yeast *Saccharomyces cerevisiae*. *Genetics* 1999;152:509–18

12

The control of mammalian female meiosis and the factors that influence chromosome segregation

P.A. Hunt

INTRODUCTION

The human female is extraordinarily susceptible to meiotic errors. At least 15–20% of all human conceptions are chromosomally abnormal, typically as a result of errors in chromosome segregation during oogenesis[1]. The consequences of these errors to human health are profound. The most common type of abnormality, aneuploidy, is the leading cause of mental retardation and pregnancy failure in our species. It has been known for more than 50 years that the likelihood of aneuploidy increases strikingly with the age of the mother, yet the basis of this maternal age effect, as well as its contribution to the age-related decrease in fertility in women, remains unknown. Improved culture conditions and new methods for the analysis of single cells have made studies of human oocytes matured *in vitro* possible, thus providing direct access to aneuploidy at its inception (i.e. during the meiotic divisions). In addition, both naturally occurring and engineered mouse mutations have provided new insight into the control of the meiotic divisions and into the factors that influence chromosome segregation. This review summarizes recent data from both studies in the human and experimental studies in the mouse, describes how these data have influenced our thinking about human aneuploidy and presents important directions for future research.

THE BIOLOGY OF MAMMALIAN FEMALE MEIOSIS

Meiosis is a specialized cell division consisting of one round of DNA synthesis followed by two cell divisions. Although the meiotic process is initiated in the fetal ovary, before birth all oocytes become arrested in prophase of the first meiotic division. Resumption and completion of the first meiotic division normally occurs only in the sexually mature animal after the oocyte and the ovarian follicle that enclose it have undergone extensive growth. During this growth phase, known as folliculogenesis, the oocyte acquires the ability to resume and complete the meiotic divisions and to undergo fertilization and the early cleavage divisions.

The first meiotic division (MI) has several unique features (Figure 1). Homologous chromosomes pair and initiate recombination in the fetal ovary during prophase of MI. The process of recombination, involving the physical exchange of DNA between homologous chromosomes, not only ensures that no two gametes are genetically identical, but also creates physical associations (chiasmata) between homologs at the sites of recombination. The completion of MI, which occurs in the adult ovary just prior to ovulation, involves the segregation of homologous chromosomes and reduces the number of chromosomes in the cell by one-half (Figure 1). A second meiotic spindle is formed immediately after the completion of MI but the cell arrests at metaphase of the second meiotic division (MII). The completion of MII is triggered by sperm entry at fertilization, and chromosome segregation is essentially the same as a mitotic division, with the segregation of sister chromatids (Figure 1).

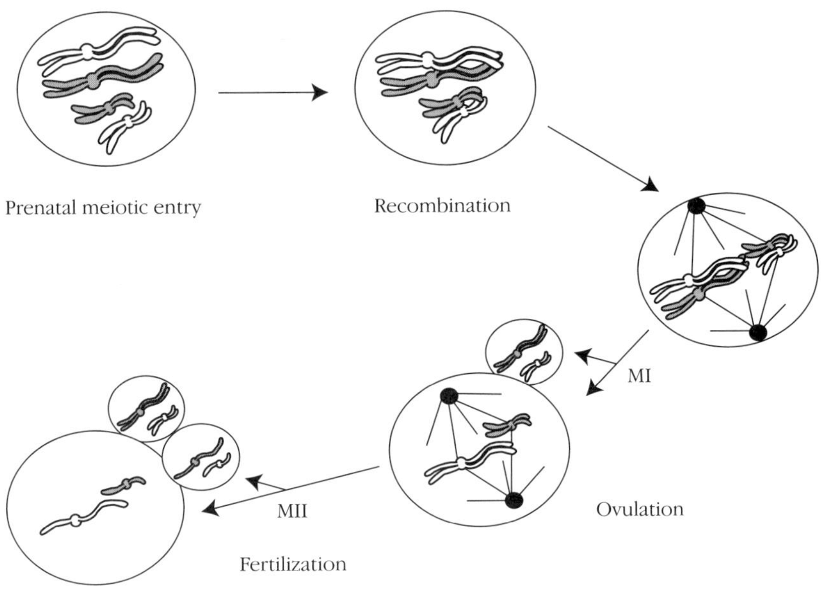

Figure 1 The female meiotic divisions. The first meiotic division is initiated during fetal development. During prophase of MI, homologous chromosomes pair and initiate genetic recombination. The cell then enters an extended period of meiotic arrest which, in the human female, can last for over 40 years. In the ovaries of a sexually mature female, quiescent oocytes initiate an extended growth phase, which culminates in the resumption and completion of MI just prior to ovulation of the mature oocyte. The completion of MI results in the segregation of one homolog to the first polar body and the retention of the other in the oocyte. At MII, the homolog that remains in the oocyte undergoes a second division, during which one chromatid is segregated to the second polar body and the other is retained in the oocyte

THE ROLE OF RECOMBINATION IN MEIOTIC CHROMOSOME SEGREGATION

Mis-segregation of homologous chromosomes at the first meiotic division in females is the major cause of human meiotic non-disjunction[2]. The sites of recombination, or chiasmata, are thought to function in two ways to ensure the proper segregation of homologs at the first meiotic division: first, by maintaining the homologous chromosomes in a paired orientation that promotes their capture by opposite spindle poles and, second, by counterbalancing the forces directing homologous centromeres towards opposite spindle poles, thus allowing the congression of the chromosomes to the spindle equator[3] (reviewed in references 4 and 5).

The role of recombination in ensuring proper chromosome segregation at MI is convincingly illustrated in recombination-deficient mutations. In yeast and *Drosophila*, a number of different mutations have been described that reduce the level of recombination, and all show a corresponding increase in the incidence of meiotic non-disjunction. Furthermore, in studies of spontaneous non-disjunction in yeast and *Drosophila*, abnormally positioned recombination events, or chiasmata (e.g. either too close to the centromere or too close to the telomeres), also increase the likelihood of non-disjunction[5,6].

In the human as well, recent data from several laboratories indicate that alterations in genetic recombination are an important contributor to non-disjunction. That is, reductions in recombination are associated with all human trisomies thus far studied and, at least for trisomies 16 and 21, chiasmata located either too near or too far from the centromere increase the likelihood of non-disjunction. Interestingly, studies of trisomy 21 suggest that aberrant recombination is a feature of MI and MII errors involving chromosome 21 in both younger and older women[7,8]. On the basis of these observations, it has been proposed that there are two steps in maternal age-related non-disjunction[9]. The first step involves the establishment of a 'vulnerable' chiasmate configuration (e.g. a pair of homologous chromosomes that either fail to recombine or have only a single, distally placed exchange) in the fetal oocyte; the second step, which is age-dependent, involves abnormal processing of the 'vulnerable' homologous pair at metaphase I (Figure 2). If correct, this interpretation means that the non-disjunctional process is the same in younger and older women; it simply happens more frequently with age, owing to some age-related disturbance in the process.

AN EXPERIMENTAL APPROACH TO THE STUDY OF THE HUMAN MATERNAL AGE EFFECT

Studies in humans, yeast and *Drosophila* demonstrate that the position of recombination events along the length of the chromosome influences the likelihood of non-disjunction[5,6,10]. These studies, however, have not provided

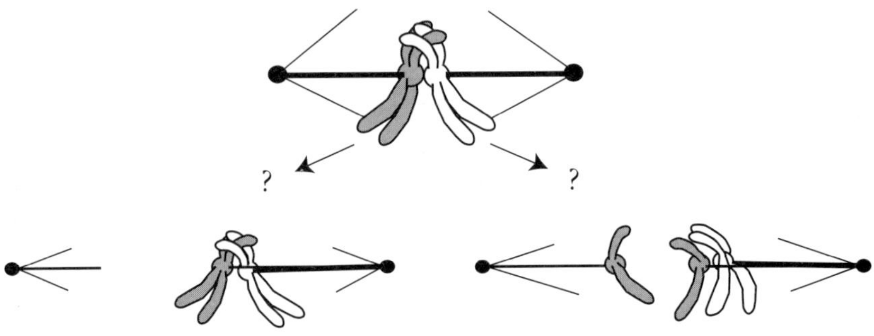

Figure 2 The site of recombination influences the likelihood of a segregation error at MI. Recombination events positioned at the distal ends of the chromosome arms increase the likelihood of a segregation error. It remains unclear, however, whether this type of exchange configuration predisposes to a true non-disjunction event (i.e. the failure of homologs to separate) or to the premature separation of sister chromatids

insight into the mechanism(s) by which chiasma position affects segregation or into the effect of maternal age on meiotic segregation in the human female. Molecular cytogenetic techniques have made possible the assessment of aneuploidy directly from the responsible cells, namely the oocytes. To understand the mechanism(s) of non-disjunctional errors in our species and the way in which age influences segregation, we initiated studies of unstimulated oocytes from women of different ages.

Over the past 4 years we have obtained nearly 600 human oocytes from surgical specimens of ovarian tissue and from follicular aspirates at the time of laparoscopic tubal ligation. This material provides access to women of a range of ages for studies of age-related changes in the meiotic process. Oocytes were recovered from unselected antral follicles, hence not all were healthy or competent to resume meiosis when placed in culture. Previous studies had suggested that approximately 50% of the oocytes recovered from unselected antral follicles spontaneously resumed meiosis when released from the follicle[11–14]. Our own data confirmed this observation. Approximately 50% of the oocytes recovered were viable and, of these, 46% meiotically matured *in vitro*.

To maximize the amount of information obtained per oocyte, we conducted sequential immunofluorescence studies to analyze the meiotic spindle and fluorescence *in situ* hybridization studies to analyze MI chromosome segregation. Our initial segregation studies were limited to four human chromosomes – 16, 18, 21 and the X – selected because cumulatively these account for nearly 60% of all clinically recognized aneuploidies. The long-term goal of these studies is to accumulate data on chromosome- and age-specific patterns of segregation that will allow us to determine why certain chromosomes are more prone to meiotic errors than others and how age affects segregation. We currently have molecular cytogenetic results on over 200 meiotic events. In those situations in which we have been able to compare our results with studies of clinically recognized human trisomies, the data have been remarkably similar[15]. Thus, studies of *in vitro* matured human oocytes appear accurately to reflect the *in vivo* situation, validating this approach as a useful tool for characterizing the underlying causes of human female non-disjunction. Our initial results demonstrate that premature separation of sister chromatids at MI (Figure 2) – recently proposed as the major mechanism of human meiotic non-disjunction[16,17] – is, indeed, responsible for a proportion of non-disjunctional events. However, our data suggest that premature separation of sister chromatids is not the only mechanism of human non-disjunction, nor is it the most common. Indeed, our preliminary results suggest that approximately 80% of all human non-disjunction involves mal-segregation of whole chromosomes, with only 20% involving premature separation of sister chromatids.

CONGRESSION FAILURE AS A BIOMARKER OF MEIOSIS IN OLDER WOMEN

We initiated immunofluorescence studies of the meiotic spindle in human oocytes as a means of accurately determining the meiotic stage of oocytes prior to segregation studies. We were, therefore, surprised when we observed gross aberrations in chromosome alignment in a significant proportion of MII arrested oocytes. The movement of the chromosomes to the spindle equator is called congression, hence we have classified this meiotic aberration as 'congression failure'. Because the oocytes in our study were from unselected antral follicles, it is possible that the high frequency of congression failure is artifactual and does not reflect the situation in the normal periovulatory follicle. However, two items of evidence suggest that this is not the case. First, the frequency of congression failure was strongly correlated with donor age; 7% of oocytes from donors under 30 years of age, 21% of those involving women of 30–39 and no less than 66% of those over 40 years displayed congression failure defects[15]. Second, strikingly similar observations have been reported by Battaglia and co-workers[18] in a small series of oocytes obtained from the periovulatory follicle. Therefore, the defects in meiotic chromosome alignment that we have termed congression failure probably reflect the *in vivo* situation, indicating that this phenotype provides an important new cytological 'biomarker' of maternal age-dependent meiotic errors.

The alignment of chromosomes at the spindle equator during metaphase is thought to facilitate the orderly segregation of the chromosomes at anaphase. Hence the age-related increase in congression failure raises an obvious question: is congression failure the underlying cause of human maternal age-related aneuploidy? Our studies suggest that the answer to this question may be yes. Although our data from direct studies of human oocytes are still preliminary, the frequency of congression failure among oocytes exhibiting an MI segregation error for one of the four chromosomes analyzed is approximately twice that observed in normal disjoining oocytes. However, this association appears to be restricted to non-disjunctional events involving older women, suggesting that other factors are involved in the origin of age-independent non-disjunction (Hunt and colleagues, unpublished).

A NEW MATERNAL AGE HYPOTHESIS

In the human female, age-related changes in the pattern of cyclicity and a decline in fertility are evident many years prior to menopause. The menopausal transition remains poorly understood. According to one hypothesis, the depletion of ovarian follicles drives the onset of menopause and the fine tuning necessary for normal cyclicity is lost when the number of follicles falls below a critical level. Alternatively, hypothalamic aging, which results in the inability to produce tight regulation of the secretion of gonadotropins, has been postulated to initiate the cascade of menopause-related events (reviewed in reference 19). Regardless of the underlying mechanism, the transition to a menopausal state is not abrupt; a striking acceleration in the rate of follicle loss occurs in the decade preceding menopause[20]. Thus, it may be that the exponential increase in meiotic non-disjunction that occurs in the mid-30s is correlated with changes in the endocrine control of reproduction that affect the process of folliculogenesis. Interestingly, the limited data available for pregnancies occurring in the first few years after menarche, when the menses are irregular, suggest that aneuploidy levels are elevated[21]. The association between age-related changes in the endocrine control of reproduction, coupled with the generalized disruption in the meiotic process evident as congression failure that we have observed in oocytes from reproductively aged human donors[15], led us to postulate that age-related aneuploidy is the result of perturbations in the process of oocyte growth. According to our hypothesis, the changing endocrine environment in the ovary causes minor alterations in the process of oocyte growth that predispose to subsequent meiotic errors.

THE MOUSE AS A MODEL FOR THE STUDY OF HUMAN ANEUPLOIDY

One of the major problems in human aneuploidy research has been the lack of a suitable animal model for experimental studies. For example, the mouse does not provide a model for the study of age-related non-disjunction *per se*, since aneuploidy is only modestly elevated in aged females. Nevertheless, the mouse does provide an experimental system for studies designed to understand the control of the meiotic divisions and the factors that influence chromosome segregation. As described below, recent murine studies conducted in our laboratory suggest that mammalian female meiosis lacks an important cell cycle control mechanism to detect aberrant chromosome behaviors at metaphase that could lead to segregation errors at anaphase[22].

The fidelity of cell division is ensured by cell cycle checkpoints that regulate transition points in the cell cycle. These cell cycle surveillance mechanisms function to detect mistakes and inhibit cell cycle progression under conditions that would result in grave errors in cell division (reviewed in references 23–25). Of particular interest from the standpoint of chromosome segregation is the checkpoint that operates at the metaphase–anaphase transition. This checkpoint has been described as a spindle assembly or a chromosome-mediated checkpoint, since defects in either spindle formation (reviewed in reference 26) or the alignment of chromosomes at metaphase[27–30] can delay the onset of anaphase. By ensuring that all chromosomes are properly attached to spindle microtubules and aligned at the mid-zone of the bipolar spindle before the cell proceeds into anaphase, this cell cycle control mechanism functions to prevent the mis-segregation of chromosomes to daughter cells.

On the basis of recent studies, we have suggested that this checkpoint is only partially functional in mammalian female meiosis[31]. Specifically, studies in our laboratory[31] and by others[32–35] have demonstrated that the presence of an intact and stable spindle is a prerequisite for anaphase onset. The congression of all the chromosomes to the spindle equator, however, is not, since the presence of unaligned chromosomes at the first meiotic division does not delay the onset of anaphase[22,36,37] (also P.A. Hunt, unpublished). The lack of a sensitive mechanism for monitoring chromosome alignment and ensuring that all chromosomes form a stable bipolar attachment to the spindle and align at the spindle equator prior to anaphase onset has major implications. First, the lack of a mechanism to detect chromosome behaviors at metaphase that would lead to segregation errors at anaphase provides a reason for the high error rate during female meiosis. Second, the lack of this quality control mechanism suggests that cells exhibiting congression failure at MI would not be prohibited from initiating anaphase; thus an increase in the frequency of congression failure – as we have observed in our studies of human oocytes – should be correlated with an increased incidence of MI non-disjunction.

Although our studies of human oocytes suggest that congression failure is a common feature of oocytes from women over 35 years of age, evidence that the inability to align chromosomes at the spindle equator does not delay anaphase onset is virtually impossible to obtain from studies of human oocytes. In addition, although the level of non-disjunction is higher among oocytes that exhibit congression failure at MII, it is impossible in our studies to demonstrate that congression failure at MI impairs chromosome segregation at anaphase of the first meiotic division. Finally, the most important question – what causes congression failure? – is simply not amenable to study in the human. Therefore, we have been using the mouse as an experimental model system to address these questions.

Because we hypothesized that age-associated alterations in the growth environment of human oocytes affect the meiotic process, we initiated meiotic analyses of three situations in the mouse where the growth process of the oocyte is altered:

(1) *XY sex-reversed female mice produced on the C57BL/6 background provide an example of a mouse mutant with a folliculogenesis defect.* These XY females carry structurally normal X and Y chromosomes but are sex reversed, owing to an effect of the genetic background[38]. XY females exhibit abnormalities in folliculogenesis, including loss of oocytes in the medullary region of the ovary during early development[39] and subtle defects in the cumulus cells, oocyte and zona pellucida in mature follicles[40]. Although the meiotic capability of the oocyte remains intact, the disturbance in folliculogenesis results in the production of oocytes that are incapable of supporting embryonic development[41].

(2) *The LHβ transgenic mouse provides an example of folliculogenesis in an altered endocrine environment.* A transgenic mouse with an altered LHβ gene that results in significantly elevated serum luteinizing hormone (LH) levels has recently been produced[42]. Female carriers of the transgene develop hormonal alterations (including elevated LH, an elevated LH/follicle stimulating hormone (FSH) ratio, elevated testosterone and estradiol, and an altered testosterone/estradiol ratio) which lead to precocious puberty, a disruption in folliculogenesis and infertility[43]. Although LH hypersecretion results in rapid depletion of primordial follicles[44], embryo transfer experiments have demonstrated that the oocytes produced by LHβ transgenic females are developmentally competent[45].

(3) *In vitro oocyte culture provides an example of oocyte growth in the virtual absence of hormonal stimulus.* Recently, several culture systems have been developed to support the *in vitro* growth and maturation of murine oocytes derived from immature follicles. Oocytes from oocyte–granulosa complexes isolated from preantral follicles of neonatal mice[46,47], from intact primary follicles[48] or from primordial follicles[49] can be successfully grown, matured and fertilized *in vitro* and, upon transfer to foster mothers, can give rise to liveborn offspring. Although oocytes grown in the existing culture systems become competent to complete meiosis, undergo fertilization and support embryonic development, the available evidence suggests that they are not the equivalent of oocytes that develop *in vivo* (reviewed in reference 50). In the culture system developed by John Eppig, theca cells are excluded, hence oocyte growth proceeds in the absence of the major steroidogenic cells of the follicle.

The results of our studies of human oocytes led us to postulate that human age-related aneuploidy is the result of a decline in the process of folliculogenesis[15]. We predicted that perturbations in the growth process would result in meiotic aberrations even in a species that does not exhibit a strong maternal age effect. Meiotic studies of oocytes from XY sex-reversed mice, of oocytes from LHβ transgenic females and of oocytes obtained from the *in vitro* culture system developed by Eppig support this hypothesis. Despite differences in the underlying etiology and in the frequency and types of meiotic disturbances observed, we have observed a significant increase in meiotic aberrations in all three situations. Moreover, the *predominant* abnormality in all three mouse models is congression failure (Hunt and colleagues, unpublished).

THE FUTURE

Our studies of human oocytes suggest that the inability to align chromosomes accurately on the meiotic spindle may be an important underlying cause of the age-dependent increase in meiotic errors. Concurrent studies in the mouse suggest that cells exhibiting congression failure initiate anaphase without delay but have an increased likelihood of chromosome segregation errors. These studies provide support for the hypothesis that female meiosis lacks a stringent chromosome-mediated checkpoint control mechanism and that this difference in cell cycle control results in a higher error rate in female meiosis. They do not, however, provide insight into the effect of age on the meiotic process in the human female. To test the hypothesis that congression failure is a reflection of alterations in the growth process of the mammalian oocyte, we have been conducting meiotic studies of oocytes obtained from different situations in the mouse where the growth environment is known to be abnormal. The results of these studies provide evidence that perturbations in the growth process can have a dramatic impact on meiotic chromosome segregation. Although these results are tantalizing, a number of important questions remain to be addressed. What is the link between the hormonal control of folliculogenesis and the target (i.e. the meiotic spindle and/or the kinetochore) that results in the inability to align chromosomes on the meiotic spindle? If, as we have hypothesized, female meiosis lacks a chromosome-mediated checkpoint control mechanism, what is the molecular basis of the lack of this control mechanism? Is this difference in cell cycle control unique to meiosis or are the early embryonic cleavage divisions similarly subject to unique cell cycle control mechanisms?

ACKNOWLEDGEMENTS

Our studies of human oocytes have been supported by National Institutes of Health grant HD31866. I am grateful to the members of my laboratory – past and present – for their technical and intellectual input and to Terry Hassold for helpful discussions and comments on the manuscript.

REFERENCES

1. Jacobs PA. The chromosome complement of human gametes. *Oxford Rev Reprod Biol* 1992;14:48–72
2. Hassold T, Hunt PA, Sherman S. Trisomy in humans: incidence, origin and etiology. *Curr Opin Genet Dev* 1993;3:398–403
3. Nicklas RB. Chromosome segregation mechanisms. *Genetics* 1974;78:205–13
4. Carpenter ATC. Chiasma function. *Cell* 1994;77:959–62
5. Hawley RS. Exchange and chromosome segregation in eukaryotes. In Kucherlapati R, Smith G, eds. *Genetic Recombination.* Washington, DC: American Society of Microbiology, 1988:497–525
6. Moore DP, Orr-Weaver TL. Chromosome segregation during meiosis: building an unambivalent bivalent. In Handel MA, ed. *Meiosis and Gametogenesis*. San Diego: Academic Press, 1998:263–99
7. Sherman S, Petersen M, Freeman S, *et al*. Non-disjunction of chromosome 21 in maternal meiosis I: evidence for a maternal age-dependent mechanism involving reduced recombination. *Hum Mol Genet* 1994;3:1529–35
8. Lamb NE, Feingold E, Savage A, *et al*. Characterization of susceptible chiasma configurations that increase the risk for maternal non-disjunction of chromosome 21. *Hum Mol Genet* 1997;6:1391–9
9. Lamb N, Freeman SB, Savage-Austin A, *et al*. Non-disjunction of chromosome 21: evidence for initiation of all maternal errors during meiosis I. *Nature Genet* 1996; 14:400–5
10. Hassold T, Merrill M, Adkins K, *et al.* Recombination and maternal age-dependent non-disjunction: molecular studies of trisomy 16. *Am J Hum Genet* 1995;57:867–74
11. Gras L, McBain J, Trounson A, Kola I. The incidence of chromosomal aneuploidy in stimulated and unstimulated (natural) uninseminated human oocytes. *Hum Reprod* 1992;7:1396–401
12. Jagiello G, Ducayen M, Fang J-S, Graffeo J. Cytogenetic observations in mammalian oocytes. In Pearson PL, Lewis KR, eds. *Chromosomes Today.* New York: John Wiley, 1976:43–63
13. Uebele-Kallhardt B-M. *Human Oocytes and their Chromosomes: An Atlas.* Berlin: Springer-Verlag, 1978
14. Van Blerkom J. Extrinsic and intrinsic influences on human oocyte and early embryonic developmental potential. In Wasserman PM, ed. *Elements of Mammalian Fertilization*. Boca Raton: CRC Press, 1990:81–109
15. Volarcik K, Sheean L, Goldfarb J, *et al*. The meiotic competence of *in vitro* matured human oocytes is influenced by donor age: evidence that folliculogenesis is compromised in the reproductively aged ovary. *Hum Reprod* 1998;13:154–60
16. Angell RR. Predivision in human oocytes at meiosis I: a mechanism for trisomy formation in man. *Hum Genet* 1991;86:383–7
17. Angell RR, Xian J, Keith J, *et al*. First meiotic abnormalities in human oocytes: mechanism of trisomy formation. *Cytogenet Cell Genet* 1994;65:194–202
18. Battaglia DE, Goodwin P, Klein NA. Influence of maternal age on meiotic spindle assembly in oocytes from naturally cycling women. *Hum Reprod* 1996;11:2217–22
19. Wise PM, Krajnak KM, Kashon ML. Menopause: the ageing of multiple pacemakers. *Science* 1996;273:67–70
20. Richardson SJ, Nelson JF. Follicular depletion during the menopausal transition. *Ann NY Acad Sci* 1990;592:13–20
21. Hassold T, Jacobs P. Trisomy in man. *Ann Rev Genet* 1984;18:69–97

22. LeMaire-Adkins R, Radke K, Hunt PA. Lack of checkpoint control at the metaphase–anaphase transition: a mechanism of meiotic non-disjunction in mammalian females. *J Cell Biol* 1997;139:1611–19
23. Murray A. Cell cycle checkpoints. *Curr Opin Cell Biol* 1994;6:872–6
24. Elledge SJ. Cell cycle checkpoints: preventing an identity crisis. *Science* 1996;274: 1664–71
25. Page AW, Orr-Weaver TL. Stopping and starting the meiotic cell cycle. *Curr Biol* 1997;7:23–31
26. Wells WAE. The spindle-assembly checkpoint: aiming for a perfect mitosis, every time. *Trends Cell Biol* 1996;6:228–34
27. Rieder CL, Schultz A, Cole R, Sluder G. Anaphase onset in vertebrate somatic cells is controlled by a checkpoint that monitors sister kinetochore attachment to the spindle. *J Cell Biol* 1994;127:1301–10
28. Li X, Nicklas RB. Mitotic forces control a cell-cycle checkpoint. *Nature (London)* 1995;373:630–2
29. Rieder CL, Cole RW, Khodjakov A, Sluder G. The checkpoint delaying anaphase in response to chromosome monoorientation is mediated by an inhibitory signal produced by unattached kinetochores. *J Cell Biol* 1995;130:941–8
30. Wells WAE, Murray AW. Aberrantly segregating centromeres activate the spindle assembly checkpoint in budding yeast. *J Cell Biol* 1996;133:75–84
31. Woods LM, Hodges C, Baart E, *et al*. Chromosomal control of meiotic spindle assembly: abnormal meiosis I in female *Mlh1* mutant mice. *J Cell Biol* 1999;145:1395–406
32. Eichenlaub-Ritter U, Boll I. Nocodazole sensitivity, age-related aneuploidy, and alterations in the cell cycle during maturation of mouse oocytes. *Cytogenet Cell Genet* 1989;52:170–6
33. Pesty A, Lefevre B, Kubiak J, *et al*. Mouse oocyte maturation is affected by lithium via the polyphosphoinositide metabolism and the microtubule network. *Mol Reprod Dev* 1994;38:187–99
34. Eichenlaub-Ritter U, Betzendahl I. Chloral hydrate induced spindle aberrations, metaphase I arrest and aneuploidy in mouse oocytes. *Mutagenesis* 1995;10:477–86
35. Can A, Albertini DF. Stage specific effects of carbendazim (MBC) on meiotic cell cycle progression in mouse oocytes. *Mol Reprod Dev* 1997;46:351–62
36. Hunt PA, LeMaire R, Embury P, *et al*. Analysis of chromosome behavior in intact mammalian oocytes: monitoring the segregation of a univalent chromosome during mammalian female meiosis. *Hum Mol Genet* 1995;4:2007–12
37. Yin H, Cukurcam S, Betzendahl I, *et al*. Trichlorfon exposure, spindle aberrations and non-disjunction in mammalian oocytes. *Chromosoma* 1998;107:514–22
38. Eicher E, Washburn L, Whitney B, Morrow K. *Mus poschiavinus* Y chromosome in the C57BL/6J murine genome causes sex reversal. *Science* 1982;217:535–7
39. Taketo-Hosotani T, Nishioka Y, Nagamine CM, *et al*. Development and fertility of ovaries in the B6.Y DOM sex-reversed female mouse. *Development* 1989;107: 95–105
40. Vanderhyden BC, Macdonald EA, Merchant-Larios H, *et al*. Interactions between the oocyte and cumulus cells in the ovary of the B6.Y^{TIR} sex-reversed female mouse. *Biol Reprod* 1997;57:641–6
41. Merchant-Larios H, Clarke HJ, Taketo T. Developmental arrest of fertilized eggs from the B6.YDOM sex-reversed female mouse. *Dev Genet* 1994;15:435–42
42. Risma KA, Clay CM, Nett TM, *et al*. Targeted overexpression of luteinizing hormone in transgenic mice leads to infertility, polycystic ovaries, and ovarian tumors. *Proc Natl Acad Sci USA* 1995;92:1322–6

43. Risma KA, Hirshfield AN, Nilson JH. Elevated luteinizing hormone in prepubertal transgenic mice causes hyperandrogenemia, precocious puberty, and substantial ovarian pathology. *Endocrinology* 1997;138:3540–7
44. Flaws JA, Abbud R, Mann RJ, *et al*. Chronically elevated luteinizing hormone depletes primordial follicles in the mouse ovary. *Biol Reprod* 1997;57:1233–7
45. Mann RJ, Keri RA, Nilson JH. Transgenic mice with chronically elevated LH are infertile due to anovulation, defects in uterine receptivity, and midgestation pregnancy failure. *Endocrinology* 1999;140:2592–601
46. Eppig JJ, Schroeder AC. Capacity of mouse oocytes from preantral follicles to undergo embryogenesis and development to live young after growth, maturation, and fertilization *in vitro*. *Biol Reprod* 1989;41:268–76
47. Eppig JJ, Wigglesworth K, O'Brien MJ. Comparison of embryonic developmental competence of mouse oocytes grown with and without serum. *Mol Reprod Dev* 1992;32:33–40
48. Spears N, Boland NI, Murray AA, Gosden RG. Mouse oocytes derived from *in vitro* grown primary ovarian follicles are fertile. *Hum Reprod* 1994;9:527–32
49. Eppig JJ, O'Brien MJ. Development *in vitro* of mouse oocytes from primordial follicles. *Biol Reprod* 1996;54:197–207
50. Eppig JJ, O'Brien MJ, Wigglesworth K. Mammalian oocyte growth and development *in vitro*. *Mol Reprod Dev* 1996;44:260–73

13

The potential role of the oocyte in follicle development and ovarian aging

U. Vitt, M. Hayashi and A.J.W. Hsueh

THE FATE OF A FOLLICLE: INITIAL RECRUITMENT AND SUBSEQUENT DEMISE OR OVULATION

Each ovarian follicle has a unique developmental fate. Although neighboring follicles could exert influences on each other, development of individual follicles is not clearly synchronized and several follicles at the same stage of development do not necessarily end up on the same developmental path. During early life, a fixed number of primordial ovarian follicles are endowed with one oocyte surrounded by a single layer of granulosa cells. In humans, the initial primordial follicle pool is in the range of 1–2 million. Although most of these follicles remain dormant or arrested, some of them start to grow, owing to a process here called initial recruitment. The number of follicles starting to grow is related to the number of primordial follicles still remaining in the quiescent pool at a specific point in time[1,2]. In rats, all follicles at the early antral stage undergo atresia mediated by apoptosis before the onset of puberty[3]. After puberty, a small number of early antral follicles escape apoptotic demise as the result of stimulation by circulatory follicle stimulating hormone (FSH). These follicles grow into antral follicles under gonadotropin and local hormone stimulation. A few of the antral follicles eventually reach the preovulatory stage and ovulate in response to the preovulatory gonadotropin surge. After the release of the matured oocyte, the somatic cells in the follicle become luteinized and form the corpus luteum that secretes hormones essential for the maintenance of pregnancy.

THE UNIQUE CHARACTERISTICS OF THE OOCYTE AND THE POTENTIAL ROLE OF THE FEMALE GAMETE IN FOLLICLE DEVELOPMENT

The mammalian oocyte represents a unique cell type in the body (Table 1). Oocytes have a prolonged lifespan; some of them can survive in women for decades before undergoing ovulation as in preovulatory follicles or, more

Table 1 Unique features of the oocyte

1.	Large size (100-fold growth in size)
2.	Prolonged lifespan (decades in the human)
3.	Undergoes meiosis
4.	Close communication with cumulus and other follicle cells (gap junctions)
5.	Mechanisms for sperm penetration and polyspermy block
6.	Maternal transcripts for fertilization and early embryo development into a whole organism

likely, degeneration as in atretic follicles. In addition, oocytes remain dormant during most of their lifespan and are arrested at the dictyate stage of the prophase of meiosis before germinal vesicle breakdown is initiated by the preovulatory gonadotropin surge[4]. Furthermore, the oocyte contains maternal transcripts necessary for sperm pronucleus formation, syngamy and the early steps of embryogenesis[5], and largely contributes to the formation of the zona pellucida important for polyspermy block.

During follicle development, the female germ cell undergoes tremendous growth, reaching a 100-fold increase in cell volume. Associated with oocyte growth are pronounced biochemical and morphological changes[6,7]. The extremely large size of these cells probably necessitates their metabolic coupling to surrounding follicular cells[8]. Earlier studies have demonstrated a close communication between the oocyte and the surrounding cumulus cells through gap junctions that allow the exchange of small molecules such as cAMP and ions[9]. These gap junctions are essential for oocyte growth[10]. During oocyte growth, these cells acquire cell cycle proteins important for meiosis, a process unique for germ cells[11]. Connexin 37-deficient mice, which fail to form gap junctions between oocytes and granulosa cells, do not achieve meiotic competence. Furthermore, the ovaries of these mutant mice lack large antral follicles and display numerous inappropriate corpora lutea[12]. These results indicate that communication between the oocyte and cumulus cells is important for appropriate oocyte and follicle development. However, growth of the follicle up to the preantral stage seems to be unaffected by the lack of gap junctions in mutant mice. Therefore, control of these early stages of folliculogenesis by the oocyte can be achieved only by secretion of paracrine factors.

Several reports have suggested the role of the oocyte as a hormone-producing cell capable of secreting paracrine factors to regulate the development of the surrounding somatic cells (Table 2). Conditioned media from the oocyte promote the proliferation of granulosa cells[13], enable FSH-induced cumulus expansion[14–17] and enhance hyaluronic acid synthesis by cumulus cells[15]. Therefore, the oocyte influences the mucification procedure of the surrounding cumulus that occurs late during folliculogenesis and is essential for successful fertilization.

Cumulus cells surrounding the oocyte are less differentiated than the highly differentiated granulosa cells closest to the basal lamina, and show lower steroid production and luteinizing hormone (LH) receptor levels. The less differentiated status of the cumulus cells is probably necessary for

Table 2 Cumulus/granulosa cell functions regulated by oocyte-secreted factor(s)

	Removal of oocyte	*Oocyte factor(s)*	*References*
Proliferation	↓	↑	13
FSH-induced cumulus expansion	↓	↑	14–17
Synthesis of hyaluronic acid	↑	↑	15
Luteinization (morphology)	↑	?	19
Progesterone production	↑	↓	20,21
Estradiol production	↑↓*	?	20(porcine) 21(murine)*
FSH-induced progesterone production	↑	?	20
Expression of LH receptors	↑	↓	22

*Porcine oocytectomy leads to an increase in estradiol production, whereas in mice it leads to a decrease

optimal oocyte development, whereas the highly differentiated mural granulosa cells are essential for steroidogenesis as well as the follicle rupture that is induced by the preovulatory LH surge. Therefore, it has been suggested that oocyte factors might inhibit granulosa cell differentiation and would therefore be responsible for the formation of two distinct subpopulations of cumulus and mural granulosa cells[18]. Early morphological studies indicated that removal of the oocyte leads to luteinization of the surrounding granulosa cells[19]. Recent studies have shown that removal of the oocyte leads to increased progesterone production and expression of LH receptors by surrounding cumulus or granulosa cells. It is of importance that both functional parameters in cumulus and granulosa cells were inhibited by oocyte-secreted factors[20–22]. Although the inhibitory influence of the oocyte on progesterone production has consistently been found in studies using different species, this is not the case for estradiol production. In the pig, the removal of the oocyte from the cumulus–oocyte complex led to an increase in estradiol production by cumulus cells[20], whereas in the mouse the removal of the oocyte resulted in lower estradiol production by the remaining cumulus[21].

In summary, the oocyte secretes one or more factors that inhibit luteinization and maintain the neighboring cumulus cells in a less differentiated state. It is becoming clear that the oocyte not only depends on the supporting follicular cells for development but plays an active role in controlling the growth and differentiation of the surrounding somatic cells in the same follicle. It is possible that the genetic makeup of an individual oocyte could determine the secretion of oocyte hormones, which, in turn, may regulate the growth and differentiation of the surrounding somatic cells.

THE EFFECTS OF OOCYTE-DERIVED GROWTH DIFFERENTIATION FACTOR-9 ON FOLLICLE GROWTH AND MATURATION

The role of endocrine hormones (FSH and LH), local growth factors and cytokines[23–25] in ovarian follicle development has been extensively studied and reviewed. Although these studies serve as the basis for formulating the present clinical protocols of ovarian stimulation by gonadotropins[26] and provide information on the variations in the intraovarian hormonal milieu, only recent studies have emphasized the role of oocyte hormones in the regulation of follicle development.

Growth differentiation factor-9 (GDF-9), a member of the transforming growth factor (TGF)-β gene family, was found to be expressed exclusively in the oocyte, suggesting its unique role in follicle development[27]. It is noteworthy that mutant mice with GDF-9 gene deletion exhibit a major defect in follicle development, showing the arrest of all follicles beyond the primary follicle stage[28]. On the basis of these findings, we generated recombinant GDF-9 and specific anti-GDF-9 antibodies. It was demonstrated that GDF-9 is expressed in oocytes throughout different stages of follicle development and that recombinant GDF-9 stimulates inhibin-α production in ovarian explant cultures[29]. Furthermore, GDF-9 significantly increased the diameter of preantral rat follicles under serum-free culture conditions and enhanced FSH-induced follicular growth (Figure 1).

The results of studies dealing with the regulation of cumulus and granulosa cell functions by GDF-9 are summarized in Table 3. In addition to the ability

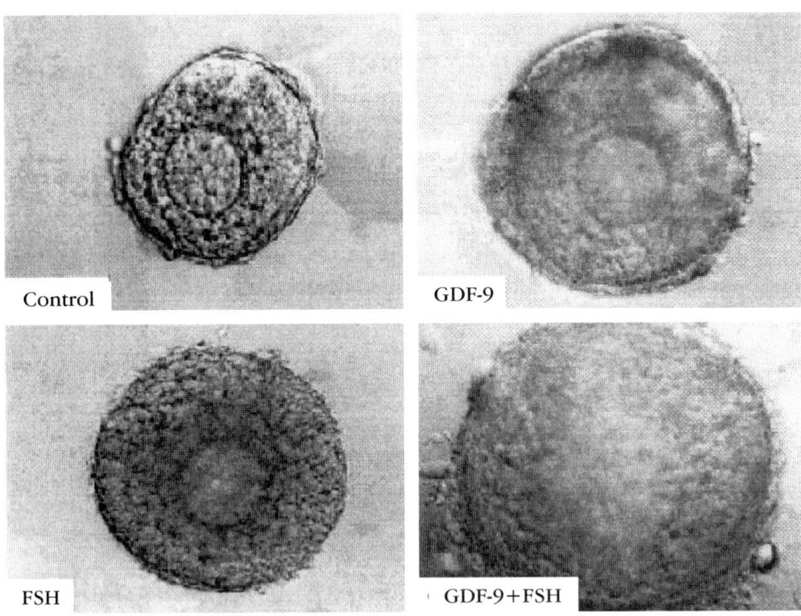

Figure 1 Growth differentiation factor-9 (GDF-9) stimulation of preantral follicle growth. Preantral follicles were dissected from the ovaries of neonatal rats at 14 days of age and cultured in serum-free conditions with or without GDF-9 and follicle stimulating hormone (FSH). GDF-9 and FSH both increased follicle diameter during 48 h of culture. GDF-9 also enhanced follicular growth induced by FSH. Reprinted with permission from reference 29

Table 3 Effects of growth differentiation factor-9 (GDF-9) on cumulus/granulosa cell function

	GDF-9	*References*
Proliferation	↑	31
FSH-induced cumulus expansion	↑	30
Hyaluronan synthase-2	↑	30
Luteinization (morphology)	?	
Progesterone production	↑	30 and 31
Estradiol production	↑	31
FSH-induced progesterone production	↓	31
FSH-induced estradiol production	↓	31
Expression of LH receptors	↓	31

of GDF-9 to enhance preantral follicle growth and inhibin-α production[29], a recent study showed that treatment with GDF-9 enhances FSH-induced cumulus expansion and expression of hyaluronan synthase-2[30]. Our recent study[31] also showed that GDF-9 treatment increased thymidine incorporation and the number of cultured granulosa cells. These results are consistent with the observed effects of oocyte conditioned media on cumulus cell maturation (Table 2). Although treatment with GDF-9 alone was shown to enhance progesterone production, we also found that GDF-9 decreased FSH-induced steroidogenesis and expression of LH receptors by cultured granulosa cells. The latter is again consistent with the observed effects of oocyte-conditioned media on granulosa and cumulus cell function. These results indicate that the oocyte, via secretion of GDF-9, could enhance follicle growth by increasing the granulosa cell number; by inhibiting the differentiation of the closely associated cumulus cells, it could lead to the formation of two distinct subpopulations of granulosa cells.

To date, the receptors for GDF-9 are unknown. Other members of the TGF-β family have been shown to bind to a family of serine/threonine receptor kinases that fall into two classes: type I and type II. Binding of homo- and heterodimers of different family members leads to the association of these two receptor types, phosphorylation of the type I receptor by the type II receptor and subsequent signalling events[32]. It has been shown that bone morphogenetic proteins (BMP)-2, -4 and -7, which are closely related to GDF-9, interact with the same type I receptors for signal transduction and also share a common type II receptor[33,34]. Furthermore, BMP-2 and -4 are believed to use the activin type I receptor for signalling[35]. It is not known whether GDF-9 binds to its own specific receptor or to other receptors of the TGF-β superfamily shown to be expressed by granulosa cells[36].

Recently, GDF-9B (also known as BMP-15), a protein similar to GDF-9 in structure, has been found to be co-expressed with GDF-9 in oocytes[37,38]. Owing to their structural characteristics, the possibility of non-covalent heterodimer formation between GDF-9 and GDF-9B has been discussed[38]. Heterodimers of different BMPs have been shown to have bioactivity higher than, and/or distinct from, homodimers[39]. If dimers are indeed formed

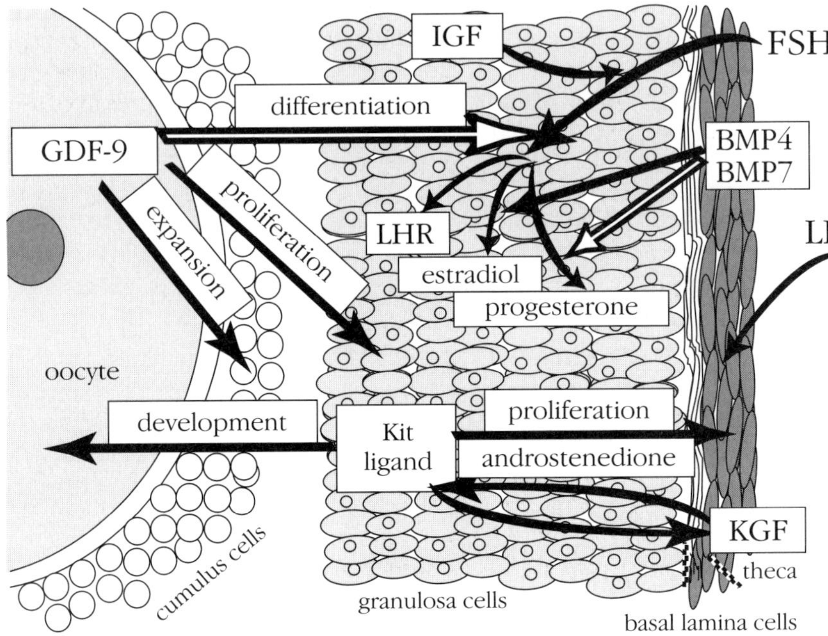

Figure 2 Regulation of follicle development by paracrine hormones. Stimulatory and inhibitory effects are indicated by filled and empty arrows, respectively. In addition to endocrine hormones follicle stimulating hormone (FSH) and luteinizing hormone (LH) that stimulate the differentiation of granulosa and theca cells, growth differentiation factor-9 (GDF-9) of oocyte origin inhibits FSH-induced progesterone and estrogen production, and LH receptor (LHR) expression by granulosa cells. In contrast, GDF-9 stimulates granulosa cell proliferation and cumulus expansion. Insulin-like growth factors (IGF) are expressed in all cell types of the follicle and are believed to enhance FSH action in granulosa cells. Kit ligand is produced by granulosa cells and leads to oocyte growth but maintains meiotic arrest and enhances theca cell proliferation and androstenedione production. The expression of Kit ligand in granulosa cells is enhanced by keratinocyte growth factor (KGF), and Kit ligand enhances KGF expression by theca cells. Bone morphogenetic proteins (BMP)-4 and -7 were shown to be expressed in theca cells and their corresponding receptors in the granulosa cells. Both BMPs enhanced and reduced FSH-induced estrogen and progesterone production, respectively

between GDF-9 and GDF-9B, the heterodimers could have unique functions not found for either GDF-9 or GDF-9B.

Multiple paracrine growth factors and cytokines secreted by granulosa and theca cells have been reported[23,24]. The presence of different insulin-like growth factors (IGFs) as well as their binding proteins has been reviewed in earlier studies. IGFs are expressed in all follicular cell types and are believed to enhance FSH effects[40]. In addition to oocyte-secreted GDF-9, which acts on follicle somatic cells, granulosa cell-derived Kit ligand enhances oocyte growth and maintains meiotic arrest[41]. Kit ligand also stimulates theca cell proliferation and androstenedione production and was shown to be essential for specific stages of follicular development[42]. The expression of Kit ligand in granulosa cells is enhanced by theca cell-derived keratinocyte growth factor (KGF)[43]. In addition, treatment with KGF enhances preantral follicle growth *in vitro*[44]. Recent studies also indicate the expression in theca cells of BMP-4 and -7, which are closely related to GDF-9, as well as the expression of receptors for these proteins in granulosa cells. Furthermore, both BMPs influenced FSH-induced granulosa cell steroidogenesis *in vitro*[36]. The paracrine actions of these growth factors present in the follicle are summarized in Figure 2.

INITIAL FOLLICLE RECRUITMENT IS A DETERMINING FACTOR IN OVARIAN AGING. GDF-9 ANTAGONISTS AS FOLLICLE PRESERVATION PILLS?

With the large wave of 'baby boomers' reaching menopause in the next decade, studies on the mechanism of this important physiological process have gained additional momentum. These studies, however, are hampered by the lengthy duration of the menopausal process. Although experimental primate models should provide the best approach to understanding the menopause in humans, this model also suffers from the long reproductive lifespan of these animals. Instead, findings based on the more practical rodent models have been extrapolated to the human situation. Because menopause is associated with the near exhaustion of the follicle pool, it is generally believed that the depletion of follicles in the ovary signals human menopause[45].

Mainly based on rodent studies, the hypothesis has been put forward that the initial recruitment of the ovarian follicle is a determining factor in follicle depletion[2]. Most primordial follicles that have initiated growth continue to develop into primary, secondary and antral follicles. At the antral stage, the majority of follicles undergo atretic degeneration through apoptosis. Because minimal primordial follicle demise has been observed, the initiation of primordial follicle growth becomes the determining factor in follicle pool depletion, and thus the onset of menopause[46]. GDF-9 and related oocyte factors are essential for these early stages of follicle recruitment. The availability of recombinant GDF-9 provides an opportunity to achieve accelerated ovarian aging in rodents, thus substantiating the role of this oocyte factor in follicle pool depletion. In addition, future investigations on ovarian receptors for GDF-9 could allow the design of GDF-9 antagonists and offer the possibility of delaying the menopause following pharmacological intervention in initial follicle recruitment.

REFERENCES

1. Faddy MJ, Gosden RG. A mathematical model of follicle dynamics in the human ovary. *Hum Reprod* 1995;10:770–5
2. Hirshfield AN. Relationship between the supply of primordial follicles and the onset of follicular growth in rats. *Biol Reprod* 1994;50:421–8

3. Hsueh AJW, Billig H, Tsafriri A. Ovarian follicle atresia: a hormonally controlled apoptotic process. *Endocr Rev* 1994;15:707–24
4. Downs SM, Daniel SA, Eppig JJ. Induction of maturation in cumulus cell-enclosed mouse oocytes by follicle-stimulating hormone and epidermal growth factor: evidence for a positive stimulus of somatic cell origin. *J Exp Zool* 1988;245:86–96
5. Picton H, Briggs D, Gosden R. The molecular basis of oocyte growth and development. *Mol Cell Endocrinol* 1998;145:27–37
6. Anderson E. Comparative aspects of the ultrastructure of the female gamete. *Int Rev Cytol* 1974;(suppl):1–70
7. Wassarman PM, Josefowicz WJ. Oocyte development in the mouse: an ultrastructural comparison of oocytes isolated at various stages of growth and meiotic competence. *J Morphol* 1978;156:209–35
8. Herlands RL, Schultz RM. Regulation of mouse oocyte growth: probable nutritional role for intercellular communication between follicle cells and oocytes in oocyte growth. *J Exp Zool* 1984;229:317–25
9. Lawrence TS, Beers WH, Gilula NB. Transmission of hormonal stimulation by cell-to-cell communication. *Nature (London)* 1978;272:501–6
10. Eppig JJ. A comparison between oocyte growth in coculture with granulosa cells and oocytes with granulosa cell–oocyte junctional contact maintained *in vitro*. *J Exp Zool* 1979;209:345–53
11. Wassarman PM, Schultz RM, Letourneau GE. Protein synthesis during meiotic maturation of mouse oocytes *in vitro*. Synthesis and phosphorylation of a protein localized in the germinal vesicle. *Dev Biol* 1979;69:94–107
12. Simon AM, Goodenough DA, Li E, *et al*. Female infertility in mice lacking connexin 37. *Nature (London)* 1997;385:525–9
13. Vanderhyden BC, Telfer EE, Eppig JJ. Mouse oocytes promote proliferation of granulosa cells from preantral and antral follicles *in vitro*. *Biol Reprod* 1992;46: 1196–204
14. Buccione R, Vanderhyden BC, Caron PJ, *et al*. FSH-induced expansion of the mouse cumulus oophorus *in vitro* is dependent upon a specific factor(s) secreted by the oocyte. *Dev Biol* 1990;138:16–25
15. Salustri A, Ulisse S, Yanagishita M, *et al*. Hyaluronic acid synthesis by mural granulosa cells and cumulus cells *in vitro* is selectively stimulated by a factor produced by oocytes and by transforming growth factor-beta. *J Biol Chem* 1990;265:19517–23
16. Vanderhyden BC, Caron PJ, Buccione R, *et al*. Developmental pattern of the secretion of cumulus expansion-enabling factor by mouse oocytes and the role of oocytes in promoting granulosa cell differentiation. *Dev Biol* 1990;140:307–17
17. Eppig JJ, Peters AH, Telfer EE, *et al*. Production of cumulus expansion enabling factor by mouse oocytes grown *in vitro*: preliminary characterization of the factor. *Mol Reprod Dev* 1993;34:450–6
18. Eppig JJ. Intercommunication between mammalian oocytes and companion somatic cells. *BioEssays* 1991;13:569–74
19. Nekola MV, Nalbandov AV. Morphological changes of rat follicular cells as influenced by oocytes. *Biol Reprod* 1971;4:154–60
20. Coskun S, Uzumcu M, Lin YC, *et al*. Regulation of cumulus cell steroidogenesis by the porcine oocyte and preliminary characterization of oocyte-produced factor(s). *Biol Reprod* 1995;53:670–5
21. Vanderhyden BC, Tonary AM. Differential regulation of progesterone and estradiol production by mouse cumulus and mural granulosa cells by a factor(s) secreted by the oocyte. *Biol Reprod* 1995;53:1243–50

22. Eppig JJ, Wigglesworth K, Pendola F, *et al.* Murine oocytes suppress expression of luteinizing hormone receptor messenger ribonucleic acid by granulosa cells. *Biol Reprod* 1997;56:976–84
23. Adashi EY. The potential relevance of cytokines to ovarian physiology: the emerging role of resident ovarian cells of the white blood cell series. *Endocr Rev* 1990;11: 454–64
24. Adashi EY. Intraovarian peptides. Stimulators and inhibitors of follicular growth and differentiation. *Endocrinol Metab Clin North Am* 1992;21:1–17
25. Hsueh AJW, Adashi EY, Jones PB, *et al.* Hormonal regulation of the differentiation of cultured ovarian granulosa cells. *Endocr Rev* 1984;5:76–127
26. Fauser BC, Van Heusden AM. Manipulation of human ovarian function: physiological concepts and clinical consequences. *Endocr Rev* 1997;18:71–106
27. McGrath SA, Esquela AF, Lee SJ. Oocyte-specific expression of growth/differentiation factor-9. *Mol Endocrinol* 1995;9:131–6
28. Dong J, Albertini DF, Nishimori K, *et al.* Growth differentiation factor-9 is required during early ovarian folliculogenesis. *Nature (London)* 1996;383:531–5
29. Hayashi M, McGee EA, Min G, *et al.* Recombinant growth differentiation factor-9 (GDF-9) enhances growth and differentiation of cultured early ovarian follicles. *Endocrinology* 1999;140:1236–44
30. Elvin JA, Clark AT, Wang P, *et al.* Paracrine actions of growth differentiation factor-9 in the mammalian ovary. *Mol Endocrinol* 1999;13:1035–48
31. Vitt VA, Hayashi M, Klein C, *et al.* Growth differentiation factor-9 stimulates proliferation but suppresses the follicle-stimulating hormone-induced differentiation of cultured granulosa cells from small antral and preovulatory rat follicles. *Biol Reprod* 2000;62:370–77
32. Massague J. TGF-beta signal transduction. *Annu Rev Biochem* 1998;67:753–91
33. ten Dijke P, Yamashita H, Sampath TK, *et al.* Identification of type I receptors for osteogenic protein-1 and bone morphogenetic protein-4. *J Biol Chem* 1994; 269:16985–8
34. Liu F, Ventura F, Doody J, *et al.* Human type II receptor for bone morphogenic proteins (BMPs): extension of the two-kinase receptor model to the BMPs. *Mol Cell Biol* 1995;15:3479–86
35. Ebendal T, Bengtsson H, Soderstrom S. Bone morphogenetic proteins and their receptors: potential functions in the brain. *J Neurosci Res* 1998;51:139–46
36. Shimasaki S, Zachow RJ, Li D, *et al.* A functional bone morphogenetic protein system in the ovary. *Proc Natl Acad Sci USA* 1999;96:7282–7
37. Laitinen M, Vuojolainen K, Jaatinen R, *et al.* A novel growth differentiation factor-9 (GDF-9) related factor is coexpressed with GDF-9 in mouse oocytes during folliculogenesis. *Mech Dev* 1998;78:135–40
38. Dube JL, Wang P, Elvin J, *et al.* The bone morphogenetic protein 15 gene is X-linked and expressed in oocytes. *Mol Endocrinol* 1998;12:1809–17
39. Suzuki A, Kaneko E, Maeda J, *et al.* Mesoderm induction by BMP-4 and -7 heterodimers. *Biochem Biophys Res Commun* 1997;232:153–6
40. Adashi EY, Resnick CE, D'Ercole AJ, *et al.* Insulin-like growth factors as intraovarian regulators of granulosa cell growth and function. *Endocr Rev* 1985;6:400–20
41. Manova K, Huang EJ, Angeles M, *et al.* The expression pattern of the c-kit ligand in gonads of mice supports a role for the c-kit receptor in oocyte growth and in proliferation of spermatogonia. *Dev Biol* 1993;157:85–99
42. Yoshida H, Takakura N, Kataoka H, *et al.* Stepwise requirement of c-kit tyrosine kinase in mouse ovarian follicle development. *Dev Biol* 1997;184:122–37

43. Parrott JA, Skinner MK. Thecal cell–granulosa cell interactions involve a positive feedback loop among keratinocyte growth factor, hepatocyte growth factor, and Kit ligand during ovarian follicular development. *Endocrinology* 1998;139:2240–5
44. McGee EA, Chun SY, Lai S, *et al*. Keratinocyte growth factor promotes the survival, growth, and differentiation of preantral ovarian follicles. *Fertil Steril* 1999;71:732–8
45. Faddy MJ, Gosden RG. A model conforming the decline in follicle numbers to the age of menopause in women. *Hum Reprod* 1996;11:1484–6
46. Gosden RG, Faddy MJ. Ovarian ageing, follicular depletion, and steroidogenesis. *Exp Gerontol* 1994;29:265–74

14

Mitochondrial dysfunction and ovarian aging

J.M. Cummins

INTRODUCTION

In this review, I discuss the role of mitochondrial DNA in the aging ovary. The process of oogenesis is intimately involved with the transmission, possible selection and clonal amplification of the mitochondrial genome, and there is growing evidence that this interacts with the overall life cycle and with reproductive aging. As relatively little is known in detail about the way mitochondria interact with aging processes in the ovary in general, I concentrate on mitochondrial inheritance and function in the oocyte and embryo. For more comprehensive accounts of the role of the mitochondrion in the life cycle, and in particular cytoplasmic inheritance and its role in development and performance in livestock animals, see reference 1. For reviews of the role of mitochondria in disease and aging in general, see references 2 and 3. I have recently reviewed the role of mitochondria in reproduction[4]. For a discussion on the implications of cytoplasmic inheritance on epigenesis and genome imprinting, interested readers should consult recent reviews by John and Surani[5] and Latham[6].

ORIGINS OF MITOCHONDRIAL DNA

Mitochondria are probably derived from purple bacteria by an endosymbiotic process that gave the ancestral eukaryotes a means of exploiting oxygen[7]. This process could have arisen through symbiotic association of an anaerobic, hydrogen-dependent host with a symbiont that was able to respire, but that generated molecular hydrogen as a waste product of anaerobic metabolism[8]. There is much current discussion regarding the route of capture, and the mode by which ancestral cells discarded the bacterial capsule and derived a double-membrane nucleus[9,10]. The ancestral mitochondrion most probably resembled the present day *Rickettsia*, an endosymbiont of crab lice and the cause of human typhoid fever[10]. In contemporary eukaryotes, mitochondria have sacrificed much of their genome to the somatic cell nucleus. They act as subservient organelles, managing the hazardous business of oxidative phosphorylation in the cytoplasm, sequestered away from the sensitive 'master' nuclear genome.

Human mitochondria exist as a set of semi-autonomous organelles, each with several copies of their own restricted genome of 16.6 kb. This codes for 13 components of the oxidative phosphorylation pathway, two ribosomal RNAs and 22 transfer RNAs. More than 200 control genes (some estimate over 1000) are found in the nucleus[9,11]. Control is therefore complicated, involving much exchange of information between the nucleus and the many copies of mitochondrial DNA (mtDNA) in each cell's cytoplasm[11,12].

Mitochondria possess the machinery for recombination and DNA repair[13,14]. However, in general the lack of protective histones means that mtDNA mutations persist on average about 20 times more frequently than in nuclear DNA[15,16]. Mutations can take the form of single or multiple base pair replacements or modifications. Replication errors can also generate deletions by internal recombination, generally around tandem repeat 'hot spots'. Mutations and deletions are central factors in aging and mitochondrial disease progression (see below). The high mutation rate also means that nuclear genes have to evolve rapidly in concert with those of the mitochondria to maintain effective oxidative phosphorylation[17]. This also has implications for cloning technology and cytoplasmic transfer: at least one report documents altered growth and reduced muscular performance in heteroplasmic construct mice where there is a mismatch between nuclear and mtDNA[18]. While most mutations are probably lethal in embryogenesis, some survive; there is a wide range of mitochondrial diseases associated with point mutations and deletions. These are generally neuromuscular disorders that are non-Mendelian in inheritance, progressive and lethal[3]. Some groups are working towards gene therapy in mitochondrial diseases[19] and are studying the mode of inheritance in oocytes[20].

One central concept in the context of the aging oocyte is that the endosymbiotic origins of mitochondria and the evolution of aerobic metabolism in eukaryotes probably formed the basis for the evolution of active cell death. In metazoan organisms, this manifests mainly as programmed cell death, or apoptosis[21]. Mitochondria play a central role as the orchestrators of apoptosis in many systems, and in this review I concentrate on their possible influence in steering the destiny of female germ cells.

MITOCHONDRIAL DNA: INHERITANCE AND AMPLIFICATION IN THE GERM CELL LINEAGE

With very rare exceptions, mitochondria and other cytoplasmic factors such as centrioles and chloroplasts are inherited uniparentally in eukaryotic organisms[22,23]. The mechanisms that ensure uniparental inheritance are extremely diverse and have probably evolved separately many times[22]. The evolutionary reasons for this are obscure. Hurst and Hamilton[24] have suggested that it may have evolved to avoid lethal genome conflict among subservient yet essential organelles. The asymmetric life history between maternally and paternally derived mitochondrial DNA may be central to the evolution of two genders, with their complementary life histories[25].

A general rule seems to be that organisms are generally intolerant of heteroplasmy. Work with cytoplast and karyoplast transfers in cattle and mice has shown unpredictable outcomes. In many cases (but not all), there is a tendency for non-random and tissue-specific drift towards a dominant mitochondrial genome in the animals that result[26–34]. It is significant that, in the ten most famous animals cloned by nuclear transfer (Dolly and her cohort), there is no evidence of heteroplasmy. Thus, the mitochondria that may have accompanied the donor nuclei clearly did not survive[35]. Whether this is active elimination, as occurs with the sperm[4], or whether this is merely a passive or stochastic process is a fascinating topic for future research.

In mammals, sperm mitochondria enter the egg at fertilization but do not generally survive more than 2–3 days[4,36]. They are apparently tagged with ubiquitin during spermatogenesis and this is exposed by disulfide bond reduction in the glutathione-rich environment of the early embryo (Sutovsky, personal communication)[37,38]. The recognition mechanism is unknown but must be species-specific, as paternal mtDNA can survive in interspecies hybrids[39–42]. Reports of rare maternal–paternal human mtDNA recombination indicate that occasionally sperm mitochondria can evade this surveillance mechanism and fuse with an oocyte's mitochondrion[43,44]. This is not necessarily surprising, as mitochondrial fusion can occur during late oogenesis. In pigs, mitochondrial numbers are reduced by fusion to two-thirds, and mean organelle volume increases three-fold[1,45]. If such fusion or aggregation of mitochondria during late oogenesis is normal, then sperm mitochondria may become incorporated in this process. Those most likely to be captured would be those in the neck region. These disperse soon after sperm entry, to allow for spindle microtubule catalysis by the sperm centrosome – a process essential for normal male and female pronuclear apposition in non-murine mammals[23,46].

The life of mitochondria in the human germline has been reviewed by Jansen and de Boer[47], who based their work on published electron micrographs. In the earliest premigratory germ cells that have been studied, there are probably fewer than ten mitochondria. Moreover, the cells are rich in glycogen, suggesting a reliance on anaerobic metabolism, thus possibly 'sparing the mitochondria from oxidative challenge to mtDNA integrity'[47]. Mitochondria increase to around 200 in each oogonium and they take on an arched form that looks quiescent. They change from a random cytoplasmic distribution during leptotene, and move towards a perinuclear location during zygotene. They then migrate towards a pole of the cell during diplotene to form Balbiani's vitelline body[48]. During the replication of germ cells in the first half of pregnancy, mitochondria increase in number exponentially, but they do not change appearance. Most proliferation occurs close to the nucleus[49,50]. The overall number of oocytes falls from 2 million at birth to around 300 000 at menarche[51], and each resting primordial oocyte contains about 6000 mitochondria. The rapid cytoplasmic growth of the oocytes recruited for ovulation means that, when mature, mitochondrial numbers have increased to 100 000 to 400 000 in humans but each probably only contains one copy of mtDNA[47,52]. At this stage the mitochondria remain in a congregated form in the body of Balbiani[48]. The oocyte at fertilization is known to possess defined axes and gradients, which probably predetermine later cleavage planes, and even the cytoplasmic region that will later form the inner cell mass[53–55]. This process is significantly affected by blood flow and oxygen availability in the enlarging preovulatory follicle[56–58]. However, whether a particular subset of mitochondria is spatially defined at this stage is not known; moreover, eggs can survive the redistribution of organelles by centrifugation[59]. Following fertilization (in hamsters), mitochondria tend to cluster around the nuclei and in the cytocortex, indicating that these regions are particularly in need of local oxidative energy[60]. In mice, the preovulatory oocyte has around 92 500 mitochondria. Approximately 11% of the molecules are in a catenated form and there is no evidence of replication, which does not start until the egg cylinder stage at day 6.5[61–63].

It is generally assumed that mitochondria in the oocyte are relatively quiescent in early development. However, the requirements for growth during the preovulatory period mean that the needs for oxidative phosphorylation and ATP are relatively high[56]; indeed, meiotic arrest is maintained by high intracytoplasmic cAMP levels[64]. Little appears to be known about the status of oxidative phosphorylation in relation to atresia in the fetal oocytes.

EVOLUTIONARY SIGNIFICANCE OF THE MITOCHONDRIAL BOTTLENECK

A healthy complement of founding mitochondria is essential for embryonic growth and fitness after fertilization. This is apparently accomplished by a stringent genetic bottleneck in early embryogenesis[4,26,27,47,65]. This may be reinforced by the selective elimination of oogonia with defective mtDNA (see below). A genetic consequence of this is that non-deleterious mutations in germ cells can become rapidly 'fixed' in subsequent generations[66]. Various lines of evidence indicate that mitochondria in oogonia and the early embryo are quiescent and hence relatively unlikely to engender damaging reactive oxygen species (ROS)[67]. Indeed, as pointed out earlier, replication of mtDNA in the mouse embryo does not start until the egg cylinder stage at day 6.5[61–63]. One report suggests that all mtDNA in the mature human may effectively be derived from clonal expansion of a single precursor copy[68], but others report higher source numbers in mice[27]. The evidence linking oocyte atresia with specific mtDNA defects – as opposed to simple aging – is scarce[20,69,70]. Nevertheless, this is an area that deserves more research, as it may give insight into the diminishing fertility of the mammalian oocyte with age[47,71].

As asexually reproducing genomes are subject to relatively high mutation rates, mitochondria are especially liable to Müller's ratchet, the inexorable accumulation of deleterious mutations[72]. There are good theoretical grounds for arguing that a strict numerical bottleneck can counteract this, particularly if there is selection for mitochondrial fitness at the same stage of the life cycle[73,74]. In this model, Bergstrom and Pritchard[73] found that a bottleneck acts against deleterious mutations by increasing the variance in fitness between oocytes. Moreover, a selective bottleneck in theory leads to improved mitochondrial performance and can slow the progression of the ratchet.

AGING AND MITOCHONDRIA

Mitochondria play an important role in aging and neurodegenerative disorders. Deletions and mutations accumulate preferentially in post-mitotic tissues such as the heart and the central nervous system[2,75–77]. This is because, in rapidly dividing tissues, cell lines that accumulate lethal threshold levels of mtDNA die and are eliminated from the pool. Post-mitotic tissues have no such way of eliminating 'bad' mitochondria, which can therefore accumulate and eventually lead to irreparable damage. Laboratories attempting to quantify mtDNA damage generally concentrate on major deletions such as the 'common' 4977-bp deletion seen in the human, but this is purely for convenience, as it gives an unambiguous signal after amplification by the polymerase chain reaction (PCR)[78,79]. On a cautionary note, we have recently developed a competitive PCR assay for rat and human mtDNA deletions, and have found that conventional approaches can be very inaccurate. One technique using serial dilution overestimates the amount of the 'common' deletion up to 1000-fold[80]. Long PCR is a technique that couples conventional PCR with a 3′5′ exonuclease to amplify most of the mitochondrial genome. This has been used to detect multiple deletions in aging tissues[81–84]. It is now clear that the genome undergoes extensive fragmentation with aging. In very old human individuals, the amount of wild-type intact mtDNA may be down to only 11% of the total. Interestingly, specific mtDNA haplotypes are also significantly associated with long life in humans[85].

Life expectancy within a species is closely correlated with overall nuclear DNA repair efficiency and inversely with mtDNA damage. For example, mtDNA mutation and general body tumor formation rates are approximately 40-fold higher in mice than in humans[86]. While mitochondria obviously play only a part in the aging story[87], it seems clear that they hold many of the keys to life cycle dynamics through their mode of inheritance, and through tissue-specific control of energy production. There are also intriguing effects of maternal mitochondrial genotypes on human lifespan and susceptibility to disease[88].

AGING AND FEMALE REPRODUCTION

The general decline in mammalian female reproductive performance with age has been documented for many years[71,89]. For humans, declining fecundity is related to a reduction in the frequency of intercourse, and to a decrease in the numbers of primordial follicles. Towards the end of full reproductive life, follicular recruitment and ovulation occur earlier; there is a short follicular phase and total cycle length, even though ovarian steroid secretion remains normal[91]. There are also increases in the rate of aneuploidy, due primarily to non-disjunction in the second meiotic division[91–93]. Increasing maternal age is also associated with increasing rates of trisomy, dizygotic twinning and obstetric complications, decreased ratios of male to female infants and increases in maternally inherited mitochondrial diseases[94–97]. Loss of fertility in the oocyte precedes onset of the menopause, and has even been described as the 'oopause'[47,98]. This is clearly seen in donor oocyte programs, where both meiotic competence and the success of pregnancy reflect the age of the donor and not the recipient[99–101]. One can also identify cytoplasmic as well as nuclear factors in aging oocytes[102–104]. Some groups have experimented with cytoplasmic and germinal vesicle transfer, as a means of rejuvenating the oocyte in cases of poor embryo quality, or repeated failure of zygotes to develop *in vitro*[105–107].

Humans are almost unique among mammals in having a genetically programmed period of female infertility that precedes physical senescence. The menopause is a trait that is apparently only shared with Pilot whales and is thought to be very ancient in Hominid evolution[108]. Cessation of ovulation is thought to have given early humans an advantage, by facilitating transgenerational cultural transmission (the 'grandmother hypothesis')[109]. It is a good example of how, in evolutionary terms, investment in reproductive performance may be 'traded off' for investment in longevity[110,111]. Indeed, it is striking that, in *Caenorhabditis elegans*, lifespan is controlled by germline signals acting via an insulin/insulin-like growth factor (IGF) pathway that is known to regulate the aging of this organism. Mutants with reduced activity of the insulin/IGF-1 receptor homolog DAF-2 live twice as long as normal[112].

For the pituitary–gonadal axis, the menopause involves increases in pituitary gonadotropins and decreases in the secretion and synthesis of ovarian progesterone and estrogen. The ovary also shows atrophic changes including a thinner cortex, decreases in the numbers of primordial follicles and increases in the numbers of corpora albicantes and fibrous tissues[113].

THE AGING OOCYTE, MITOCHONDRIA, APOPTOSIS AND ATRESIA

The vast majority of oocytes undergo atresia in fetal life, so from a peak of 7 million in mid-gestation human females are born with about 2 million, and this declines to half a million at puberty[51]. Of these, only a few are ever released. Oocytes are maintained at the dictyate (4N) stage of meiosis prophase I, so that they are all genetically identical and there is no potential for genome conflict[114]. The earliest signs of atresia in the human ovary are nuclear degeneration, mitochondrial damage and vacuolization and dilatation of the endoplasmic reticulum. This may spread to the surrounding follicle cells, leading to true follicular (as opposed to oocyte) atresia[115]. Some germ cells may be lost by active extrusion to the celom from the fetal gonad. Survival of oocytes appears to depend critically on the establishment of a basal lamina surrounding the primordial follicle (reviewed by Motta and colleagues[115]). In human females, recruitment of follicles into the growth phase declines from about 15/day in young women, to 1/day in women aged 40. This steady decline continues into the menopause[116], which is triggered when the mean number of remaining follicles is in the order of 1100[117].

Krakauer and Mira[118] have data showing a strong cross-species positive correlation between the restriction imposed on the mitochondrial genome variance by the bottleneck, and the mean numbers of offspring produced. There is a similar but negative correlation between the rate of oocyte atresia and the minimum number of mitochondria in the founding germ cells. The net effect of the bottleneck, as Bergstrom and Pritchard[73] have pointed out (discussed above), is to amplify any genetic differences between oocytes in terms of mitochondrial genomes. They hypothesize that atresia may be a mechanism for eliminating defective mitochondria.

If this hypothesis is correct, then a key to oocyte atresia may lie in the central role that mitochondria play in the initiation of apoptosis and in regulating calcium metabolism. Apoptosis is clearly implicated in other aspects of the ovarian cycle[119–121], but what about the oocyte itself?

It is now well established that leakage of cytochrome C from dying mitochondria is a key triggering event in the cascade leading to apoptosis[122]. The outer membranes of mitochondria, the endoplasmic reticulum and the nuclear envelope express the protein Bcl-2 on their surface. Bcl-2 binds a molecule of the protein Apaf-1, which is bound in turn to a molecule of caspase 9. This is one of a family of over a dozen caspase proteases – cysteine proteases that share a conserved active site and cleave proteins at very precise sites[123]. Internal cell signals cause Bcl-2 to release the heterodimer of Apaf-1 and caspase 9, which aggregate in the cytosol. Caspase 9 cleaves and, in so doing, activates other caspases in an expanding cascade of proteolytic activity leading to digestion of structural proteins in the cytoplasm, degradation of chromosomal DNA and ultimate cell death[124,125]. Returning to the mitochondrion, it appears that cytochrome C release is controlled by two sets of proteins. Those of the Bcl-2 family inhibit cytochrome C release[126], whereas proteins that promote death (Bax and Bak) stimulate opening of a voltage-dependent channel (porin) causing water to enter the mitochondrion, which swells and dies, allowing intraorganelle factors to escape[127].

Bcl-2 also regulates calcium transport across the mitochondrial wall[128,129] and helps regulate the mitochondrial membrane potential. Breakdown in this potential is accompanied by release of damaging ROS that are normally controlled by antioxidant systems such as superoxide dismutase[130]. Homeostasis between cell death and cell proliferation thus probably relies on heterodimerism between Bcl-2 and Bax[131]. It is also modulated by nitric oxide derived from nitric oxide synthase, as knockout mice for this gene product show significant reductions in ovulatory efficiency and meiotic maturation, with many oocytes undergoing apoptosis[132].

Mitochondrial death thus involves the following sequence of events:

(1) Collapse of the mitochondrial transmembrane potential;
(2) Uncoupling of the respiratory chain and release of damaging ROS;
(3) Hyperproduction of superoxide anions;
(4) Disruption of mitochondrial biogenesis;
(5) Outflow of matrix calcium and glutathione;
(6) Release of soluble intermembrane proteins.

These ultimately lead to caspase activation with secondary endonuclease activation and consequent oligonucleosomal DNA fragmentation[133,134]. Rosse and associates[135] found that, in cells transiently transfected with the gene for Bax, the protein Bax localized to mitochondria and induced the release of cytochrome C, activation of caspase-3 and the typical events of apoptosis. On a cautionary note, they also found that cells overexpressing both Bcl-2 and Bax showed no signs of caspase activation and survived with significant amounts of cytochrome C in the cytoplasm. It is therefore possible that Bcl-2 can interfere with Bax-induced apoptosis downstream, independently of cytochrome C release.

Apoptosis is well established as the major mode of female follicle and germ cell loss across a diverse group of organisms[136,137]. It is also central to follicular atresia, to degeneration of the corpus luteum[121] and to embryo death[138]. In support of this concept, mice with targeted expression of Bcl show inhibition of follicular atresia[139] while a transgenic Bcl-2 loss-of-function mouse model showed significant reductions in germ cells colonizing the ovary[140]. Moreover, Bax-deficient female mice develop increased ovarian reserves of oocytes and show extended reproductive life[141]. Oocyte destruction caused by chemotherapy can be prevented by manipulation of apoptosis-associated signalling pathways[142], and reproductive toxicants such as anti-cancer agents and even smoking can accelerate germ cell depletion and reproductive senescence[143–145]. The machinery for apoptosis persists after ovulation and is associated with the death and fragmentation of oocytes and embryos[146,147]. Hsu and Hsueh[148] identified a novel pro-apoptotic Bcl-2 protein, Bcl-2-related ovarian killer (Bok) as well as upstream mediators for ovarian cell apoptosis. There is thus strong evidence supporting the Bcl/Bax 'rheostat' as a control mechanism for regulation of the oocyte's life cycle. However, we do not yet fully understand how apoptosis is placed in the wider context of follicular selection and dominance in the ovarian cycle[149]. Other evidence is also starting to implicate mitochondria in atretic apoptosis. Prohibitins are a family of cell-cycle regulatory inner mitochondrial membrane proteins, with potential roles in senescence, tumor suppression[150], mitochondrial inheritance[151] and lifespan[126,152]. Prohibitin immunolocalizes to the granulosa cells and oocytes of infant and juvenile rat ovaries, in the corpus luteum, as well as in follicles undergoing atresia, and may play a growth regulatory role within the ovary[153].

While mitochondria are clearly implicated in atresia, there is little direct evidence of oocyte selection that could be based on defective mtDNA. Using long PCR, Reynier and co-workers[84] found a few mtDNA rearrangements in human oocyte mitochondria. However, mitochondria in oocytes from a given donor revealed considerable heterogeneity. Keefe and colleagues[70] also found elevated levels of the 'common' 4977-bp deletion in oocytes of older women. Kitagawa and co-workers[154], using quantitative analysis, found that deleted mtDNA accumulated rapidly in the ovary at menopause while the accumulation found in abdominal muscle occurred more gradually with aging. This was confirmed by the same group when they identified the beginning of a 5-kb deletion at menopause[155]. They were unable to determine which component of the ovary contained the deletion. One possibility is that mitochondria may affect oocyte–granulosa cell interactions indirectly via calcium metabolism. Mitochondrial calcium (Ca^{2+}) homeostasis depends on close contacts with the endoplasmic reticulum and is essential in modulating organelle function[156]. Moreover, calcium signalling is intimately involved with oocyte and embryo development and the regulation of meiosis[157].

THE AGING OOCYTE, EMBRYOGENESIS AND DEVELOPMENT

There are subtle changes in oocyte cytoplasm with maternal age[158–160]. Of course, it has been known for many years that ovulated oocytes age and rapidly lose fertility both *in vivo* and *in vitro*[71]. Changes in the follicular microcirculation with age may contribute to aneuploidy[161]. Oxidative stress has been postulated as one cause of oocyte and embryo aging, through a decrease in intracellular ATP concentrations and the glutathione (GSH)/ glutathione disulfide (GSSG) ratio together with a concomitant increase in cytosolic Ca^{2+} [162]. Oocytes from older women show increases in the relative volume of mitochondria, possibly reflecting changes in oxidative phosphorylation capacity, but this is not linked to mutations in mtDNA or to functional defects of the respiratory chain enzymes[163]. Tarin and colleagues[97] have suggested that the different patterns of disease seen in offspring associated with maternal as compared to paternal aging may be explained by higher levels of oxidative stress, because their mitochondria produce higher amounts of ROS[162,164].

CONCLUSIONS AND FUTURE DIRECTIONS

While atresia and the fetal mitochondrial bottleneck appear to be linked evolutionary processes, we have yet to discover a mechanism by which 'bad' mitochondrial genomes could be selected from 'good'. The fate of germ and somatic cells in the ovary is probably decided by complex interactions between endocrine, paracrine and autocrine factors, as well as among proto-oncogenes, tumor suppressor genes, survival genes and death genes[121]. Further study of the mechanisms of ovarian apoptosis will help us understand this most mysterious phase of the life cycle. It will perhaps also enable us to develop strategies for the treatment of ovarian malfunctions, such as polycystic ovary syndrome and ovarian cancer. Understanding the dynamics of follicular growth and atresia could lead to advances in *in vitro* fertilization by permitting the growth of immature follicles *in vitro*[165]. It could also lead to better understanding of premature ovarian failure[166].

ACKNOWLEDGEMENTS

I wish to express my thanks to various colleagues who have helped in developing these thoughts: Rob Jansen, Anne Jequier, Roger Martin, Eric Shoubridge, Eric Schon, Peter Sutovsky and Jim Whelan, among others. Thanks also to Dr Egbert te Velde for inviting me to contribute and for suggesting the topic.

REFERENCES

1. Smith LC, Alcivar AA. Cytoplasmic inheritance and its effects on development and performance. *J Reprod Fertil* 1993;48(Suppl):31–43
2. Ozawa T. Genetic and functional changes in mitochondria associated with aging. *Physiol Rev* 1997;77:425–64
3. Wallace DC. Mitochondrial diseases in man and mouse. *Science* 1999;283:1482–8
4. Cummins JM. Mitochondrial DNA in mammalian reproduction. *Rev Reprod* 1998;3: 172–82
5. John RM, Surani MA. Imprinted genes and regulation of gene expression by epigenetic inheritance. *Curr Opin Cell Biol* 1996;8:348–53
6. Latham KE. Epigenetic modification and imprinting of the mammalian genome during development. *Curr Top Dev Biol* 1999;43:1–49
7. Margulis L, Sagan D. *Origins of Sex. Three Billion Years of Genetic Recombination*. New Haven: Yale University Press, 1986:258
8. Martin W, Muller M. The hydrogen hypothesis for the first eukaryote. *Nature (London)* 1998;392:37–41

9. Taanman JW. The mitochondrial genome: structure, transcription, translation and replication. *Biochim Biophys Acta Bioenerget* 1999;1401:103–23
10. Gray MW, Burger G, Lang BF. Mitochondrial evolution. *Science* 1999;283:1476–81
11. Shadel GS, Clayton DA. Mitochondrial DNA maintenance in vertebrates. *Annu Rev Biochem* 1997;68:409–35
12. Poyton RO, McEwen JE. Crosstalk between nuclear and mitochondrial genomes. *Annu Rev Biochem* 1996;65:563–607
13. Thyagarajan B, Padua RA, Campbell C. Mammalian mitochondria possess homologous DNA recombination activity. *J Biol Chem* 1996;271:27536–43
14. Bohr VA, Dianov GL. Oxidative DNA damage processing in nuclear and mitochondrial DNA. *Biochimie* 1999;81:155–60
15. Wallace DC, Ye JH, Neckelmann SN, *et al*. Sequence analysis of cDNAs for the human and bovine ATP synthase beta subunit: mitochondrial DNA genes sustain seventeen times more mutations. *Curr Genet* 1987;12:81–90
16. Pesole G, Gissi C, De Chirico A, *et al*. Nucleotide substitution rate of mammalian mitochondrial genomes. *J Mol Evol* 1999;48:427–34
17. Kenyon L, Moraes CT. Expanding the functional human mitochondrial DNA database by the establishment of primate xenomitochondrial cybrids. *Proc Natl Acad Sci USA* 1997;94:9131–5
18. Nagao Y, Totsuka Y, Atomi Y, *et al*. Decreased physical performance of congenic mice with mismatch between the nuclear and the mitochondrial genome. *Genes Genet Syst* 1998;73:21–7
19. Taylor RW, Chinnery PF, Clark KM, *et al*. Treatment of mitochondrial disease. *J Bioenerg Biomembr* 1997;29:195–205
20. Brenner CA, Wolny YM, Barritt JA, *et al*. Mitochondrial DNA deletion in human oocytes and embryos. *Mol Hum Reprod* 1998;4:887–92
21. Green DR, Reed JC. Mitochondria and apoptosis. *Science* 1998;281:1309–12
22. Birky CW. Uniparental inheritance of mitochondrial and chloroplast genes: mechanisms and evolution. *Proc Natl Acad Sci USA* 1995;92:11331–8
23. Simerly C, Wu GJ, Zoran S, *et al*. The paternal inheritance of the centrosome, the cells microtubule-organizing center, in humans, and the implications for infertility. *Nature Med* 1995;1:47–52
24. Hurst LD, Hamilton WD. Cytoplasmic fusion and the nature of sex. *Proc R Soc Lond B* 1992;247:189–94
25. Short RV. Difference between a testis and an ovary. *J Exp Zool* 1998;281:359–61
26. Jenuth JP, Peterson AC, Shoubridge EA. Tissue-specific selection for different mtDNA genotypes in heteroplasmic mice. *Nature Genet* 1997;16:93–5
27. Jenuth JP, Peterson AC, Fu K, *et al*. Random genetic drift in the female germline explains the rapid segregation of mammalian mitochondrial DNA. *Nature Genet* 1996;14:146–51
28. Meirelles FV, Smith LC. Mitochondrial genotype segregation in a mouse heteroplasmic lineage produced by embryonic karyoplast transplantation. *Genetics* 1997;145: 445–51
29. Meirelles F, Smith LC. Mitochondrial genotype segregation during preimplantation development in mouse heteroplasmic embryos. *Genetics* 1998;148:877–83
30. Steinborn R, Zakhartchenko V, Jelyazkov J, *et al*. Composition of parental mitochondrial DNA in cloned bovine embryos. *FEBS Lett* 1998;426:352–6
31. Steinborn R, Zakhartchenko V, Wolf E, *et al*. Non-balanced mix of mitochondrial DNA in cloned cattle produced by cytoplast–blastomere fusion. *FEBS Lett* 1998;426: 357–61

32. Takeda K, Takahashi S, Onishi A, *et al*. Dominant distribution of mitochondrial DNA from recipient oocytes in bovine embryos and offspring after nuclear transfer. *J Reprod Fertil* 1999;116:253–9
33. Irwin MH, Johnson LW, Pinkert CA. Isolation and microinjection of somatic cell-derived mitochondria and germline heteroplasmy in transmitochondrial mice. *Transgen Res* 1999;8:119–23
34. Hiendleder S, Schmutz SM, Erhardt G, *et al*. Transmitochondrial differences and varying levels of heteroplasmy in nuclear transfer cloned cattle. *Mol Reprod Dev* 1999;54:24–31
35. Evans MJ, Gurer C, Loike JD, *et al*. Mitochondrial DNA genotypes in nuclear transfer-derived cloned sheep. *Nature Genet* 1999;23:90–3
36. Ankel-Simons F, Cummins JM. Misconceptions about mitochondria and mammalian fertilization – implications for theories on human evolution. *Proc Natl Acad Sci USA* 1996;93:13859–63
37. Sutovsky P, Navara CS, Schatten G. Fate of the sperm mitochondria, and the incorporation, conversion, and disassembly of the sperm tail structures during bovine fertilization. *Biol Reprod* 1996;55:1195–205
38. Sutovsky P, Schatten G. Depletion of glutathione during bovine oocyte maturation reversibly blocks the decondensation of the male pronucleus and pronuclear apposition during fertilization. *Biol Reprod* 1997;56:1503–12
39. Gyllensten U, Wharton D, Wilson AC. Maternal inheritance of mitochondrial DNA during backcrossing of two species of mice. *J Hered* 1985;76:321–4
40. Gyllensten U, Wharton D, Josefsson A, *et al*. Paternal inheritance of mitochondrial DNA in mice. *Nature (London)* 1991;352:255–7
41. Kaneda H, Hayashi JI, Takahama S, *et al*. Elimination of paternal mitochondrial DNA in intraspecific crosses during early mouse embryogenesis. *Proc Natl Acad Sci USA* 1995;92:4542–6
42. Shitara H, Hayashi J, Takahama S, *et al*. Maternal inheritance of mouse mtDNA in interspecific hybrids – segregation of the leaked paternal mtDNA followed by the prevention of subsequent paternal leakage. *Genetics* 1998;148:851–7
43. Eyre-Walker A, Smith NH, Maynard Smith J. How clonal are human mitochondria? *Proc R Soc Lond B* 1999;266:477–84
44. Hagelberg E, Goldman N, Lió P, *et al*. Evidence for mitochondrial DNA recombination in a human population of island Melanesia. *Proc R Soc Lond B* 1999;266:485–92
45. Cran DG. Qualitative and quantitative structural changes during pig oocyte maturation. *J Reprod Fertil* 1985;74:237–45
46. Manandhar G, Simerly C, Salisbury JL, *et al*. Centriole and centrin degeneration during mouse spermiogenesis. *Cell Motil Cytoskel* 1999;43:137–44
47. Jansen RPS, de Boer K. The bottleneck: mitochondrial imperatives in oogenesis and ovarian follicular fate. *Mol Cell Endocrinol* 1998;145:81–8
48. Pozo J, Corral E, Pereda J. Subcellular structure of prenatal human ovary: mitochondrial distribution during meiotic prophase. *J Submicrosc Cytol Pathol* 1990;22:601–7
49. Gondos B, Westergaard L, Byskov AG. Initiation of oogenesis in the human fetal ovary: ultrastructural and squash preparation study. *Am J Obstet Gynecol* 1986;155:189–95
50. Davis AF, Clayton DA. *In situ* localization of mitochondrial DNA replication in intact mammalian cells. *J Cell Biol* 1996;135:883–93
51. Baker TG. Oogenesis and ovulation. In Austin CR, Short RV, eds. *Reproduction in Mammals. Book 1. Germ Cells and Fertilization*, 2nd edn. Cambridge: Cambridge University Press, 1982:17–45

52. Chen X, Prosser R, Simonetti S, *et al*. Rearranged mitochondrial genomes are present in human oocytes. *Am J Hum Genet* 1995;57:239–47
53. Antczak M, Van Blerkom J. Oocyte influences on early development: the regulatory proteins leptin and STAT3 are polarized in mouse and human oocytes and differentially distributed within the cells of the preimplantation stage embryo. *Mol Hum Reprod* 1997;3:1067–86
54. Edwards RG, Beard HK. Oocyte polarity and cell determination in early mammalian embryos. *Mol Hum Reprod* 1997;3:863–905
55. Gardner RL. The early blastocyst is bilaterally symmetrical and its axis of symmetry is aligned with the animal–vegetal axis of the zygote in the mouse. *Development* 1997;124:289–301
56. Van Blerkom J, Davis PW, Lee J. ATP content of human oocytes and developmental potential and outcome after *in-vitro* fertilization and embryo transfer. *Hum Reprod* 1995;10:415–24
57. Van Blerkom J, Antczak M, Schrader R. The developmental potential of the human oocyte is related to the dissolved oxygen content of follicular fluid – association with vascular endothelial growth factor levels and perifollicular blood flow characteristics. *Hum Reprod* 1997;12:1047–55
58. Van Blerkom J. Epigenetic influences on oocyte development competence: perifollicular vascularity and intrafollicular oxygen. *J Assist Reprod Genet* 1998;15: 226–34
59. Cran DG. The distribution of organelles in mammalian oocytes following centrifugation prior to injection of foreign DNA. *Gamete Res* 1987;18:67–76
60. Barnett DK, Kimura J, Bavister BD. Translocation of active mitochondria during hamster preimplantation embryo development studied by confocal laser scanning microscopy. *Dev Dynam* 1996;205:64–72
61. Pikó L, Taylor KD. Amounts of mitochondrial DNA and abundance of some mitochondrial gene transcripts in early mouse embryos. *Dev Biol* 1987;123:364–74
62. Pikó L, Matsumoto L. Numbers of mitochondria and some properties of mitochondrial DNA in the mouse egg. *Dev Biol* 1976;49:1–10
63. Taylor KD, Pikó L. Mitochondrial biogenesis in early mouse embryos – expression of the mRNAs for subunits IIV, VB, and VIIC of cytochrome C oxidase and subunit 9 (p1) of H+-ATP synthase. *Mol Reprod Dev* 1995;40:29–35
64. Eppig JJ. Coordination of nuclear and cytoplasmic oocyte maturation in eutherian mammals. *Reprod Fertil Dev* 1996;8:485–9
65. Marchington DR, Hartshorne GM, Barlow D, *et al*. Homopolymeric tract heteroplasmy in mtDNA from tissues and single oocytes – support for a genetic bottleneck. *Am J Hum Genet* 1997;60:408–16
66. Olivo PD, Van de Walle MJ, Laipis PJ, *et al*. Nucleotide sequence evidence for rapid genotypic shifts in the bovine mitochondrial DNA D-loop. *Nature (London)* 1983;306:400–2
67. Allen JF. Separate sexes and the mitochondrial theory of ageing. *J Theor Biol* 1996;180:135–40
68. Blok RB, Gook DA, Thorburn DR, *et al*. Skewed segregation of the mtDNA nt 8993 (T→G) mutation in human oocytes. *Am J Hum Genet* 1997;60:1495–501
69. Chen X, Prosser R, Simonetti S, *et al*. Deleted mitochondrial DNA molecules are present in normal human ova. *Neurology* 1994;44:A336
70. Keefe DL, Niven-Fairchild T, Powell S, *et al.* Mitochondrial deoxyribonucleic acid deletions in oocytes and reproductive ageing in women. *Fertil Steril* 1995;64: 577–83

71. Adams CE. Reproductive senescence. In Austin CR, Short RV, eds. *Reproduction in Mammals. Book 4. Reproductive Fitness*, 2nd edn. Cambridge: Cambridge University Press, 1984:210–33
72. Müller HJ. The relation of recombination to mutational advance. *Mutat Res* 1964;1:2–9
73. Bergstrom CT, Pritchard J. Germline bottlenecks and the evolutionary maintenance of mitochondrial genomes. *Genetics* 1998;149:2135–46
74. Bergstrom CT, McElhany P, Real LA. Transmission bottlenecks as determinants of virulence in rapidly evolving pathogens. *Proc Natl Acad Sci USA* 1999;96:5095–100
75. Wallace DC. Mitochondrial DNA in ageing and disease. *Sci Am* 1997;277:40–7
76. Wallace DC. Mitochondrial genetics: a paradigm for ageing and degenerative diseases? *Sc NY* 1992;256:628–32
77. Cortopassi GA, Wong A. Mitochondria in organismal ageing and degeneration. *Biochim Biophys Acta* 1999;1410:183–93
78. Soong NW, Arnheim N. Detection and quantification of mitochondrial DNA deletions. *Methods Enzymol* 1996;264:421–31
79. Zhang C, Peters LE, Linnane AW, *et al*. Comparison of different quantitative PCR procedures in the analysis of the 4977-bp deletion in human mitochondrial DNA. *Biochem Biophys Res Commun* 1996;223:450–5
80. Ahmed F, Kougianos E, Cummins JM, *et al*. Single-step method for the determination of the amount of the common deletion in mitochondrial DNA. *Biotechniques* 1999;26:290–6
81. Fromenty B, Carrozzo R, Shanske S, *et al*. High proportions of mtDNA duplications in patients with Kearns–Sayre-syndrome occur in the heart. *Am J Med Genet* 1997;71: 443–52
82. Fromenty B, Manfredi G, Sadlock J, *et al*. Efficient and specific amplification of identified partial duplications of human mitochondrial DNA by long PCR. *Biochim Biophys Acta Gene Struct Express* 1996;1308:222–30
83. Melov S, Shoffner JM, Kaufman A, *et al*. Marked increase in the number and variety of mitochondrial DNA rearrangements in ageing human skeletal muscle. *Nucleic Acids Res* 1995;23:4122–6
84. Reynier P, Chretien MF, Savagner F, *et al*. Long PCR analysis of human gamete mtDNA suggests defective mitochondrial maintenance in spermatozoa and supports the bottleneck theory for oocytes. *Biochem Biophys Res Commun* 1998;252:373–7
85. De Benedictis G, Rose IG, Carrieri G, *et al*. Mitochondrial DNA inherited variants are associated with successful ageing and longevity in humans. *FASEB J* 1999;13:1532–6
86. Cortopassi GA, Wang E. There is substantial agreement among interspecies estimates of DNA repair activity. *Mech Ageing Dev* 1996;91:211–8
87. Holliday R. *Understanding Ageing*. Cambridge: Cambridge University Press, 1995:207
88. Korpelainen H. Genetic maternal effects on human life span through the inheritance of mitochondrial DNA. *Hum Hered* 1999;49:183–5
89. Foote RH. The gametogenic function of the ageing ovary in the mammal. In Blandau RJ, ed. *Ageing Gametes. Their Biology and Pathology*. Basel: S Karger, 1975:179–200
90. Klein NA, Soules MR. Endocrine changes of the perimenopause. *Clin Obstet Gynecol* 1998;41:912–20
91. Tietze C. Reproductive span and rate of reproduction among Hutterite women. *Fertil Steril* 1957;8:89–97
92. Dailey T, Dale B, Cohen J, *et al*. Association between non-disjunction and maternal age in meiosis-II human oocytes. *Am J Hum Genet* 1996;59:176–84
93. Eichenlaub-Ritter U. Genetics of oocyte ageing. *Maturitas* 1998;30:143–69
94. Hassold TJ, Jacobs PA. Trisomy in man. *Annu Rev Genet* 1984;18:69–97

95. Berkowitz GS, Skovron ML, Lapinski RH, *et al.* Delayed childbearing and the outcome of pregnancy. *N Engl J Med* 1990;322:659–64
96. Finch CE. The evolution of ovarian oocyte decline with ageing and possible relationships to Down syndrome and Alzheimer disease. *Exp Gerontol* 1994;29:299–304
97. Tarin JJ, Brines J, Cano A. Long-term effects of delayed parenthood. *Hum Reprod* 1998;13:2371–6
98. Jansen RPS. Older ovaries: ageing and reproduction. *Med J Aust* 1995;162:623–4
99. Volarcik K, Sheean L, Goldfarb J, *et al.* The meiotic competence of *in-vitro* matured human oocytes is influenced by donor age: evidence that folliculogenesis is compromised in the reproductively aged ovary. *Hum Reprod* 1998;13:154–60
100. Sauer MV. Pregnancy wastage and reproductive ageing: the oocyte donation model. *Curr Opin Obstet Gynecol* 1996;8:226–9
101. Sauer MV. The impact of age on reproductive potential: lessons learned from oocyte donation. *Maturitas* 1998;30:221–5
102. Lim AS, Tsakok MF. Age-related decline in fertility: a link to degenerative oocytes? *Fertil Steril* 1997;68:265–71
103. Dorland M, van Kooij RJ, te Velde ER. General ageing and ovarian ageing. *Maturitas* 1998;30:113–18
104. Van Blerkom J, Sinclair J, Davis P. Mitochondrial transfer between oocytes: potential applications of mitochondrial donation and the issue of heteroplasmy. *Hum Reprod* 1998;13:2857–68
105. Alikani M, Cohen J, Tomkin G, *et al.* Human embryo fragmentation *in vitro* and its implications for pregnancy and implantation. *Fertil Steril* 1999;71:836–42
106. Cohen J, Scott R, Alikani M, *et al.* Ooplasmic transfer in mature human oocytes. *Mol Hum Reprod* 1998;4:269–80
107. Lanzendorf SE, Mayer JF, Toner J, *et al.* Pregnancy following transfer of ooplasm from cryopreserved–thawed donor oocytes into recipient oocytes. *Fertil Steril* 1999;71:575–7
108. Peccei JS, Austad SN. A hypothesis for the origin and evolution of menopause. *Maturitas* 1995;21:83–9
109. Hawkes K, O'Connell JF, Jones NGB, *et al.* Grandmothering, menopause, and the evolution of human life histories. *Proc Natl Acad Sci USA* 1998;95:1336–9
110. Perls TT, Alpert L, Fretts RCC. Middle-aged mothers live longer. *Nature (London)* 1997;389:133
111. Kirkwood TB. Ovarian ageing and the general biology of senescence. *Maturitas* 1998;30:105–11
112. Hsin H, Kenyon C. Signals from the reproductive system regulate the lifespan of *C. elegans*. *Nature (London)* 1999;399:362–6
113. Burger HG. The endocrinology of the menopause. *J Steroid Biochem Mol Biol* 1999;69:31–5
114. Mira A. Why is meiosis arrested? *J Theor Biol* 1998;194:275–87
115. Motta PM, Nottola SA, Familiari G, *et al.* Ultrastructure of human reproduction from folliculogenesis to early embryo development. A review. *Ital J Anat Embryol* 1995;100:9–72
116. Leidy LE, Godfrey LR, Sutherland MR. Is follicular atresia biphasic? *Fertil Steril* 1998;70:851–9
117. Gosden RG, Faddy MJ. Biological bases of premature ovarian failure. *Reprod Fertil Dev* 1998;10:73–8
118. Krakauer DC, Mira A. Mitochondria and germ-cell death. *Nature (London)* 1999;400: 125–6

119. Gosden R, Spears N. Programmed cell death in the reproductive system. *Br Med Bull* 1997;53:644–61
120. Kaipia A, Hsueh AJ. Regulation of ovarian follicle atresia. *Annu Rev Physiol* 1997;59: 349–63
121. Amsterdam A, Gold RS, Hosokawa K, *et al.* Crosstalk among multiple signaling pathways controlling ovarian cell death. *Trends Endocrinol Metab* 1999;10:255–62
122. Shimizu S, Narita M, Tsujimoto Y. Bcl-2 family proteins regulate the release of apoptogenic cytochrome c by the mitochondrial channel VDAC [see comments]. *Nature (London)* 1999;399:483–7
123. Garcia-Calvo M, Peterson EP, Rasper DM, *et al*. Purification and catalytic properties of human caspase family members. *Cell Death Differ* 1999;6:362–9
124. Jacobson MD, Weil M, Raff MC. Programmed cell death in animal development. *Cell* 1997;88:347–54
125. Nagata S. Apoptosis by death factor. *Cell* 1997;88:355–65
126. Dell'Orco RT, McClung JK, Jupe ER, *et al*. Prohibitin and the senescent phenotype. *Exp Gerontol* 1996;31:245–52
127. Martinou JC. Apoptosis. Key to the mitochondrial gate. *Nature (London)* 1999;399: 411–12
128. Baffy G, Miyashita T, Williamson JR, *et al*. Apoptosis induced by withdrawal of interleukin-3 (IL-3) from an IL-3-dependent hematopoietic cell line is associated with repartitioning of intracellular calcium and is blocked by enforced Bcl-2 oncoprotein production. *J Biol Chem* 1993;268:6511–19
129. Murphy AN, Bredesen DE, Cortopassi G, *et al*. Bcl-2 potentiates the maximal calcium uptake capacity of neural cell mitochondria. *Proc Natl Acad Sci USA* 1996;93: 9893–8
130. Kiningham KK, Oberley TD, Lin S-M, *et al*. Overexpression of manganese superoxide dismutase protects against mitochondrial-initiated poly(ADP-ribose) polymerase-mediated cell death. *FASEB J* 1999;13:1601–10
131. Kroemer G, Zamzami N, Susin SA. Mitochondrial control of apoptosis. *Immunol Today* 1997;18:44–51
132. Jablonka-Shariff A, Olson LM. The role of nitric oxide in oocyte meiotic maturation and ovulation: meiotic abnormalities of endothelial nitric oxide synthase knock-out mouse oocytes. *Endocrinology* 1998;139:2944–54
133. Zamzami N, Hirsch T, Dallaporta B, *et al*. Mitochondrial implication in accidental and programmed cell death: apoptosis and necrosis. *J Bioenerg Biomembr* 1997;29: 185–93
134. Trbovich AM, Hughes FM Jr, Perez GI, *et al*. High and low molecular weight DNA cleavage in ovarian granulosa cells: characterization and protease modulation in intact cells and in cell-free nuclear autodigestion assays. *Cell Death Differ* 1998;5: 38–49
135. Rosse T, Olivier R, Monney L, *et al*. Bcl-2 prolongs cell survival after Bax-induced release of cytochrome C. *Nature (London)* 1998;391:496–9
136. Morita Y, Tilly JL. Oocyte apoptosis: like sand through an hourglass. *Dev Biol* 1999;213:1–17
137. Tilly JL. Apoptosis and ovarian function. *Rev Reprod* 1996;2:162–72
138. Warner CM, Cao W, Exley GE, *et al*. Genetic regulation of egg and embryo survival. *Hum Reprod* 1998;13(Suppl 3):178–90
139. Morita Y, Perez GI, Maravei DV, *et al*. Targeted expression of Bcl-2 in mouse oocytes inhibits ovarian follicle atresia and prevents spontaneous and chemotherapy-induced oocyte apoptosis *in vitro*. *Mol Endocrinol* 1999;13:841–50

140. Ratts VS, Flaws JA, Kolp R, *et al.* Ablation of bcl-2 gene expression decreases the numbers of oocytes and primordial follicles established in the post-natal female mouse gonad. *Endocrinology* 1995;136:3665–8
141. Perez GI, Robles R, Knudson CM, *et al.* Prolongation of ovarian lifespan into advanced chronological age by Bax-deficiency. *Nature Genet* 1999;21:200–3
142. Perez GI, Knudson CM, Leykin L, *et al.* Apoptosis-associated signaling pathways are required for chemotherapy-mediated female germ cell destruction. *Nature Med* 1997;3:1228–32
143. Tilly JL. Molecular and genetic basis of normal and toxicant-induced apoptosis in female germ cells. *Toxicol Lett* 1998;103:497–501
144. te Velde ER, Dorland M, Broekmans FJ. Age at menopause as a marker of reproductive ageing. *Maturitas* 1998;30:119–25
145. Borman SM, VanDePol BJ, Kao S, *et al.* A single dose of the ovotoxicant 4-vinylcyclohexene diepoxide is protective in rat primary ovarian follicles. *Toxicol Appl Pharmacol* 1999;158:244–52
146. Perez GI, Tao XJ, Tilly JL. Fragmentation and death (a.k.a. apoptosis) of ovulated oocytes. *Mol Hum Reprod* 1999;5:414–20
147. Juriscova A, Varmuza S, Casper RF. Programmed cell death and human embryo fragmentation. *Mol Hum Reprod* 1996;2:93–8
148. Hsu SY, Hsueh AJ. Intracellular mechanisms of ovarian cell apoptosis. *Mol Cell Endocrinol* 1998;145:21–5
149. Baka SG, Toth TL, Veeck LL, *et al.* Evaluation of the spindle apparatus of *in vitro* matured human oocytes following cryopreservation. *Hum Reprod* 1995;10: 1816–20
150. Steglich G, Neupert W, Langer T. Prohibitins regulate membrane protein degradation by the m-AAA protease in mitochondria. *Mol Cell Biol* 1999;19:3435–42
151. Berger KH, Yaffe MP. Prohibitin family members interact genetically with mitochondrial inheritance components in *Saccharomyces cerevisiae. Mol Cell Biol* 1998;18: 4043–52
152. Coates PJ, Jamieson DJ, Smart K, *et al.* The prohibitin family of mitochondrial proteins regulate replicative lifespan. *Curr Biol* 1997;7:607–10
153. Thompson WE, Powell JM, Whittaker JA, *et al.* Immunolocalization and expression of prohibitin, a mitochondrial associated protein within the rat ovaries. *Anat Rec* 1999;256:40–8
154. Kitagawa T, Suganuma N, Nawa A, *et al.* Rapid accumulation of deleted mitochondrial deoxyribonucleic acid in postmenopausal ovaries. *Biol Reprod* 1993;49:730–6
155. Suganuma N, Kitagawa T, Nawa A, *et al.* Human ovarian ageing and mitochondrial DNA deletion. *Horm Res* 1993;39:16–21
156. Brini M, Pinton P, King MP, *et al.* A calcium signaling defect in the pathogenesis of a mitochondrial DNA inherited oxidative phosphorylation deficiency. *Nature Med* 1999;5:951–4
157. Tesarik J. Calcium signaling in human preimplantation development: a review. *J Assist Reprod Genet* 1999;16:216–20
158. Van Blerkom J. Occurrence and developmental consequences of aberrant cellular organization in meiotically mature human oocytes after exogenous ovarian hyperstimulation. *J Electron Microsc Tech* 1990;16:324–46
159. Van Blerkom J. Developmental failure in human reproduction associated with preovulatory oogenesis and pre-implantation embryogenesis. In Van Blerkom J, Motta P, eds. *Ultrastructure of Human Gametogenesis and Embryogenesis.* Dordrecht: Kluwer, 1989:125–80

160. Van Blerkom J. Morphodynamics of nuclear and cytoplasmic reorganization during the resumption of arrested meiosis in the mouse oocyte. *Prog Clin Biol Res* 1989;294:33–51
161. Gaulden ME. Maternal age effect: the enigma of Down syndrome and other trisomic conditions. *Mutat Res* 1992;296:69–88
162. Tarin JJ. Potential effects of age-associated oxidative stress on mammalian oocytes/embryos. *Mol Hum Reprod* 1996;2:717–24
163. Muller-Hocker J, Schafer S, Weis S, *et al.* Morphological–cytochemical and molecular genetic analyses of mitochondria in isolated human oocytes in the reproductive age. *Mol Hum Reprod* 1996;2:951–8
164. Tarin JJ. Aetiology of age-associated aneuploidy – a mechanism based on the free radical theory of ageing. *Hum Reprod* 1995;10:1563–5
165. Salha O, Abusheika N, Sharma V. Dynamics of human follicular growth and *in-vitro* oocyte maturation. *Hum Reprod Update* 1998;4:816–32
166. Bondy CA, Nelson LM, Kalantaridou SN. The genetic origins of ovarian failure. *J Women's Health* 1998;7:1225–9

15

Transgenic animal models and ovarian function

A.P.N. Themmen and A.L.L. Durlinger

INTRODUCTION

Ovarian aging can be seen in terms of quality; that is, the chance of reproductive success decreases as women reach the fourth decade of life, and becomes reduced to very low levels after 40 years of age[1], even though recruited and growing follicles are present. In ovarian aging the interplay between the ovary and the brain is very important[2]. Classical experiments in the rodent model show that aged ovaries placed under the kidney capsule in young cycling animals show a recommencement of estrous cycling and ovulations, indicating that the aging effect is not exclusive to the ovary. Furthermore, aging effects in the central nervous system lead to changes in the hypothalamic rhythms and in cycle irregularities[2]. However, in middle-aged rats it has been shown that both the ovary and the hypothalamus may contribute to the selective rise in follicle stimulating hormone (FSH) that accompanies decreased reproductive function in these animals[3–5]. In addition, the number of remaining primordial follicles in the ovary is correlated with reproductive success. Therefore, the study of the regulation of the follicular dynamics in the ovary is of great importance to our understanding of the process of ovarian aging.

Many factors and genes are involved in the correct functioning of the ovary: the recruitment of the primordial follicles, their subsequent growth, maturation and differentiation into the Graafian follicle, and successful ovulation. As a consequence, there is a multiplicity of candidates to study, to increase our knowledge of the physiological processes that are important for female fertility. Many of these factors may also contribute to the phenomenon of ovarian failure[6]. In addition, some characteristics of ovarian aging are unique to the human – the experimental animals that are most useful in the study of reproductive processes do not show all the aspects of ovarian aging as do humans; this complicates endeavors to develop animal models to study the process. However, the animal studies are essential to indicate those factors and genes that are promising targets for investigation in clinical studies.

This review highlights some of the recently developed transgenic animals that show phenotypes that are related to processes also operative in reproductive aging in women.

OVARIAN DEVELOPMENT

An illuminating example of factors that have effects on ovarian function at different periods during development and function of the ovary is stem cell factor (also known as kit-ligand) produced by the Steel (*Sl*) locus in the mouse. *Sl* together with the tyrosine kinase receptor for stem cell factor, encoded by the locus White Spotting (*W*) are essential for the migration and proliferation of primordial germ cells, and loss-of-function mutations in those loci cause infertility in both sexes, since the primordial germ cells never reach the gonadal primordium and fail to divide[7]. However, some mutations in *Sl* that do not cause complete inactivity of the growth factor, but rather aberrant regulation of expression, cause a less severe effect on ovarian development. In such mutants the ovary contains follicles, and primordial follicle formation has occurred, although these female mice are infertile, since their ovaries contain fewer oocytes and folliculogenesis is blocked at an early stage, with one layer of cuboidal granulosa cells (Sl^{pan} locus)[8], or at an even later stage (Sl^{con} locus)[9]. This difference in the timing of follicular arrest is correlated with the strength of the effect of the mutation on the expression of stem cell factor and clearly indicates that stem cell factor is involved in the regulation of primordial germ cell migration and proliferation, as well as in early follicular growth. In this respect it is of interest that added stem cell factor in cultured 4-day-old rat ovaries induces primordial follicle growth, suggesting that stem cell factor is involved in the control of primordial follicle recruitment[10].

Another gene that has an important function early in ovarian development and in the determination of primordial germ cell number is *Zfx*[11]. In the mouse, this X-chromosomal gene has two homologs on the Y chromosome (*Zfy* and *Zfy2*) and a processed derived gene on chromosome 10 (*Zfa*). The ZFX/ZFY proteins may have a role in sex differentiation or spermatogenesis. *Zfx null* mice were derived by homologous recombination and were smaller, were less viable and had fewer germ cells, similar to the phenotype found in human XO females (Turner's syndrome). Detailed examination of the developing ovaries revealed that neonatal *Zfx null* mice already show a stark reduction in the number of oocytes, and this is probably the result of a 50% reduction in the number of primordial germ cells present in the urogenital ridge early in development (11.5 d.p.c.). The relationship between growth and germ cell number may be explained by an effect of Zfx on growth of the epiblast and in that manner on the number of cells of the epiblast that are committed to the germ cell lineage[11]. In this respect, it is of interest to note that BMP-4, a member of the transforming growth factor-β (TGF-β) superfamily (see below) has been shown to play a role in the process of the determination of the size of the founding population of primordial germ cells in the allantois[12,13]. Adult female *Zfx null* mice showed decreased fertility and premature ovarian failure, i.e. the number of oocytes fell to less than 100 per ovary at 18 weeks.

ATRESIA

After the migration of the primordial germ cells to the gonadal ridge and their subsequent proliferation, the vast majority of germ cells are lost in an apoptotic process called atresia, either before follicle formation, or afterwards during the continuous influx of primordial follicles into the growing pool[14]. The effects of atresia on ovarian lifespan have been studied in a set of transgenic mouse lines[15–17] that changed the expression of two proteins that play an essential role in apoptosis in general: Bcl-2 and Bax. The Bcl-2 protein is an anti-apoptotic protein (death-repressor), which was illustrated by the phenotype of the Bcl-2 *null* mouse line that showed massive apoptosis in the thymus and spleen[18]. Analysis of the ovaries of the Bcl-2 *null* mice revealed primordial follicle-like structures without an oocyte, indicating germ cell loss as a result of apoptosis, accompanied by an expected decrease in primary and small preantral follicles[15]. This loss-of-function experiment was complemented by a gain-of-function study in which expression of Bcl-2 was targeted to growing oocytes under the control of the zona pellucida protein-3 promoter[16]. No increases in numbers of remaining primordial or primary follicles were observed in these transgenic animals, probably because the transgene is expressed in growing follicles only, and therefore does not affect the survival of oocytes in primordial follicles. However, a decrease in atresia in small preantral follicles was observed, indicating an effect of Bcl-2 slightly later[16]. The central role of the death-promoting protein Bax in ovarian atresia was illustrated by the phenotype of Bax *null* mice[17]. Primordial follicle numbers in adult Bax *null* mice were greatly enhanced, culminating in prolongation of the ovarian lifespan into advanced chronological age (20–22 months), although these aged mice failed to become pregnant, probably as a result of hypothalamic–pituitary aging.

MEMBERS OF THE TGF-β FAMILY OF GROWTH AND DIFFERENTIATION FACTORS

Several members of the TGF-β superfamily of growth and differentiation factors are expressed in the ovary. Well-known examples are of course the inhibins and activins involved in both the feedback FSH regulation by the ovary and the intraovarian processes[19]; anti-Müllerian hormone (AMH, see below)[20,21], and also growth factors such as bone and morphogenetic protein-3 (BMP-3)[22] and a complete system of BMP-4 and -7 with their receptors, are present in the ovary[23].

Recently, the role of yet another TGF-β family member, growth/differentiation factor 9 (GDF-9), has been examined in great detail. GDF-9 was cloned in a hunt for TGF-β-like factors involved in mouse development and was found to be specifically expressed in mouse and human oocytes of early primary follicles starting at the 3a stage[24–26]. The subsequently developed GDF-9 *null* mouse line revealed a block in follicle development at the primary follicle stage, with one layer of granulosa cells (stage 3b) accompanied by high luteinizing hormone (LH) and FSH levels[27,28], strongly suggesting an essential role for GDF-9 in early primary follicle development. However, in two elegant studies, Elvin and co-workers[29,30] showed that GDF-9 has a broader role in the regulation of follicular development. Thus, in the absence of GDF-9 in the GDF-9 *null* animals theca cell markers, such as 17-hydroxylase and c-kit (stem cell factor receptor) were absent, whereas the granulosa cell products α-inhibin and stem cell factor (Kit ligand) were up-regulated, indicating a direct regulatory effect of GDF-9 on these intraovarian growth factors[30]. In addition, although the granulosa cells in the blocked stage 3b follicles did not divide, they did not go into apoptosis and, upon loss of the oocyte, even formed a corpus luteum-like steroidogenic cluster of cells, although some non-luteal cell markers remained (α-inhibin and aromatase)[30].

In keeping with these observations in the GDF-9 *null* mouse model, GDF-9 stimulated the growth of rat preantral follicles *in vitro* and the production of α-inhibin in neonatal ovary explants[31]. However, the effects of GDF-9 were not confined to the early preantral follicles. In subsequent *in vitro* experiments[29], GDF-9 was found to mimic several of the effects that had been previously attributed to oocyte-produced factor(s). Thus, GDF-9 can induce several key ovarian genes, such as *StAR* (steroidogenic acute regulatory protein; involved in progesterone production which is also stimulated by GDF-9), and the enzymes hyaluronan synthase 2 (HAS2) and cyclo-oxygenase 2 (COX2), while expression of the LH receptor and urokinase plasminogen activator (uPA) were suppressed. Most importantly, with the use of cumulus complexes from which the oocyte had been removed, GDF-9 could be shown to cause cumulus expansion. These observations show that GDF-9, one of the several TGF-β family members produced in the ovary, has an important role at several stages of follicular development: GDF-9 is essential for the development of early primary follicles, is involved in the regulation of theca cell differentiation characteristics and induces an important process in successful fertilization – cumulus expansion. The importance of the growth-stimulatory effects of GDF-9 on early follicles complements the role of the pituitary gonadotropin FSH, which has similar growth effects on later follicles. Ablation of FSH signalling in FSH[32] or FSH receptor[33] *null* mice results in a block at the early tertiary follicle stage, showing that FSH is not essential for early follicular growth. Recently, a close homolog of GDF-9, GDF-9B (also called BMP-15) was identified[26,34]. GDF-9B shows a similar expression pattern to GDF-9, although the onset of GDF-9B expression in the oocyte appears to be later during follicular development.

AMH is also a TGF-β family member. It is produced by the fetal Sertoli cells in the developing testis and signals the regression of the Müllerian ducts, the *anlagen* of the female internal sex organs, in the male fetus. AMH is also expressed in the postnatal ovary in preantral (from the primary stage onward) and small antral follicles, but completely disappears in the larger antral follicles and in Graafian follicles[20,21]. An inhibitory effect of AMH on FSH-induced granulosa cell parameters has been demonstrated[35]. Notwithstanding the absence of a clear ovarian effect in the AMH and AMH type II receptor *null* mice[36,37], we decided to investigate follicular dynamics in AMH *null* mouse ovaries in detail[38].

Ovaries of AMH *null* mice and their heterozygous and wild-type littermates were examined at 25 days, 4 months and 13 months of age. These ages were chosen to represent three different stages in the reproductive life of the female mouse. At 25 days of age, female mice are prepubertal and do not have estrous cycles; at 4 months of age, the females are at the height of their reproductive life; and at 13 months of age, the females have almost reached reproductive cessation[39]. Ovaries of 4-month-old AMH *null* mice were found to be significantly larger (23 ± 3 mg; mean weight ± SEM) than the ovaries from heterozygous (18 ± 1 mg) and wild-type mice (13 ± 1 mg). Detailed follicle counting in the sectioned ovaries from these 4-month-old mice revealed that this weight increase was caused by an almost three-fold increase in the number of small follicles, i.e. preantral and small antral follicles with a diameter less than 310 μm. The number of larger follicles was very small in females of all

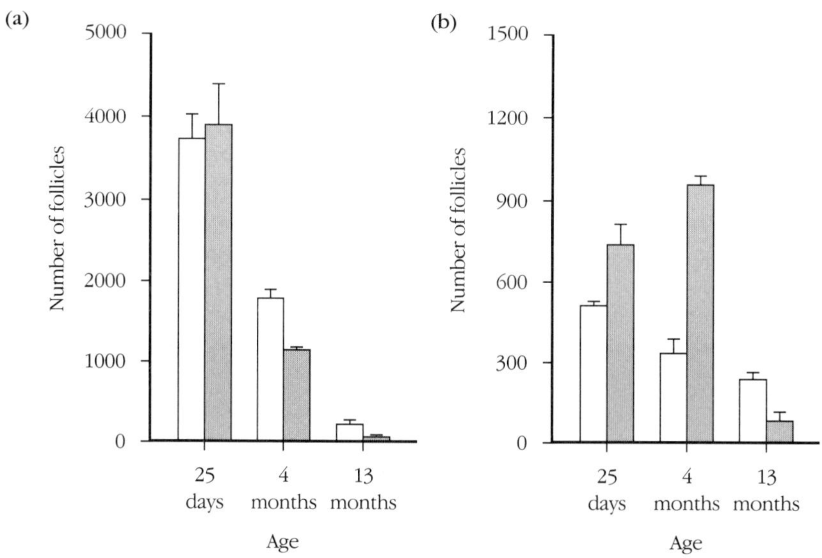

Figure 1 Ablation of anti-Müllerian hormone (AMH) expression resulted in increased primordial follicle depletion and increased small follicular growth. Ovaries of AMH *null* and wild-type mice at the indicated ages were sectioned, and the numbers of primordial (a) and preantral and small antral growing follicles (b) were determined. Open bars, wild-type animals; hatched bars, AMH *null* animals

three ages. This was expected, since in immature 25-day-old animals growing follicles become atretic before they reach this stage of follicular development[40]. The cycling animals of 4 and 13 months of age were killed on the day of estrus, a time point during the estrous cycle when no large follicles have yet developed[41,42]. The increase in the number of small follicles at 4 months was accompanied by a large decrease in the number of primordial follicles. This effect of the absence of AMH on growing follicles in the ovary was already apparent in prepubertal animals (25 days old). In the aged animals, almost all primordial follicles were lost, which also resulted in a paucity of growing small follicles (Figure 1). It is of interest to note that, in almost all females heterozygous for the AMH *null* mutation, the number of follicles fell in between the numbers found in wild-type and AMH *null* females. For other gene knockout animal models, such as activin *null* mice or FSH *null* mice[32,43], such a gene dosage effect has not been reported. Moreover, Müllerian duct regression in male AMH *null* mice occurred to the same extent as in heterozygous males[36]. The AMH gene dose dependency observed in the present study may indicate that ovarian AMH production or secretion is not under stringent feedback control, but rather depends on the intrinsic activity of the gene itself.

Thus, AMH plays an important role in primordial follicle recruitment, such that more primordial follicles are recruited in AMH *null* mice than in wild-type mice. Consequently, the ovaries of AMH *null* females show a relatively early depletion of their stock of primordial follicles and the female AMH *null* mouse therefore provides a useful model to study the regulation of primordial follicle recruitment and the relationship between follicular dynamics and ovarian aging.

This short overview of some of the recently developed transgenic mouse models reveals that, in addition to classical hormones such as FSH and LH, many different factors are of essence in correct ovarian functioning. Such factors are good candidates for the study of the demise of primordial follicles in the human ovary that accompanies ovarian aging and menopause.

REFERENCES

1. te Velde ER, Scheffer GJ, Dorland M, *et al*. Developmental and endocrine aspects of normal ovarian ageing. *Mol Cell Endocrinol* 1998;145:67–73
2. Wise PM, Smith MJ, Dubal DB, Wilson ME, Krajnak KM, Rosewell KL. Neuroendocrine influences and repercussions of the menopause. *Endocr Rev* 1999;20:243–8
3. Knobil E. The neuroendocrine control of the menstrual cycle. *Recent Prog Horm Res* 1980;36:53–88
4. DePaolo LV, Chappel SC. Alterations in the secretion and production of follicle-stimulating hormone precede age-related lengthening of estrous cycles in rats. *Endocrinology* 1986;118:1127–33
5. DePaolo LV. Age-associated increases in serum follicle-stimulating hormone levels on estrus are accompanied by a reduction in the ovarian secretion of inhibin. *Exp Aging Res* 1987;13:3–7

6. Bondy CA, Nelson LM, Kalantaridou SN. The genetic origins of ovarian failure. *J Womens Health* 1998;7:1225–9
7. Besmer P, Manova K, Duttlinger R, *et al*. The kit-ligand (steel factor) and its receptor c-kit/W: pleiotropic roles in gametogenesis and melanogenesis. *Development* 1993;(suppl):125–37
8. Huang EJ, Manova K, Packer AI, *et al*. The murine steel panda mutation affects kit ligand expression and growth of early ovarian follicles. *Dev Biol* 1993;157:100–9
9. Bedell MA, Brannan CI, Evans EP, *et al*. DNA rearrangements located over 100 kb 5′ of the Steel (Sl)-coding region in Steel-panda and Steel-contrasted mice deregulate Sl expression and cause female sterility by disrupting ovarian follicle development. *Genes Dev* 1995;9:455–70
10. Parrott JA, Skinner MK. Kit-ligand/stem cell factor induces primordial follicle development and initiates folliculogenesis. *Endocrinology* 1999;140:4262–71
11. Luoh SW, Bain PA, Polakiewicz RD, *et al*. Zfx mutation results in small animal size and reduced germ cell number in male and female mice. *Development* 1997;124:2275–84
12. Lawson KA, Dunn NR, Roelen BA, *et al*. Bmp4 is required for the generation of primordial germ cells in the mouse embryo. *Genes Dev* 1999;13:424–36
13. McLaren A. Signaling for germ cells. *Genes Dev* 1999;13:373–6
14. Hsueh AJ, Billig H, Tsafriri A. Ovarian follicle atresia: a hormonally controlled apoptotic process. *Endocr Rev* 1994;15:707–24
15. Ratts VS, Flaws JA, Kolp R, *et al*. Ablation of bcl-2 gene expression decreases the numbers of oocytes and primordial follicles established in the post-natal female mouse gonad. *Endocrinology* 1995;136:3665–8
16. Morita Y, Perez GI, Maravei DV, *et al*. Targeted expression of Bcl-2 in mouse oocytes inhibits ovarian follicle atresia and prevents spontaneous and chemotherapy-induced oocyte apoptosis *in vitro*. *Mol Endocrinol* 1999;13:841–50
17. Perez GI, Robles R, Knudson CM, *et al*. Prolongation of ovarian lifespan into advanced chronological age by Bax-deficiency. *Nature Genet* 1999;21:200–3
18. Veis DJ, Sorenson CM, Shutter JR, Korsmeyer SJ. Bcl-2-deficient mice demonstrate fulminant lymphoid apoptosis, polycystic kidneys, and hypopigmented hair. *Cell* 1993;75:229–40
19. Matzuk MM, Kumar TR, Shou W, *et al*. Transgenic models to study the roles of inhibins and activins in reproduction, oncogenesis, and development. *Recent Prog Horm Res* 1996;51:123–54; discussion 155–7
20. Baarends WM, Uilenbroek JT, Kramer P, *et al*. Anti-mullerian hormone and anti-mullerian hormone type II receptor messenger ribonucleic acid expression in rat ovaries during postnatal development, the estrous cycle, and gonadotropin-induced follicle growth. *Endocrinology* 1995;136:4951–62
21. Baarends WM, van Helmond MJ, Post M, *et al*. A novel member of the transmembrane serine/threonine kinase receptor family is specifically expressed in the gonads and in mesenchymal cells adjacent to the mullerian duct. *Development* 1994;120:189–97
22. Jaatinen R, Rosen V, Tuuri T, Ritvos O. Identification of ovarian granulosa cells as a novel site of expression for bone morphogenetic protein-3 (BMP-3/osteogenin) and regulation of BMP-3 messenger ribonucleic acids by chorionic gonadotropin in cultured human granulosa–luteal cells. *J Clin Endocrinol Metab* 1996;81:3877–82
23. Shimasaki S, Zachow RJ, Li D, *et al*. A functional bone morphogenetic protein system in the ovary. *Proc Natl Acad Sci USA* 1999;96:7282–7
24. Pedersen T. Follicle growth in the immature mouse ovary. *Acta Endocrinol (Copenh)* 1969;62:117–32

25. McGrath SA, Esquela AF, Lee SJ. Oocyte-specific expression of growth/differentiation factor-9. *Mol Endocrinol* 1995;9:131–6
26. Laitinen M, Vuojolainen K, Jaatinen R, *et al.* A novel growth differentiation factor-9 (GDF-9) related factor is co-expressed with GDF-9 in mouse oocytes during folliculogenesis. *Mech Dev* 1998;78:135–40
27. Dong J, Albertini DF, Nishimori K, *et al.* Growth differentiation factor-9 is required during early ovarian folliculogenesis. *Nature (London)* 1996; 383:531–5
28. Carabatsos MJ, Elvin J, Matzuk MM, Albertini DF. Characterization of oocyte and follicle development in growth differentiation factor-9-deficient mice. *Dev Biol* 1998; 204:373–84
29. Elvin JA, Clark AT, Wang P, *et al.* Paracrine actions of growth differentiation factor-9 in the mammalian ovary. *Mol Endocrinol* 1999;13:1035–48
30. Elvin JA, Yan C, Wang P, *et al.* Molecular characterization of the follicle defects in the growth differentiation factor 9-deficient ovary. *Mol Endocrinol* 1999;13:1018–34
31. Hayashi M, McGee EA, Min G, *et al.* Recombinant growth differentiation factor-9 (GDF-9) enhances growth and differentiation of cultured early ovarian follicles. *Endocrinology* 1999;140:1236–44
32. Kumar TR, Wang Y, Lu N, Matzuk MM. Follicle stimulating hormone is required for ovarian follicle maturation but not male fertility. *Nature Genet* 1997;15:201–4
33. Dierich A, Sairam MR, Monaco L, *et al.* Impairing follicle-stimulating hormone (FSH) signaling *in vivo*: targeted disruption of the FSH receptor leads to aberrant gametogenesis and hormonal imbalance. *Proc Natl Acad Sci USA* 1998;95:13612–17
34. Dube JL, Wang P, Elvin J, *et al.* The bone morphogenetic protein 15 gene is X-linked and expressed in oocytes. *Mol Endocrinol* 1998;12:1809–17
35. di Clemente N, Goxe B, Rémy JJ, *et al.* Effect of AMH upon aromatase activity and LH receptors of granulosa cells of rat and porcine immature ovaries. *Endocrine* 1994;2: 553–8
36. Behringer RR, Finegold MJ, Cate RL. Mullerian-inhibiting substance function during mammalian sexual development. *Cell* 1994;79:415–25
37. Mishina Y, Rey R, Finegold MJ, *et al.* Genetic analysis of the Mullerian-inhibiting substance signal transduction pathway in mammalian sexual differentiation. *Genes Dev* 1996;10:2577–87
38. Durlinger ALL, Kramer P, Karels B, *et al.* Control of primordial follicle recruitment by anti-mullerian hormone in the mouse ovary. *Endocrinology* 1999;140:5789–96
39. Gosden RG, Laing SC, Felicio LS, *et al.* Imminent oocyte exhaustion and reduced follicular recruitment mark the transition to acyclicity in ageing C57BL/6J mice. *Biol Reprod* 1983;28:255–60
40. Sander HJ, Meijs-Roelofs HM, van Leeuwen EC, *et al.* Inhibin increases in the ovaries of female rats approaching first ovulation: relationships with follicle growth and serum FSH concentrations. *J Endocrinol* 1986;111:159–66
41. Welschen R, Rutte M. Ovulation in adult rats after treatment with pregnant mare serum gonadotrophin during oestrus. *Acta Endocrinol (Copenh)* 1971;68:41–9
42. Osman P. Rate and course of atresia during follicular development in the adult cyclic rat. *J Reprod Fertil* 1985;73:261–70
43. Matzuk MM, Kumar TR, Bradley A. Different phenotypes for mice deficient in either activins or activin receptor type II. *Nature (London)* 1995;374:356–60

16

Premature ovarian failure

Y.M. van Kasteren

INTRODUCTION

At the age of 40 years, 1% of all women have already gone through their menopause[1]. About 10% of all women evaluated for secondary amenorrhea will be diagnosed to have premature ovarian failure (POF)[2,3]. Apart from the usual climacteric symptoms they suffer from the psychological burden of feeling old prematurely. For many POF patients reproductive failure is one of the most troublesome features of the disease. In the era of assisted reproductive technology (ART), oocyte donation offers a realistic option. Nevertheless, the primary intention of infertile women (and men) was, and still is, to reproduce with their own gametes.

PREMATURE OVARIAN FAILURE

Definition

The definition still gives rise to controversy on three issues: the inclusion of primary or secondary amenorrhea, the duration of amenorrhea and the level of serum follicle stimulating hormone (FSH). Coulam[4] defined POF as cessation of ovarian function after puberty and before the age of 40, and after normal development of secondary sexual characteristics. This definition excludes cases of hypergonadotropic primary amenorrhea. These cases should be labelled as primary gonadal failure[4].

Duration of amenorrhea is another point of controversy. Originally, the definition stated 'menopause at or before age 40', meaning that the diagnosis could be made only in retrospect, 12 months after the last menstrual period. Currently, most authors use the definition of amenorrhea of 4–6 months, some even only 2 months[5]. The serum level of FSH, by which POF is defined, varies from > 10 IU/l to > 40 IU/l[6]. Most authors use a serum FSH level of > 40 IU/l. Often ovarian failure will develop gradually, with the same waxing and waning of the hormonal status and the clinical picture as in the normal perimenopausal period, until a true postmenopausal status has been established. Therefore, every cut-off level will be arbitrary.

It seems likely that the four known entities – ovarian dysgenesis (no development of secondary sexual characteristics), primary ovarian failure (primary hypergonadotropic amenorrhea with at least some development of secondary sexual characteristics), premature ovarian failure (secondary hypergonadotropic amenorrhea) and incipient ovarian failure (regular menstrual cycles, with elevated early follicular FSH and infertility) – form a continuous spectrum. Any separation will be artificial. However, for research purposes it is important to define criteria as strictly as possible.

Etiology

Iatrogenic

Radiation exposure and chemotherapy now successfully control childhood cancers. Therefore, we will increasingly be confronted with late sequelae such as infertility due to ovarian failure[7,8]. Conway[7] reported the percentage of ovarian failure due to chemotherapy and radiation therapy to be 6% and 2%, respectively.

It is self-evident that bilateral oophorectomy will induce immediate and total ovarian failure; however, repeated and extensive ovarian surgery may also destroy the oocyte pool prematurely[8].

Infectious

It has been suggested that severe pelvic inflammatory disease (PID) and viral infection in adult life may destroy oocytes. Mumps may even induce loss of fetal oocytes[8,9].

Enzyme deficient

Galactosemia is associated with POF, possibly through destruction of oocytes by toxic metabolites[10,11]. Other authors suggest a role of aberrant glycosylation. The prevalence of galactosemia among patients with ovarian failure is 2%. Deficiency of the 17α-hydroxylase enzyme, usually with a total lack of substrate for estrogen production, causes hypergonadotropic primary amenorrhea. However, a few cases of secondary ovarian failure have been described[12].

Genetic

Patients with an abnormal karyotype constitute between 2.5 and 13.3% of POF patients[13–16]. The prevalence of an abnormal karyotype is much higher among patients with ovarian dysgenesis and primary ovarian failure[7,17].

The lack of one X chromosome (XO or Turner's syndrome) is associated with early oocyte depletion, usually, but not always, leading to primary amenorrhea. The mechanism is still unknown[18]. Patients with mosaicism karyotypes (46,XX/45,X) may develop secondary ovarian failure and can be fertile. Smaller deletions of either the short arm or the long arm of the X chromosome can also coincide with POF[19–21]. It is not clear whether this is also caused by a depletion of oocytes. Studies on breakpoints on the long arm of the X chromosome led to the concept of the 'critical region', located between Xq13 and Xq26. This region should remain intact for adequate ovarian function.

Triple X syndrome can coincide with POF, especially when a multiple mosaicism is present containing a 45,XO cell line. However, most of the triple X females will have normal ovarian function[22].

Gene mutations on the X chromosome, like the premutation of the *FRM1* gene (full mutation causes the fragile X syndrome) and the disruption of the *DIA* gene (the human homolog for the diaphanous gene in *Drosophila*), can cause premature ovarian failure by a still unknown mechanism[23–25].

Autosomes can also be involved in the development of ovarian failure. The blepharophimosis epicanthus inversus ptosis syndrome (BEPS I) is associated with primary and secondary amenorrhea. The cause of BEPS I syndrome has been mapped to the long arm of chromosome 3[26,27]. Mutation of the FSH-receptor gene on the short arm of chromosome 2 may cause a non-functional FSH receptor[28]. Mutations in the gene coding for the β-subunit of FSH on chromosome 11 create a biologically inactive FSH molecule[29,30]. In both cases normal oocytes cannot be stimulated to develop and the clinical picture of primary gonadal failure follows. This is not a cause of secondary ovarian failure. Patients with mutations in the *ATM* gene (ataxia telangiectasia) on chromosome 11q22–23 develop either primary or secondary ovarian failure due to early apoptotic degeneration of oocytes[31] (for review see reference 32).

Autoimmune

POF in association with Addison's disease, often as part of an autoimmune polyendocrinopathy syndrome (APS 1 or 2), is thought to be an autoimmune disorder[33,34] (for review see references 35 and 36). APS 1 might be linked to a defect in the *AIRE* gene on chromosome 21 (AIRE stands for 'autoimmune regulator'). The majority of these patients show specific antibodies against steroid-producing cells of the ovary and the adrenal[37–41]. Biopsies of the ovaries may show a lymphocyte and plasma cell infiltration around developing follicles in the ovaries[41,42]. Cystic enlargement may be part of the clinical picture[42], but the end stage will probably be atrophy. This was an infrequent cause of POF (1%) among a population of POF patients attending a reproductive endocrinology unit[7]. The endocrinologist, however, may encounter this form of POF more frequently.

Idiopathic

Despite the above-mentioned considerations, in the majority of POF patients a cause cannot be identified. Hence, the diagnosis is idiopathic POF. This group is probably still heterogeneous. Genetic factors may be involved.

Analogous to the male, microdeletions on the X chromosome may be detected. Recently, Devi and colleagues[43] showed that idiopathic POF patients had more XO cells per 100 cells than did controls, and they suggested a role for low-grade 46,XX/45,X mosaicism in the etiology of idiopathic POF.

Idiopathic POF may also be related to autoimmunity. This assumption is based on the following observations. First, POF without Addison's disease is associated with other endocrinopathies with a known autoimmune cause, most frequently thyroid disease[2,3,44]. Second, there is a high prevalence of non-specific and organ-specific autoantibodies in POF patients[14,45–47]. Apart from the antibodies against steroid-producing cells, which occur exclusively in autoimmune POF associated with Addison's disease, anti-ovarian antibodies have been detected in POF patients by radioimmunoassay, immunofluorescence, immunohistochemistry and enzyme-linked immunosorbent assay[48–51]. However, cross-reactivity with tubal antigens has been described[51]. Moreover, these antibodies were also detected in patients with Turner's syndrome and iatrogenic POF[51]. Some authors also found a possible relationship between ovarian antibodies and ovarian damage as caused by repeated *in vitro* fertilization (IVF) punctures[52,53]. The evidence for the existence of FSH and luteinizing hormone (LH) receptor-blocking antibodies is still scarce[54,55]. Third, changes in lymphocyte subsets have been found[47,56–58]. It has been postulated that these changes might be indicative of the central autoimmune process, with the production of autoantibodies evolving secondarily[35,36]. Recently, we performed a multicenter trial, comparing immune parameters in patients with POF and incipient ovarian failure (IOF) with controls[59]. We did not find differences in the prevalence of autoantibodies. However, we did find changes in lymphocyte subsets between all three groups, with IOF patients taking an intermediate position between controls and POF patients. The question remains, however, whether these are causative or merely epiphenomena.

Environmental factors, such as growth restriction[60], may negatively influence the migration, proliferation and maturation of oocytes prenatally. In adult life, smoking is an established environmental factor that advances age at menopause[61]. Overall, more than 60% of POF cases will be classified as idiopathic[8].

Diagnostic tests in the context of prognosis and treatment

Laparoscopy and ultrasonography

Idiopathic POF probably consists of afollicular and follicular forms. Since differentiation between these forms would be essential in evaluating therapeutic interventions, several authors have performed biopsies or wedge resections either by laparoscopy or by laparotomy. As is apparent from the studies listed in Table 1[3,62–75], about 40% of all such patients still have follicles in their ovaries. Subsequently, Mehta *et al.*[76] and others[8] confirmed by ultrasound that, in 41% of patients with POF, follicle-like structures could be visualized. Both techniques do not identify the same group of patients. Biopsies show primordial, primary and secondary follicles, whereas ultrasound identifies only antral follicles. Ultrasound will more accurately identify small antral follicles in the whole ovary, whereas biopsies may not be representative of the whole ovary. Several authors have reported pregnancies occurring in patients with negative biopsies[77,78]. Neither technique has been proven to be able to predict the potential of a patient to become pregnant. As it also has no consequences for the treatment of POF patients, diagnostic laparoscopy with ovarian biopsy has become an obsolete procedure in current practice.

Autoantibodies

The presence of autoantibodies against steroid-producing cells of adrenal and ovarian origin may indicate an autoimmune disorder. Almost all patients with POF and Addison's disease showed antibodies directed towards steroid-producing cells[36]. This form of POF is probably an autoimmune oophoritis, and may respond to corticosteroid treatment[79–81]. Autoantibodies against the thyroid and adrenal can precede the onset of disease by several years. Betterle and colleagues[82] found progression to Addison's disease in 21% of patients positive for antibodies against the adrenal cortex (ACA) and progression to subclinical stages in 29%, within a follow-up period ranging from 0.5 to 13 years. Knowledge of the presence or absence of these antibodies can be helpful in the counselling of patients. Other autoantibodies do not influence the treatment or prognosis in POF patients. However, the prevalence of ACA antibodies and/or antibodies against steroid-producing cells (SCA) varies widely, depending on the population. Betterle and associates[39]

Table 1 Results of ovarian biopsies in studies of patients with premature ovarian failure

First author	*Year of publication*	*Number of patients*	*Number of ovarian follicles*		
			None	*Few*	*Numerous*
Kinch[62]	1965	9	6	1	2
Emperaire[63]	1970	7	5	2	0
Zarate[64]	1970	7	4	3	0
Sharf[65]	1972	10	8	2	0
Starup[66]	1973	15	7	6	2
Falk[67]	1977	3	2	1	0
Duignan[68]	1978	8	3	3	2
Board[69]	1979	8	2	4	2
Rebar[70]	1982	9	5	4	0
Russell[71]	1982	19	14	0	5
Menon[72]	1984	43	27	16	0
Aiman[3]	1985	14	9	2	3
Miyaka[73]	1987	10	10	0	0
Rebar[74]	1990	12	5	7	0
Muechler[75]	1991	17	12	2	3
Total		191	119	53	19

found ACA in 10% of POF patients without other autoimmune diseases and in 20% in POF patients with other autoimmune diseases, other than Addison's disease. Almost all ACA-positive patients also showed SCA. Sotsiou and co-workers[37] found ACA in 7% of patients with autoimmune diseases other than Addison's disease, but only 19% of these ACA-positive patients showed SCA. Mignot and colleagues[45] found a prevalence of 15% for ACA (3/20) and 6% for SCA (1/16) in their population. Conway and co-workers[6] found a prevalence of 3% for ACA and 1% of SCA in a group of 97 POF patients. Van Kasteren and colleagues[83,84] found neither ACA nor SCA in the 63 POF patients participating in two randomized trials. The last three studies involved a POF population primarily recruited for reproductive issues, while the first two studies recruited patients on other grounds. Hence, it may be worthwhile to screen POF patients attending a center for endocrinology and internal diseases and it may not be worthwhile to screen POF patients attending a center for reproductive endocrinology.

Genetic screening

Genetic screening on chromosomal aberrations has no bearing on the prognosis of pregnancy or on the treatment of a POF patient. It may, however, have great bearing on the prognosis of the future fertility of daughters. The prevalence of familial cases amongst POF patients varies widely, from 4 to 31%[73,85–87]. The mode of inheritance is compatible with X-linked or autosomal dominant transmission, either maternal or paternal[85–87]. Therefore, the risk for female relatives of developing POF may be as high as 100%, whereas the standard risk is only 1%. As the prevalence of the premutation of the *FRM1* gene is 2% among sporadic cases and 8% among familial cases, screening for the premutation should be considered in all POF patients[88].

Bone mineral density

The general attitude is to advise POF patients to use hormone replacement therapy (HRT) at least until the normal expected age of menopause. However, in the absence of symptoms, the need for HRT is still open for discussion. Measuring bone mineral density (BMD) can identify patients with abnormal and normal values. Metka and colleagues[89] showed that 50% of untreated hypergonadotropic women had a pathological BMD. Moreover, Davies and co-workers[90] found that 5% of young amenorrheic women had evidence of atraumatic fractures. Thus, it is essential to measure BMD if HRT is rejected. Furthermore, women with an extremely low BMD can be detected and advised on additive treatment to HRT.

Mammography

It is not yet clear whether we should advise POF patients on HRT to undergo mammography every 2 years, as we advise the older perimenopausal women on HRT. Young women on oral contraceptives are not submitted to such a surveillance program.

A negative aspect of long-term HRT might be a slight increase in the risk of breast cancer[91]. However, almost all data on the effect of HRT concern older women on HRT. Even these data are still controversial. Specific studies on long-term aspects of HRT in POF patients are still lacking[91]. However, several authors have found a reduced risk of breast cancer with early menopause[92–95]. Thus, HRT might only increase the risk of breast cancer in POF women to normal. This assumption is supported by the data of Willis and associates[96], who found a decreased risk of fatal breast cancer in women with ever use of HRT, most pronounced in women with a natural menopause before 40 years of age. The data suggest that serial mammography can be postponed at least until after the age of 40 years.

REPRODUCTION

Recently van Kasteren and Schoemaker[97] performed a literature search to evaluate the possibility of pregnancy following diagnosis and the additional value of treatment strategies. They found 59 case reports (Table 2), eight observational studies (Table 3), nine uncontrolled studies (Table 4) and seven controlled trials (Table 5). The data of the observational studies, the uncontrolled studies and the controlled studies were used to determine the overall pregnancy rate per patient. The results of all pregnancies reported gave an impression of the live birth rate. The controlled trials were evaluated to determine the additional value of treatment.

Pregnancy and live birth

In the observational studies, 4.8% of all women became pregnant; in the uncontrolled studies, 18% became pregnant; and in the controlled studies, 1.5% became pregnant. Overall, 6.3% of all women conceived after diagnosis (Table 6). About 80% of the authors gave information on pregnancy results. A total of 112 pregnancies were available for analysis. Three pregnancies were terminated on request and five were still ongoing. Nineteen pregnancies resulted in a miscarriage, one in a stillbirth at term and one in a tubal pregnancy. Thus, 104 pregnancies resulted in the birth of 86 healthy babies (there were three twin pregnancies). No reports were found on congenital malformations or chromosomal aberrations such as trisomy 21.

Fertility treatment

The seven controlled trials tested three hypotheses. The first hypothesis was that pituitary suppression, with either gonadotropin releasing hormone agonists or estrogens, would improve ovarian responsiveness to endogenous or

Table 2 Case reports showing pregnancies after diagnosis of premature ovarian failure

Intervention	*No. of patients pregnant*
No therapy	11
Estrogens only	32
Estrogens combined	9
Other drugs	7
Total	59

Table 3 Observational studies of patients with premature ovarian failure

First author	*Year*	*No. of patients*	*No. of patients pregnant*
O'Herlihy[98]	1980	67	6
Aiman[3]	1985	35	2
Kreiner[99]	1988	86	3
Rebar[100]	1990	115	8
Eden[17]	1993	75	5
Sauer[101]	1995	200	5
Fenichel[48]	1997	47	4
Conway[7]	1997	135	4
Total		760	37

Table 4 Uncontrolled intervention trials after diagnosis of premature ovarian failure

First author	*Year*	*No. of patients*	*No. of patients pregnant*	*Therapy*
Tanaka[102]	1982	6	1	hMG
Ylostalo[103]	1982	5	3	estrogens
Menon[104]	1983	4	0	GnRH-a
Boyers[105]	1988	19	0	hMG
Ledger[106]	1989	12	0	GnRH-a
Check[107]	1990	91	19	estrogens + hMG
		9	0	GnRH-a + hMG
Buckler[108]	1993	8	0	oral contraceptives
Blumenfeld[109]	1993	15	8	corticosteroids ± GnRH-a and hMG
Corenblum[81]	1993	11	2	corticosteroids
Total		180	33	

hMG, human menopausal gonadotropin; GnRH-a, gonadotropin releasing hormone agonists

exogenous gonadotropins. The second hypothesis was that ovarian responsiveness would be improved immediately after suppression with gonadotropins or estrogens. The third hypothesis was that immunosuppressives might improve ovarian responsiveness to either endogenous or exogenous gonadotropins. None of the studies found a statistically significant difference between the two study groups. Owing to a strong variability in study design, patient selection and mode of intervention, it was not possible to combine the data of the seven studies to perform a meta-analysis. There was no evidence to indicate preference of one specific treatment or preference of treatment over no treatment. Therefore, a trial of ovulation induction should not be performed outside a research setting.

Table 5 Results of seven controlled studies of patients with premature ovarian failure

First author	*Year of publication*	*No. of patients*	*No. of patients pregnant*	*Design*	*Intervention*
Surrey[110]	1989	14	0	mixed	hMG after cyclic HRT vs. hMG + estrogens vs. hMG + GnRH-a
Nelson[111]	1992	23	1	cross-over	rebound phase after GnRH-a + cyclic HRT vs. placebo + cyclic HRT
Rosen[112]	1992	8	0	cross-over	hMG vs. no therapy in the rebound phase after cyclic HRT
Anasti[113]	1994	46	0	cross-over	rebound phase after danazol vs. rebound phase after combined HRT
van Kasteren[83]	1995	30	0	parallel groups	GnRH-a + hMG vs. placebo + hMG
Taylor[5]	1996	37	2	cross-over	estradiol vs. no therapy
van Kasteren[84]	1999	36	0	parallel groups	corticosteroids + hMG vs. placebo + hMG
Total		194	3		

hMG, human menopausal gonadotropin; HRT, hormone replacement therapy; GnRH-a, gonadotropin releasing hormone agonists

Table 6 Pregnancy rate per patient in studies of premature ovarian failure

Study type	*Number of patients*	*Pregnancy rate per patient (%)*
Observational studies	760	4.8
Uncontrolled studies	180	18.3
Controlled studies	194	1.5
Total	1134	6.4

FUTURE PERSPECTIVES

Further research should first be directed at exploring the pathogenesis of ovarian failure. This could be achieved by clinical research in patients with incipient ovarian failure and by investigating genetically engineered mouse models. Second, improvement of imaging techniques, particularly functional imaging techniques, should enable us not only to study ovarian function *in vivo*, but also to distinguish different forms of POF.

Progress in the field of cryopreservation of ovarian tissue, combined with autotransplantation and/or *in vitro* maturation and IVF, creates perspectives for conservation of reproductive potential for patients confronted with a strong possibility of developing POF in the future. Finally, xenografting of ovarian tissue offers opportunities to explore follicular growth *in vivo* and to develop techniques for alternative methods of *in vivo* maturation of human oocytes for reproduction purposes.

REFERENCES

1. Coulam CB, Adamson SC, Annegers JF. The incidence of premature ovarian failure. *Obstet Gynecol* 1986;67:604–6
2. Moraes Ruehsen M, Jones GS. Premature ovarian failure. *Fertil Steril* 1967;18: 440–61
3. Aiman J, Smentek C. Premature ovarian failure. *Obstet Gynecol* 1985;66:9–14
4. Coulam CB. Premature gonadal failure. *Fertil Steril* 1982;38:645–55
5. Taylor AE, Adams JM, Mulder JE, *et al*. A randomized, controlled trial of oestradiol replacement therapy in women with hypergonadotropic amenorrhoea. *J Clin Endocrinol Metab* 1996;81:3615–21
6. Conway GS, Kaltsas G, Patel A, *et al*. Characterization of idiopathic premature ovarian failure. *Fertil Steril* 1996;65:337–41
7. Conway GS. Premature ovarian failure. *Curr Opin Obstet Gynecol* 1997;9:202–8
8. Anasti JN. Premature ovarian failure: an update. *Fertil Steril* 1998;70:1–15
9. Morrison JC, Givens JR, Wiser WL, *et al*. Mumps oophoritis: a cause of premature menopause. *Fertil Steril* 1975;26:655–9
10. Kaufman FR, Donell GN, Roe TF, *et al*. Gonadal function in patients with galactosaemia. *J Inherit Metab Dis* 1986;9:140
11. Waggoner DD, Buist NRM, Donell GN. Long-term prognosis in galactosaemia: results of a survey of 350 cases. *J Inherit Metab Dis* 1990;13:802–18
12. Neuwinger J, Licht P, Munzer B, *et al*. Substitution with testosterone as aromatizable substrate for induction of follicular maturation, estradiol production and ovulation in a patient with 17-alpha-hydroxylase deficiency. *Exp Clin Endocrinol Diabetes* 1996;104:400–8
13. Hague WM, Tan SL, Adams J, *et al*. Hypergonadotropic amenorrhea – etiology and outcome in 93 young women. *Int J Gynaecol Obstet* 1987;25:121–5
14. Castillo S, Lopez F, Tobella L, *et al*. The cytogenetics of premature ovarian failure. *Rev Chil Obstet Ginecol* 1992;57:341–5
15. Wu RC, Kuo PL, Lin CH, *et al*. X chromosome mosaicism in patients with recurrent abortion or premature ovarian failure. *J Formos Med Assoc* 1993;92:953–6
16. Rebar W. Hypergonadotropic amenorrhea and premature ovarian failure: a review. *J Reprod Med* 1982;4:179–86
17. Eden JA. Menopause before 40 – premature, but not always permanent. *Aust NZ J Obstet Gynaecol* 1993;33:201–3
18. Singh RP, Carr DH. The anatomy and histology of XO human embryos and fetuses. *Anat Rec* 1966;155:369–83
19. Therman E, Laxova R, Susman B. The critical region on the human Xq. *Hum Genet* 1990;85:455–61
20. Sala C, Arrigo G, Torri G. Eleven X chromosome breakpoints associated with premature ovarian failure (POF) map to a 15-MB YAC contig spanning Xq21. *Genomics* 1997;40:123–31
21. Zinn AR, Tonk VS, Chen Z, *et al*. Evidence for a Turner syndrome locus at Xp11.2–p22.1. *Am J Hum Genet* 1998;63:1757–66
22. Day RW, Larson W, Wright SW. Clinical and cytogenetic studies on a group of females with XXX sex chromosome complements. *J Pediatr* 1964;64:24
23. Conway SG, Payne NN, Webb J, *et al*. Fragile X premutation screening in women with premature ovarian failure. *Hum Reprod* 1998;13:1184–7
24. Partington MW, York Moore D, Turner GM. Confirmation of early menopause in fragile X carriers. *Am J Med Genet* 1996;64:370–2

25. Bione S, Sala C, Manzini C. A human homologue of the *Drosophila* diaphanous gene is disrupted in a patient with premature ovarian failure: evidence for a preserved function in oogenesis and implications for human sterility. *Am J Genet* 1998;62:533
26. Amati P, Gasparini P, Zlotogora J, *et al*. A gene for premature ovarian failure associated with eye-lid malformation maps to chromosome 3q22–q23. *Am J Hum Genet* 1996;58:1089–92
27. Panidis B, Russo D, Vavilis D, *et al*. Familial blepharophimosis with ovarian dysfunction. *Hum Reprod* 1994;9:2034–7
28. Aittomaki K, Herva R, Stenman U, *et al*. Clinical features of primary ovarian failure caused by a point mutation in the follicle stimulating hormone receptor gene. *J Clin Endocrinol Metab* 1996;81:3722–6
29. Matthews CH, Borgato S, Beck-Peccoz P, *et al*. Primary amenorrhea and infertility due to a mutation in the beta-subunit of follicle stimulating hormone. *Nature Genet* 1993;5:83
30. Layman LC, Lee EJ, Peak DB, *et al*. Delayed puberty and hypogonadism caused by mutations in the follicle stimulating hormone beta-subunit gene. *N Engl J Med* 1997;337:607
31. Bondy AC, Nelson LM, Kalantaridou SN. The genetic origins of ovarian failure. *J Women Health* 1998;7:1225–9
32. Christine-Maitre S, Vasseur C, Portnoi M, *et al*. Genes and premature ovarian failure. *Mol Cell Endocrinol* 1998;145:75–80
33. Edmonds M, Lamki L, Killinger DW, *et al*. Autoimmune thyroiditis, adrenalitis, and oophoritis. *Am J Med* 1973;54:782–7
34. Irvine WJ, Barnes EW. Addison's disease, ovarian failure and hyperparathyroidism. *J Clin Endocrinol Metab* 1976;4:379–83
35. Weetman AP. Autoimmunity to steroid-producing cells and familial polyendocrine autoimmunity. *Baillière's Clin Endocrinol Metab* 1995;9:157–74
36. Hoek A, Schoemaker J, Drexhage HA. Premature ovarian failure and ovarian autoimmunity. *Endocr Rev* 1997;18:107–34
37. Sotsiou F, Botazzo GF, Doniach D. Immunofluorescence studies on autoantibodies to steroid-producing cells, and to germline cells in endocrine diseases and infertility. *Clin Exp Immunol* 1980;39:97–111
38. Ahonen P, Mietinnen A, Perheentupa J. Adrenal and steroidal cell antibodies in patients with autoimmune polyglandular disease type I and the risk of adrenocortical and ovarian failure. *J Clin Endocrinol Metab* 1987;64:494–500
39. Betterle C, Rossi A, Dalla Pria S, *et al*. Premature ovarian failure: autoimmunity and natural history. *Clin Endocrinol* 1993;39:35–43
40. Windquist O, Gebre-Medhin G, Gustafsson J, *et al*. Identification of the main gonadal autoantigens in patients with adrenal insufficiency and associated ovarian failure. *J Clin Endocrinol Metab* 1995;80:1717–23
41. Gloor E, Hulimann J. Autoimmune oophoritis. *Am J Clin Pathol* 1984;81:105–9
42. Sedmak DD, Hart WR, Tubbs RR. Autoimmune oophoritis: a histopathological study of involved ovaries with immunologic characterization of the mononuclear infiltrate. *Int J Gynecol Pathol* 1987;6:73–81
43. Devi AS, Metzger DA, Luciano AA, *et al*. 45,X/46,XX mosaicism in patients with idiopathic premature ovarian failure. *Fertil Steril* 1998;70:89–93
44. Alper MA, Garner PR, Seibel MM. Premature ovarian failure. Current concepts. *J Reprod Med* 1986;31:699–708
45. Mignot MH, Schoemaker J, Kleingeld M, *et al*. Premature ovarian failure. The association with autoimmunity. *Eur J Obstet Gynecol Reprod Biol* 1989;30:59–66

46. Ishizuka B, Kudo Y, Amemiya A, *et al.* Anti-nuclear antibodies in patients with premature ovarian failure. *Hum Reprod* 1999;14:70–5
47. Rabinowe SL, George KL, Ravnikar VA, *et al.* Premature menopause: monoclonal antibody defined T-lymphocyte abnormalities and antiovarian antibodies. *Fertil Steril* 1989;51:450–4
48. Fenichel P, Sosset C, Barbarino-Monnier P, *et al.* Prevalence, specificity and significance of ovarian antibodies during spontaneous premature ovarian failure. *Hum Reprod* 1997;12:2623–8
49. Luborsky JL, Vinstin J, Boyers S, *et al.* Ovarian antibodies detected by immobilized antigen immunoassay in patients with premature ovarian failure. *J Clin Endocrinol Metab* 1990;70:69–75
50. Coulam CB, Ryan RJ. Presence of circulating antibodies directed towards ovaries among women with premature ovarian failure. *Am J Reprod Immunol Microbiol* 1985;9:23–4
51. Wheatcroft NJ, Toogood AA, Li TC, *et al.* Detection of autoantibodies to ovarian antigens in women with premature ovarian failure. *Clin Exp Immunol* 1994;96:122–8
52. Barbarino-Monnier P, Gobert B, Guillet-Rosso F, *et al.* Antiovarian antibodies, repeated attempts, and outcome of *in vitro* fertilization. *Fertil Steril* 1991;56:928–32
53. Narayanan M, Nurthy PSR, Munaf SA, *et al.* Antiovarian antibodies and their effect on the outcome of assisted reproduction. *J Assist Reprod Genet* 1995;12:599–605
54. van Weissenbruch M, Hoek A, van Vliet-Beker I, *et al.* Evidence for the existence of immunoglobulins that block ovarian granulosa cell growth *in vitro*. A putative role in resistant ovary syndrome? *J Clin Endocrinol Metab* 1991;73:360–7
55. Austin GE, Coulam CB, Ryan RJ. A search for antibodies to luteinizing hormone receptors in premature ovarian failure. *Mayo Clin Proc* 1979;54:394–400
56. Mignot MH, Drexhage HA, Kleingeld M, *et al.* Premature ovarian failure: considerations of cellular immunity defects. *Eur J Obstet Gynecol Reprod Biol* 1989;30:67–72
57. Nelson LM, Kimzey RN, Merriam GR, *et al.* Increased peripheral T lymphocyte activation in patients with karyotypically normal spontaneous premature ovarian failure. *Fertil Steril* 1991;6:1082–7
58. Hoek A, van Kasteren Y, de Haan-Meuleman M, *et al.* Analysis of peripheral blood lymphocyte subsets, NK-cells and delayed type hypersensitivity type skin tests in patients with POF. *Am J Reprod Immunol* 1995;33:495–502
59. van Kasteren Y, von Blomberg M, Hoek A, *et al.* Incipient ovarian failure and premature ovarian failure show the same immunological profile. *Am J Reprod Immunol* 2000; in press
60. de Bruin JP, Dorland M, Bruinse HW, *et al.* Fetal growth retardation as a cause of impaired ovarian development. *Early Hum Dev* 1998;51:39–46
61. Kaufman DW, Slone D, Rosenberg L, *et al.* Cigarette smoking and age at natural menopause. *Am J Publ Health* 1980;70:429
62. Kinch RA, Plunkett ER, Smout MS, *et al.* Primary ovarian failure. *Am J Obstet Gynecol* 1965;91:630–41
63. Emperaire JC, Audebert A, Greenblatt RB. Premature ovarian failure. *Am J Obstet Gynecol* 1970;108:445–9
64. Zarate A, Karchmer S, Gomez E, *et al.* Premature menopause. *Am J Obstet Gynecol* 1970;106:110–14
65. Sharf M, Israeli I, Graff G. The value of ovarian biopsy in the diagnosis and treatment of amenorrhea related sterility. *Obstet Gynecol* 1972;39:89–94
66. Starup J, Sele V. Premature ovarian failure. *Acta Obstet Gynecol Scand* 1973;52:259–68

67. Falk R. Euestrogenic ovarian failure. *Fertil Steril* 1977;28:502–3
68. Duignan NM. Sex hormone levels and gonadotropin release in premature ovarian failure. *Br J Obstet Gynaecol* 1978;85:862–7
69. Board JA, Redwine AO, Moncure CW, *et al.* Identification of differing etiologies of clinically diagnosed premature menopause. *Am J Obstet Gynecol* 1979;134: 936–44
70. Rebar RW, Erickson GF, Yen SS. Idiopathic premature ovarian failure: clinical and endocrine characteristics. *Fertil Steril* 1982;37:35–41
71. Russell P, Banatyne P, Shearman RP, *et al.* Premature hypergonadotropic ovarian failure: clinicopathological study of 19 cases. *Int J Gynecol Pathol* 1982;1:185–201
72. Menon V, Logan Edwards R, Butt WR, *et al.* Review of 59 patients with hypergonadotropic amenorrhea. *Br J Obstet Gynaecol* 1984;91:63–6
73. Miyaka T, Sato Y, Takeuchi S. Implications of circulating antibodies and peripheral blood lymphocytes for the genesis of premature ovarian failure. *J Reprod Immunol* 1987;12:163–71
74. Rebar WR, Conolly HV. Clinical features of young women with hypergonadotropic amenorrhea. *Fertil Steril* 1990;53:804–10
75. Muechler EK, Huang K, Schenk E. Autoimmunity in premature ovarian failure. *Int J Fertil* 1991;36:99–103
76. Mehta AE, Matwijiw I, Lyons EA, *et al.* Noninvasive diagnosis of resistant ovary syndrome by ultrasonography. *Fertil Steril* 1992;57:56–61
77. Sutton C. The limitations of laparoscopic ovarian biopsies. *J Obstet Gynaecol Br Commonw* 1974;81:317–20
78. Polansky S, de Papp EW. Pregnancy associated with hypergonadotropic hypogonadism. *Obstet Gynecol* 1976;47:47S–51S
79. Cowchock FS, McGabe JL, Montgomery BB. Pregnancy after corticosteroid administration in premature ovarian failure (polyglandular endocrinopathy syndrome). *Am J Obstet Gynecol* 1988;158:118–19
80. Rabinowe SL, Beger ML, Welch WR, *et al.* Lymphocyte dysfunction in autoimmune oophoritis: resumption of menses with corticosteroids. *Am J Med* 1986;81:347
81. Corenblum B, Rowe T, Taylor PJ. High-dose, short-term glucocorticosteroids for the treatment of infertility resulting from premature ovarian failure. *Fertil Steril* 1993;59: 988–91
82. Betterle C, Volpato M, Rees Smith B, *et al.* Adrenal cortex and steroid 21-hydroxylase autoantibodies in adult patients with organspecific autoimmune disease: markers of low progression to clinical Addison's disease. *J Clin Endocrinol Metab* 1997;82: 932–8
83. van Kasteren YM, Hoek A, Schoemaker J. Ovulation induction in premature ovarian failure: a placebo-controlled randomized trial combining pituitary suppression with gonadotropin stimulation. *Fertil Steril* 1995;64:273–8
84. van Kasteren YM, Braat DDM, Hemrika DJ, *et al.* Corticosteroids do not influence ovarian responsiveness to gonadotropins premature ovarian failure (POF): a randomized, placebo-controlled trial. *Fertil Steril* 1999;71:90–5
85. Mattison DR, Evans MI, Schwimmer WB, *et al.* Familial premature ovarian failure. *Am J Hum Genet* 1984;36:1341–8
86. Vegetti W, Tibiletti MG, Testa G, *et al.* Inheritance in idiopathic premature ovarian failure; analysis of 71 cases. *Hum Reprod* 1988;13:1796–800
87. van Kasteren YM, Hundscheid RDL, Smits APT, *et al.* Familial idiopathic premature ovarian failure; an overrated and underestimated genetic disease? *Hum Reprod* 1999;14:2455–9

88. MacPherson J, Murray A, Webbs J, *et al*. Fragile X syndrome of POF and premutations. *J Med Genet* 1999;36:171–2
89. Metka M, Holzer G, Heytmanek G, *et al*. Hypergonadotropic hypogonadic amenorrhea (World Health Organization III) and osteoporosis. *Fertil Steril* 1992;57: 37–41
90. Davies MC, Hall ML, Jacobs HS. Bone mineral loss in young women with amenorrhea. *Br Med J* 1990;301:790–3
91. Wren BG. The breast and the menopause. In *The Menopause: Key Issues. Baillière's Clin Obstet Gynecol* 1996;10:433–68
92. Titus-Ernstoff L, Longnecker MP, Newcomb PA, *et al*. Menstrual factors in relation to breast cancer risk. *Cancer Epidemiol Biomarkers Prev* 1998;7:783–9
93. Kelsey JL, Bernstein L. Epidemiology and prevention of breast cancer. *Annu Rev Public Health* 1996;17:47–67
94. Schairer C, Persson I, Falkeborn M, *et al*. Breast cancer risk associated with gynecological surgery and indications for such surgery. *Int J Cancer* 1997;70:150–4
95. Parazinni F, Braga C, La Vecchia C, *et al*. Hysterectomy, oophorectomy in premenopause, and the risk of breast cancer. *Obstet Gynecol* 1997;90:453–6
96. Willis DB, Calle EE, Miracle-McMahill HL, *et al*. Estrogen replacement therapy and the risk of fatal breast cancer in a prospective cohort of postmenopausal women in the United States. *Cancer Causes Control* 1996;7:449–57
97. van Kasteren YM, Schoemaker J. Premature ovarian failure: a systematic review on therapeutic interventions to restore ovarian function and achieve pregnancy. *Hum Reprod* 1999;5:483–92
98. O'Herlihy C, Pepperell RJ, Evans JH. The significance of elevated FSH in young women with disorders of ovulation. *Br Med J* 1980;281:1447–50
99. Kreiner IA, Droesch K, Navott D, *et al*. Spontaneous and pharmacologically induced remissions in patients with premature ovarian failure. *Obstet Gynecol* 1988;78: 926–8
100. Rebar RW, Conolly HV. Clinical features of young women with hypergonadotropic amenorrhea. *Fertil Steril* 1990;53:804–10
101. Sauer MV. Spontaneous pregnancy in women awaiting oocyte donation. *J Reprod Med* 1995;40:630–2
102. Tanaka T, Sakuragi N, Fujimoto S, *et al*. HMG–HCG therapy in patients with hypergonadotropic ovarian anovulation: one pregnancy case report and ovulation and pregnancy rate. *Int J Fertil* 1982;27:100–4
103. Ylostalo P, Huhtaniemi I, Reinila M. Induction of ovulation with low-dose oestrogen–progestin therapy in amenorrhoeic patients. *Int J Fertil* 1982;27:153–9
104. Menon V, Logan Edwards R, Lynch SS, *et al*. Luteinizing hormone releasing hormone analogue in treatment of hypergonadotropic amenorrhea. *Br J Obstet Gynaecol* 1983;90:539–42
105. Boyers SP, Luborsky JL, DeCherney AH. Usefulness of serial measurements of serum follicle stimulating hormone, luteinizing hormone and oestradiol in patients with premature ovarian failure. *Fertil Steril* 1988;50:408–12
106. Ledger WL, Thomas EJ, Browning D, *et al*. Suppression of gonadotrophin secretion does not reverse premature ovarian failure. *Br J Obstet Gynaecol* 1989;96:196–9
107. Check JH, Nowroozi J, Chase JS, *et al*. Ovulation induction in 100 consecutive women with hypergonadotropic amenorrhea. *Fertil Steril* 1990;53:811–16
108. Buckler HM, Healy DL, Burger HG. Does gonadotropin suppression result in follicular development in premature ovarian failure? *Gynecol Endocrinol* 1993;7:123–8

109. Blumenfeld Z, Halachmi S, Peretz BA, *et al.* Premature ovarian failure – the prognostic value of autoimmunity on conception after ovulation induction. *Fertil Steril* 1993;59:750–5
110. Surrey ES, Cedars MI. The effect of gonadotropin suppression on the induction of ovulation in premature ovarian failure patients. *Fertil Steril* 1989;52:36–41
111. Nelson LM, Kimzey LM, White BJ, *et al.* Gonadotropin suppression for the treatment of karyotypically normal spontaneous premature ovarian failure: a controlled trial. *Fertil Steril* 1992;57:50–5
112. Rosen GF, Stone SC, Yee B. Ovulation induction in women with premature ovarian failure: a prospective, crossover study. *Fertil Steril* 1992;57:448–9
113. Anasti JN, Kimzey LM, Defensor RA, *et al.* A controlled study for the treatment of karyotypically normal spontaneous premature ovarian failure. *Fertil Steril* 1994;62:726–30

17

Clinical consequences of elevated follicle stimulating hormone levels in the patient treated for infertility

C.B. Lambalk, J.M. van Montfrans and C.H. de Koning

INTRODUCTION

For some time, in reproductive medicine, much attention has been given to abnormal elevation of serum follicle stimulating hormone (FSH) concentrations. In particular, during the recruitment of a new cohort of follicles, which usually takes place during the luteal–follicular transition at the time of menses, high serum FSH concentrations are associated with a low response in infertility treatment[1]. Consequently, determination of serum levels of this hormone in the early follicular phase has become routine practice in the work-up of the infertility patient. In this chapter, we first briefly summarize several general, physiological and pathophysiological aspects of variation in FSH levels in premenopausal women. Second, we critically evaluate the practical aspects of the observation of elevated FSH concentrations with respect to counselling the subfertile couple regarding the chance of pregnancy, consequences for possible further diagnostic procedures and possible therapies.

ETIOLOGY AND DIFFERENTIAL DIAGNOSIS OF ELEVATED FSH CONCENTRATIONS

Causes of fluctuations in FSH and LH concentrations

For the normal function of the ovary with respect to developing puberty and reproduction, pituitary gland secretion of luteinizing hormone (LH) and FSH is required in a well-organized way. Both hormones are glycoproteins with a common α chain and a different β chain. The half-life of both hormones depends on the level of glycosylation and varies between 20 and 60 min for LH and between 120 and 240 min for FSH. In the absence of these hormones, puberty will not develop and menstrual cycles will not occur. The secretion of these hormones is entirely dependent on regulation by luteinizing hormone releasing hormone (LHRH), which is also often referred to as gonadotropin releasing hormone (GnRH). This is a decapeptide hormone secreted by a group of about 1500 neurons in the mediobasal regions of the hypothalamus and released into the pituitary portal circulation.

Lifetime changes

In the female, long-term variations are present that depend on the time of life. At the time of birth, LH and FSH secretions are present at almost adolescent levels. This is the result of GnRH secretion by fully operational mediobasal GnRH neurons. This system becomes quiescent by the end of the first year after birth. Around this time, LH and FSH levels become undetectable, and remain so until puberty occurs, which is the result of reactivation of the GnRH neurons. The waning and waxing of this event occurs via still largely unknown mechanisms. Changes in gonadotropin secretion over puberty towards adolescence and adulthood are the most important lifetime changes of gonadotropin secretion. This situation continues until the menopause is reached. By then, the final lifetime change occurs: levels of FSH and LH become very high (increased over 50-fold) because of lack of adequate gonadal feedback mechanisms.

Changes across the cycle

In addition to these lifetime changes, a monthly variability in LH and FSH levels occurs in adult premenopausal women, and is related to the stage of their menstrual cycle. Highlights are the subtle perimenstrual increase in FSH levels for induction of follicle growth and the very high mid-cycle elevations of LH (the LH surge) for induction of first, termination of meiosis I in the oocyte; second, luteinization of granulosa cells; and third, ovulation.

Intercycle variability

It has been clearly shown by Scott and colleagues[2] that FSH levels vary considerably from cycle to cycle. In a study of 81 patients who had undergone three or more *in vitro* fertilization (IVF) attempts, the degree and potential impact of intercycle variability in basal FSH concentrations was investigated. The mean of the individual standard deviations for all 81 patients was 4.2 ± 0.4 mIU/ml. However, the patients with a mean basal FSH level of < 15 mIU/ml had a mean deviation of only 2.6 ± 0.2 mIU/ml, whereas those with a mean basal FSH level of $\geqslant 15$ mIU/ml had a mean deviation of 7.3 ± 0.7 mIU/ml. Patients with large intercycle variations responded poorly to gonadotropin stimulation independently of their basal FSH concentration.

Hourly variation

It was from the pituitary gonadotropic hormones (particularly LH) that it became clear for the first time that these were secreted episodically at intervals varying between 1 and 4 h, closely related to the synchronous episodic release of GnRH by the GnRH neurons. This synchronous episodic release of GnRH is often referred to as the hypothalamic 'pulse generator'. The 'pulsatility' is considered as a key feature of gonadotropin secretion. Under normal circumstances in which gonadotropic hormones are measurable (in both males and females), pulsatility can be observed. During the normal ovarian cycle of the human, plasma LH shows pulses about every hour in the follicular phase of the cycle and about every 4 h during the luteal phase. FSH is secreted in a similar pulsatile way throughout the cycle. After the menopause, LH and FSH pulses occur every 1–2 h.

Inter-sample variation

Variation also occurs as a result of assay variation. This variation can be substantial: up to the maximum generally acceptable coefficient of variation of around 10% as a result of within-assay errors and a similar acceptable error rate for between-assay variation.

Why measure FSH on cycle day 3?

There are a number of reasonable objections that can be made against systematically using cycle day 3 as a fixed time for measuring FSH. In fact, the menses are a rather crude reference point with respect to the endocrinology of the reproductive cycle. Nevertheless, it is a bioassay of the waning of progesterone secretion from a corpus luteum that was the result of an ovulated dominant follicle. Therefore, it is not surprising that certain endocrine parameters such as FSH measured during menses correlate well with the physiological events of the previous cycle, and, of more importance, correlate well with the events to come[3]. In our opinion, the advantages of using the rather arbitrary 'day 3' for estimating basal FSH outweighs its relative crudeness as an endocrine parameter. In the first place, it ensures uniformity with respect to sampling between the various studies of the various investigators, allowing some comparison of observations. Furthermore, there are practical advantages. The onset of menses is easily recognizable by the participating patient or volunteer; by selecting day 2 or 3, planning can take place which is convenient to the participant and sometimes crucial for the study.

Normal values

After having chosen to use basal FSH for experimental studies or patient care, each center needs to determine normal values based on its own patient population and the local available assay. This is important, because there are substantial differences between the various commercially or non-commercially developed assays to measure FSH. In our clinic we have collected over

1000 estimates of FSH concentrations on cycle day 3 in serum, taken routinely over the past few years from all new female infertility patients with a menstrual cycle. Using the Amerlite FSH assay (Amersham, UK) it appeared that the 95% upper limit for women under the age of 30 years was 8.6 IU/l (second IRP MRC 78/549). For research purposes, based on these figures, we assigned a value of > 10.0 IU/l as abnormal.

MECHANISMS CAUSING ELEVATED FSH CONCENTRATIONS

Diminished feedback

We are dealing with a classical endocrine loop between the ovary, the hypothalamus and the pituitary. Therefore, the most evident mechanism by which an increase in FSH secretion occurs is by a decrease in the activity of negative-feedback hormones. This may be due to a loss in size and quality of the cohort of follicles that are available at the time of recruitment.

Diminished feedback response

On theoretical grounds one has to consider the possibility that the end organs of feedback hormones become less sensitive to their activity.

Greater secretory drive

Finally, a greater secretory drive may be responsible for an increase in hormone secretion, provided that there are limitations in the total capacity of feedback.

PHYSIOLOGICAL FSH ELEVATIONS

Several situations in the reproductive period of the female are accompanied by temporarily elevated FSH levels. Under these circumstances, we hypothesize that re-initiation of the activity of the hypothalamic–pituitary–ovarian axis (HPO axis) after a period of prolonged quiescence is characterized by hypersecretion of FSH in temporary absence of fully operational gonadal feedback by estrogens and inhibins.

The most frequently occurring prolonged silence of the HPO axis is the prepubertal period. As already mentioned, at birth the system is entirely operational and LH and FSH secretion clearly occurs after birth, but by still largely unknown mechanisms hypothalamic GnRH secretion comes to a temporary standstill and resumes only after several years. Typically, in the first stages of the transition into puberty, only FSH secretion is measurable; after some time, nocturnal LH secretion can also be detected. By the time that the first ovulation is about to occur, FSH levels can be detected that are substantially higher than in later cycles[4]. In several conditions, recovery of activity of the HPO axis may mimic this peripubertal sequence.

Lactational amenorrhea

A physiological cause of prolonged quiescence of the HPO axis is the lactational amenorrhea that is typically the result of arrest of the hypothalamic GnRH pulse generator[5]. Indeed, Burger and colleagues[6] showed a remarkable excess of FSH secretion about 60 days postpartum in women, some of whom were already recovering from the lactation amenorrhea. It appeared that the highest FSH levels were associated with the lowest possible levels of mainly estrogen but also inhibins.

After discontinuation of oral contraceptives

A frequently occurring condition with prolonged suppression of the activity of the HPO axis in normal women is during the use of oral contraceptives[7]. In line with the proposed 'puberty mimicking' hypothesis, it is expected that the first spontaneous cycle(s) are associated with higher FSH levels. Higher FSH levels were recently demonstrated in the follicular phase of the first spontaneous cycles in women after discontinuation of oral contraceptives, in comparison to matched women who had never used this medication[8].

Aging

A normal feature in older premenopausal women is elevated FSH levels in the early follicular phase of the menstrual cycle[9]. Many, if not all, women at menopause have experienced some prior period that can be characterized as occult, imminent or incipient ovarian failure. By definition, this is the period prior to menopause with regular menstrual cycles, without climacteric signs but with elevated FSH levels in the early follicular phase of the cycle[9,10].

In patients with imminent ovarian failure, studies of the pulsatile pattern of FSH and LH, the response to GnRH and ovarian feedback may be informative on the mechanisms and causes of the altered FSH concentrations. We studied these features on the 3rd day of the menstrual cycle in 13 subfertile patients with elevated basal FSH values (> 10.0 IU/l) and in 16 controls. Not only FSH levels but also LH concentrations were higher in these patients than in controls. This was found to be due to increased FSH and LH pulse amplitude with a strong increase in response to GnRH. The frequencies of FSH and LH pulses were similar. The concentrations of inhibin A and inhibin B were lower in patients with elevated basal FSH concentrations, while estradiol concentrations were unchanged.

Apparently, the increased secretion of gonadotropins in patients with imminent ovarian failure is a result of impaired ovarian feedback. The higher

LH and FSH responses to GnRH in these patients indicate that a decline in secretion of other ovarian factors such as gonadotropin surge inhibiting factor (GnSIF) could also play a role in the endocrine (patho)physiology of imminent ovarian failure[11]. As mentioned earlier, in addition to a decline of ovarian feedback, an increase of the ovarian threshold for FSH may also contribute to the occurrence of higher serum FSH levels. Indeed, in a recent experiment we found evidence that this is the case. Six patients with elevated early follicular phase FSH levels and regular menses and 13 controls received an LHRH agonist in order to desensitize the pituitary, resulting in blockade of endogenous LH and FSH secretion. Subsequently, recombinant FSH was given intravenously with a very slowly increasing dosage and simultaneous very close monitoring of ovarian activity and serum FSH levels. With this technique we were able to determine the lowest (threshold) serum level of FSH at which ongoing follicular growth was initiated. It appeared that in patients with imminent ovarian failure, the lowest levels of FSH upon which follicular growth occurred were significantly higher than in controls (median FSH threshold 6.75 vs. 4.65 IU/l, respectively; $p = 0.023$).

In conclusion, elevated FSH levels in the patient with imminent ovarian failure are the result of an increase in the ovarian FSH requirement in combination with a decrease in ovarian feedback.

Spuriously elevated FSH

When high levels of FSH are found with normal LH levels and no cycle abnormalities, one explanation may be the presence of heterological antibodies in the serum of the patient that interfere with the assay. In a recent series of about 30 patients, we found three such cases. In all, there was no parallelism after the serum was diluted and prepared with polyethyleneglycol, which removes all immunoglobulins, resulting in normal FSH levels. Therefore, when abnormally high FSH values are found, this should be a standard additional procedure for ruling out false elevations. Since the heterological antibodies interfere with the compounds of the assay kit, another assay could be used in such cases.

Familial dizygotic twinning

Several studies have shown increased plasma gonadotropin levels in mothers of dizygotic twins[12–14]. In the case of hereditary dizygotic twinning it appears that elevated FSH levels are associated with an increase in number of FSH pulses in the early follicular phase[15]. These pulses appear to be FSH pulses without a concurrent LH pulse. We observed no changes in LH secretion and both the LH and the FSH responses of the pituitary to GnRH were unchanged. There were no indications of a difference in mode of ovarian feedback since inhibin A, inhibin B and estradiol levels were unchanged.

These data indicate that some neuroendocrine mechanism is involved in the generation of higher FSH levels in hereditary twinning. Because of the clearly observed solitary FSH pulses without a concomitant LH pulse, we hypothesize that in this situation an extra releasing hormone is responsible for FSH release: FSH-RH. On the other hand, we did not find a difference in any of the parameters of pulsatile LH and FSH secretion when postmenopausal women from hereditary dizygotic twinning families were compared to controls. This was probably due to difficulties in observing subtle differences in pulsatile FSH secretion within the rather fluctuating hormonal pattern that is a characteristic of the postmenopausal state. Given this observation, we suggest as an alternative explanation for our findings in premenopausal mothers of dizygotic twins that their hypothalamic–pituitary system has a lower responsiveness to ovarian feedback hormones.

PATHOPHYSIOLOGICAL FSH ELEVATIONS

Recovery from weight loss or stress amenorrhea

A condition mimicking puberty might be the recovery from hypothalamic amenorrhea after a period of weight loss or stress. The cause of this type of amenorrhea is entirely attributable to deficient activity of the GnRH pulse generator[16]. The recovery of gonadotropin secretion results from re-initiation of this system. Currently, there are no data available providing evidence that FSH hypersecretion occurs under the circumstances of recovery from weight loss or from stress amenorrhea. On the other hand, it was demonstrated by Braat and Schoemaker[17] that induction of ovulation with exogenously administered pulses of GnRH in these patients led to higher FSH levels in the first treatment cycle, compared to subsequent treatment cycles. The elevated FSH concentrations were associated with multiple follicle growth and an increased incidence of multiple pregnancies.

Intoxication

The best example of the fact that intoxications can influence FSH concentration is the deleterious effect of smoking. Current smoking is associated with signs of accelerated development of diminished ovarian reserve, as shown by the clomiphene challenge test[18]. According to a study by Cooper and coworkers[19], FSH concentrations were 66% higher in active smokers and 39% in passive smokers compared to controls.

Iatrogenic causes

One of the most frequently occurring iatrogenic causes of an increase in basal FSH levels is unilateral ovariectomy. It was clearly shown in a study by

Khalifa and colleagues[20] that women with one ovary had significantly elevated FSH concentrations compared to controls. They also showed that the total number of follicles retrieved during IVF treatment in these women was significantly decreased, which probably mirrors the relationship between basal FSH concentration and size of the available cohort. Nevertheless, in this particular study there was no difference in pregnancy outcome.

PRACTICAL CONSEQUENCES

Implications of elevated FSH levels for fecundity in the patient treated for infertility

Several studies have been published indicating a poor pregnancy prognosis in patients with elevated basal FSH concentrations undergoing IVF or other assisted reproduction technology (ART) programs. These studies have prompted many subfertility clinics to include screening for elevated basal FSH concentrations in the basic subfertility evaluation of patients. We have recently investigated the predictive value of elevated basal FSH concentrations in a general population of patients with subfertility. In a nested case–control study, we performed long-term follow-up in 50 consecutive patients with elevated basal FSH concentrations (> 10.0 IU/l) and in 50 age-matched controls. These patients all underwent a routine subfertility evaluation, and treatment was initiated to address the specific cause of subfertility (if identified). In this population, a minority of the patients received ART treatment. The results of the study were that the pregnancy rate in the group with elevated basal FSH concentrations was not significantly different from that in the control group. Therefore, elevated basal FSH concentrations had no additional value for the prognosis in this population of patients with subfertility. It appears that screening for elevated basal FSH concentrations identifies too many false-positive test results, and that other factors causing impaired fecundity obscure the effect of elevated basal FSH concentrations. However, many clinics use the basal FSH test and some even counsel patients towards adoption in the case of elevated basal FSH concentrations. We have the opinion that this practice is not evidence based and certainly does not serve the patient's best interests. Screening for elevated basal FSH concentrations should not be performed in patients who will not undergo any assisted reproduction treatment.

Need for further diagnostics?

When a careful history is taken and spuriously elevated FSH levels are ruled out, no further diagnostic procedures are needed in non-pregnant patients with this finding. When they become pregnant, however, there are reasons to consider (non-invasive) prenatal diagnosis.

Elevated basal FSH concentrations in relation to trisomy-21 pregnancies

Two recently published articles have drawn attention to a relationship between the risk for aneuploidies during pregnancy and signs of a diminished ovarian reserve. Our group has studied basal FSH concentrations in women with a history of a pregnancy with a fetus with Down's syndrome (trisomy 21)[21]. This study identified elevated mean basal FSH concentrations in women with a history of a Down's syndrome pregnancy, and an increased number of women with basal FSH concentrations over 11.5 IU/l in the Down's syndrome group. Nasseri and colleagues[22] investigated basal FSH and estradiol concentrations in women with a history of a spontaneous abortion containing an aneuploid conception. They found an increased number of women with elevated basal FSH or estradiol concentrations in the group of women with a history of a chromosomally aneuploid conception. The two studies thus identify an age-independent relationship between signs of a diminished primordial follicle pool and the occurrence of aneuploid conceptions.

These findings may have consequences for women with elevated basal FSH concentrations who become pregnant. The calculated odds ratio for having elevated basal FSH concentrations in women with a history of a Down's syndrome pregnancy was 3.0. Since the incidence of Down's syndrome conceptions is relatively low, the odds ratio of 3.0 may in theory be used to estimate the risk of a Down's syndrome pregnancy in women with elevated basal FSH levels. Women with elevated basal FSH concentrations who achieve pregnancy should be warned that they may have an increased risk of an aneuploid pregnancy. However, since currently available screening tests and diagnostic tests to identify chromosomal abnormalities during pregnancy have relatively good test characteristics, the presence of elevated basal FSH concentrations before pregnancy will probably not replace any of the currently available screening or diagnostic tests.

Therapeutic considerations

Elevated basal FSH concentrations found in an early stage of the infertility work-up does not rule out the possibility of pregnancy. Fecundity in patients with elevated basal FSH concentrations was not different from that in patients with normal FSH levels. Therefore, when elevated FSH is substantiated in the fertility patient, a full fertility diagnostic work-up is justified or even mandatory. Furthermore, in the infertility patient with elevated FSH levels any fertility treatment should be applied on the basis of abnormal findings. For instance, this would suggest tubal surgery or IVF in case of tubal pathology, or insemination or IVF in case of male or cervical factor, in patients with elevated basal FSH concentrations just as in patients with normal values.

In older patients undergoing any of the assisted reproduction techniques, the daily dose of FSH is often increased and combined with early follicular phase initiation of GnRH agonist to employ the so-called flare-up. The benefit of these strategies with respect to increasing the number of oocytes retrieved or the number of pregnancies produced has been questioned[23]. The question is whether there would be any advantage to administering 2 extra ampules of FSH (150 IU) to a patient with a basal FSH level of, for example, 15 IU/l during an IVF cycle, leading to an additional 4-UL/l serum FSH increase, since these patients have an endogenous FSH secretion comparable to approximately 5 ampules per day. On the other hand, considering that lower doses of FSH are routinely given to young women in order to prevent ovarian hyperstimulation syndrome, an increase of the dose in older patients may be justified. To date, there have been no good experimental data that substantiate any usefulness of administering this additional FSH in IVF hyperstimulation protocols in patients with imminent ovarian failure.

At this time, many IVF clinics consider discontinuation of IVF after one cycle in patients with high FSH levels and low response, because of expected disappointing results. This expectation may be justified when a limited number of three cycles are available, resulting in a limited number of oocytes, with subsequent limitations in selection of oocytes. The only way to compensate for this would be to increase the number of IVF cycles, which is exactly the opposite of current practice. Of course, this would be a very time-consuming approach, with a heavy burden for the patient. On the other hand, since additional FSH administration would probably not yield many more additional oocytes, perhaps prolonged IVF procedures in the natural cycle are an option in this type of patient.

Finally, in view of our observation that more than half of the patients with elevated FSH levels and an ovulatory cycle become pregnant, we feel that an oocyte donation procedure seems almost unethical and should not be offered immediately at this stage. From the recipient's point of view, there is no reason to advance this procedure instead of waiting until sustained anovulation occurs. Technically, the only justifiable reason for proceeding to oocyte donation immediately after measurement of an elevated FSH concentration would be the availability and age of a suitable oocyte donor.

SUMMARIZING CONCLUSIONS

In patients with imminent ovarian failure, elevated basal FSH concentrations reflect diminished feedback and an increase of the ovarian threshold for FSH. In familial dizygotic twinning, elevated basal FSH concentrations reflect an increase of the pituitary secretory drive. In a general population of patients with subfertility, the predictive value of serum FSH concentration regarding subfertility is limited, and screening for elevated basal FSH concentrations should therefore not be used in the regular work-up of all infertility patients. The occurrence of trisomy-21 pregnancies is associated with a three-fold increased risk of having elevated FSH concentrations (> 11.5 IU/l). This observation implies that women with elevated FSH concentrations may have an increased risk for a chromosomally abnormal pregnancy.

REFERENCES

1. Scott RTJ, Hofmann GE. Prognostic assessment of ovarian reserve. *Fertil Steril* 1995; 63:1–11
2. Scott RT, Hofmann GE, Oehninger S, *et al.* Intercycle variability of day 3 follicle-stimulating hormone levels and its effect on stimulation quality in *in vitro* fertilization. *Fertil Steril* 1990;54:297–302
3. Hall JE, Schoenfeld DA, Martin KA, *et al.* Hypothalamic GnRH and FSH dynamics during the luteal–follicular transition. *J Clin Endocrinol Metab* 1992;74:600–7
4. Wennink JM, Delemarre-van de Waal HA, Schoemaker R, *et al.* Luteinizing hormone and follicle stimulating hormone secretion patterns in girls throughout puberty measured using highly sensitive immunoradiometric assays. *Clin Endocrinol Oxf* 1990;33: 333–44
5. Tay CC, Glasier AF, McNeilly AS. Effect of antagonists of dopamine and opiates on the basal and GnRH-induced secretion of luteinizing hormone, follicle stimulating hormone and prolactin during lactational amenorrhoea in breastfeeding women. *Hum Reprod* 1993;8:532–9
6. Burger HG, Hee JP, Mamers P, *et al.* Serum inhibin during lactation: relation to the gonadotrophins and gonadal steroids. *Clin Endocrinol Oxf* 1994;41:771–7
7. Hemrika DJ, Slaats EH, Kennedy JC, *et al.* Pulsatile luteinizing hormone patterns in long term oral contraceptive users. *J Clin Endocrinol Metab* 1993;77:420–6
8. Jernstrom H, Knutsson M, Olsson H. Temporary increase of FSH levels in healthy, nulliparous, young women after cessation of low-dose oral contraceptive use. *Contraception* 1995;52:51–6
9. Sherman BM, Korenman SG. Hormonal characteristics of the human menstrual cycle throughout reproductive life. *J Clin Invest* 1975;55:699–706
10. Ahmed Ebbiary NA, Lenton EA, Cooke ID. Hypothalamic–pituitary ageing: progressive increase in FSH and LH concentrations throughout the reproductive life in regularly menstruating women. *Clin Endocrinol Oxf* 1994;41:199–206
11. de Koning J. Gonadotrophin surge-inhibiting/attenuating factor governs luteinizing hormone secretion during the ovarian cycle: physiology and pathology. *Hum Reprod* 1995;10:2854–61
12. Martin NG, Olsen ME, Theile H, *et al.* Pituitary–ovarian function in mothers who have had two sets of dyzygotic twins. *Fertil Steril* 1984;41:878–80
13. Martin NG, Robertson DM, Chenevix Trench G, *et al.* Elevation of follicular phase inhibin and luteinizing hormone levels in mothers of dizygotic twins suggests non-ovarian control of human multiple ovulation. *Fertil Steril* 1991;56:469–74
14. Nylander PP. Serum levels of gonadotrophins in relation to multiple pregnancy in Nigeria. *Br J Obstet Gynaecol* 1973;80:651–3
15. Lambalk CB, Boomsma DI, de Boer L, *et al.* Increased levels and pulsatility of follicle stimulating hormone in mothers of hereditary dizygotic twins. *J Clin Endocrinol Metab* 1998;83:481–6
16. Cameron JL, Nosbisch C. Suppression of pulsatile luteinizing hormone and testosterone secretion during short term food restriction in the adult male rhesus monkey *(Macaca mulatta)*. *Endocrinology* 1991;128:1532–40

17. Braat DD, Schoemaker J. Endocrinology of gonadotropin-releasing hormone induced cycles in hypothalamic amenorrhea: the role of the pulse dose. *Fertil Steril* 1991;56: 1054–9
18. Sharara FI, Beatse SN, Leonardi MR, *et al*. Cigarette smoking accelerates the development of diminished ovarian reserve as evidenced by the clomiphene citrate challenge test. *Fertil Steril* 1994;62:257–62
19. Cooper GS, Baird DD, Hulka BS, *et al*. Follicle-stimulating hormone concentrations in relation to active and passive smoking. *Obstet Gynecol* 1995;85:407–11
20. Khalifa E, Toner JP, Muasher SJ, *et al*. Significance of basal follicle stimulating hormone levels in women with one ovary in a program of *in vitro* fertilization. *Fertil Steril* 1992;57:835–9
21. Van Montfrans JM, Dorland M, Oosterhuis GJE, *et al*. Increased concentrations of follicle-stimulating hormone in mothers of children with Down's syndrome. *Lancet* 1999;353:1853–4
22. Nasseri A, Mukherjee T, Grifo JA, *et al*. Elevated day 3 serum follicle stimulating hormone and/or estradiol may predict fetal aneuploidy. *Fertil Steril* 1999;71:715–18
23. Levy T, Ben-Rafael Z. Low- versus high-dose human menopausal gonadotropin in an *in vitro* fertilization–embryo transfer program. *J Assist Reprod Genet* 1995;12:235–8

18

Oocyte quality versus endometrium quality in *in vitro* fertilization

C. Simón, J.C. Martin and A. Pellicer

INTRODUCTION

Since the introduction of *in vitro* fertilization (IVF), substantial improvement has been made in ovulation induction, oocyte retrieval, fertilization capability and embryonic development. However, the end-point, which is the improvement of implantation and pregnancy rates after transferring three or four embryos, remains below physiological expectations. It has been estimated that implantation in the human is efficient in no more than 30% of cases[1]. Considering that only one embryo is present in natural cycles, this gives us a 30% implantation rate. The responsibility for this low implantation efficiency has to be shared between the embryo (30% of the blastocysts are morphologically abnormal at the time of implantation *in vivo*[2]) and a defective embryonic–endometrial dialog (30% of early pregnancy losses occur before the expected time of menstruation[3]).

This implantation efficiency seems to be very poor when compared with other animal species, but is still unachievable using assisted reproduction technologies (ART). Implantation ability is reduced in ovum donation programs (18% implantation rate) in which hormone replacement therapy (HRT) is used to prepare the endometrium. It is even lower during controlled ovarian hyperstimulation (COH) used for IVF, in which the implantation rate is no more than 12% per embryo[4], resulting in 50% and 30% pregnancy rate per transfer, respectively[4]. We know from basic studies that the success of embryonic implantation relies upon a perfect dialog between good-quality embryos and a receptive endometrium.

Here, using different approaches, we analyze the endometrium as part of the clinical implantation process. Our results suggest that the main reason for these disappointing results is the quality of the endometrial factor, which is affected during pharmacological treatments used in ART (HRT and COH).

UTERINE RECEPTIVITY

Uterine receptivity is lower during COH used for IVF, compared to HRT and natural cycles[5]. This is not surprising, considering that drugs used in ovulation induction, aimed to recruit more oocytes, produce supraphysiological levels of steroid hormones which, in turn, induce morphological[6,7] and biochemical[8] endometrial changes relevant to uterine receptivity.

A comparison between standard IVF and donor oocyte cycles reveals that COH, necessary to produce multiple embryos in IVF, leads to a less receptive endometrium, inhibiting embryo implantation[5]. This finding is not new; it is known that COH inhibits embryo implantation in mice[9] and rats[10]. The concept was further proved when embryo implantation data from regular IVF patients were compared with those obtained from anonymous donors to HRT-treated recipients[5]. In this study, IVF patients' characteristics were matched to those of the oocyte donors, and similar ovarian stimulation protocols were used. Better implantation and pregnancy rates were achieved in the HRT group, suggesting that COH inhibits embryo implantation in IVF by decreasing endometrial receptivity.

INCREASING ENDOMETRIAL RECEPTIVITY WHILE KEEPING THE SAME EMBRYONIC FACTOR

We and others have consistently found lower implantation rates per embryo replaced in those patients undergoing IVF with a high response to gonadotropins[11–14], although this contrasts with other reports, where a high response was associated with no change[15,16] or increased implantation[17].

We have previously demonstrated that high serum estradiol levels (> 3000 pg/ml) on the day of human chorionic gonadotropin (hCG) administration in high-responder patients, regardless of the number of oocytes retrieved and serum progesterone levels, were detrimental to uterine receptivity without affecting embryo quality[13]. Indeed, pregnancy and implantation rates in recipients of embryos derived from the oocytes of high responders were similar to those of normal responders[13]. Furthermore, we documented an increase in serum estradiol levels during the preimplantation period in high responders compared to normal responders, suggesting that there is an abnormal endocrine milieu that might be responsible for impaired implantation[14].

Following this research line, and considering that very high levels of serum estradiol during the preimplantation period are deleterious for endometrial receptivity, we undertook a study to determine whether uterine receptivity (implantation and pregnancy rates) may be improved in high-responder patients undergoing IVF by using a step-down regimen, which aims to decrease estradiol levels during the preimplantation period[18].

This study included a total of 91 IVF cycles corresponding to 86 high-responder patients undergoing at least one previously failed IVF attempt with three to four good-quality embryos transferred and, on the day of hCG administration, an estradiol level of > 3000 pg/ml. These were classified as high responders, as previously described[19]. In the following cycle, 24 patients were treated in 29 cycles by using a step-down principle previously used for other clinical situations[20], and 62 patients were treated in 62 cycles by using the same standard protocol as in the previous cycle.

As a result of this regimen, estradiol levels on the day of hCG administration were significantly lower in patients undergoing step-down treatment compared to their own previous failed cycle (1919 ± 477 vs. 5770 ± 650 pg/ml; $p = 0.001$). In patients undergoing the same standard protocol as in the previously failed cycle, the levels were similar (5271 ± 613 vs. 4035 ± 489 pg/ml). A comparison between the step-down regimen and the standard protocol in the following cycle is presented in Table 1. Estradiol levels on the day of hCG administration were significantly lower in the step-down regimen compared to the standard protocol (1919 ± 477 vs. 5271 ± 613 pg/ml; $p = 0.001$), as well as throughout the preimplantation period.

The major problem within the step-down protocol was to determine the individual follicle stimulating hormone (FSH) threshold in clinical practice, since the threshold for administered FSH may differ up to tenfold for different patients. For this reason, five cycles (17.2%) were cancelled because the FSH threshold was not reached and follicle development was arrested, as demonstrated by an abrupt 80% estradiol decline.

As expected, the number of oocytes collected was lower in the step-down regimen compared to the standard protocol (18.1 ± 2.1 vs. 23.1 ± 1.6; $p = 0.001$). Similar fertilization rates were obtained (74.2% vs. 76.1%) and the number of good-quality embryos transferred was also similar (3.3 ± 0.2 vs. 3.4 ± 0.2). However, implantation and pregnancy rates were significantly

Table 1 Reproductive outcome of cycles using the step-down regimen versus the standard protocol in *in vitro* fertilization. Values are expressed as mean ± SE unless otherwise indicated

	Step-down regimen (*n* = 24)	*Standard protocol* (*n* = 62)	*p Value*
Age (years)	31.6 ± 1.2	33.8 ± 0.3	NS
No. of previous failed cycles	1.2 ± 0.1	1.0 ± 0.0	0.02
GnRH analog treatment (days)	22.9 ± 0.7	20.5 ± 0.9	NS
Days of treatment	10.6 ± 0.1	9.6 ± 0.2	NS
Ampules of gonadotropins	22.4 ± 0.8	31.6 ± 1.6	NS
Estradiol level (pg/ml)	1919 ± 477	5271 ± 613	0.001
No. of oocytes	18.1 ± 2.1	23.1 ± 1.6	0.001
Fertilization rate (%)	74.2	76.1	NS
No. of embryos transferred	3.3 ± 0.2	3.4 ± 0.2	NS
No. of embryos frozen	2.5 ± 0.7	3.1 ± 0.5	NS
Pregnancy rate (%)	64.2	24.2	0.0002
Implantation rate (%)	29.3	8.5	0.02
Hyperstimulated patients (%)	0	12.9	0.04

GnRH, gonadotropin releasing hormone

improved in patients undergoing the step-down regimen compared to those stimulated with the standard protocol (29.3% and 64.2% vs. 8.5% and 24.2%, respectively; $p = 0.02$ and $p = 0.0002$, respectively)[18].

IMPROVING EMBRYONIC FACTOR WHILE KEEPING ENDOMETRIAL RECEPTIVITY

Based on our previous work[21,22], we have developed a clinical program in which embryos were co-cultured with autologous endometrial epithelial cells (AEEC) until the blastocyst stage and then transferred back to the patient. To investigate the effect of the endometrial factor in patients with implantation failure, co-culture with AEEC was clinically applied in patients with implantation failure, defined as at least three previously failed cycles with three to four good-quality embryos transferred in either IVF (with their own oocytes) or oocyte donation, compared to a routine day-2 transfer in patients with implantation failure.

Our study design facilitated the dissecting out of the contribution of the endometrial and embryonic factors to the implantation process by comparing the efficacy of blastocyst transfer on a fixed day in different models of uterine receptivity. Ovum donation is an optimal model of uterine receptivity, because the endometrium of the recipient is artificially prepared by sequential administration of estrogen and progesterone at physiological levels[23,24], whereas ovulation-induction drugs used in IVF induce a suboptimal receptivity model.

A comparison of IVF and ovum donation cycles in patients with implantation failure undergoing co-culture of embryos with AEEC and transfer at the blastocyst stage compared to day-2 transfer, in terms of number of patients, number of cycles, number of previous failed cycles, age and infertility etiology is presented in Table 2.

In 80 oocyte donation cycles, 6.8 ± 0.2 embryos per cycle started co-culture, resulting in 61.2% blastocyst formation; 2.3 ± 0.1 blastocysts were transferred and 38 pregnancies were obtained (implantation and pregnancy rates being 32.7% and 54.3%, respectively). Eight miscarriages (21%), 18 ongoing pregnancies and 12 live births were recorded. Nine cycles were cancelled (12.5%), owing to embryonic development failure. In patients with implantation failure undergoing day-2 embryo transfer, implantation and pregnancy rates were significantly lower compared to those undergoing blastocyst transfer (4.5% and 13.3%, respectively)[25] ($p < 0.01$) (Table 3).

In 168 IVF cycles, 8.1 ± 0.3 embryos started co-culture, resulting in 49.2% blastocyst formation; 2.3 ± 0.1 blastocysts were transferred and 30 clinical pregnancies (20.2%) with an implantation rate of 11.9% were obtained. Six miscarriages (20%), one ectopic pregnancy (3.3%), eight ongoing pregnancies and 15 live births were recorded. Fifteen cycles were cancelled (9%),

Table 2 Comparison between *in vitro* fertilization (IVF) and ovum donation patients with implantation failure who had embryos co-cultured with autologous endometrial epithelial cells (AEEC) and who underwent blastocyst transfer and those who underwent routine day-2 transfer. Where applicable, values are mean ± SD

	IVF		*Ovum donation*	
	AEEC blastocyst transfer	*Day-2 transfer*	*AEEC blastocyst transfer*	*Day-2 transfer*
No. of patients	127	20	57	15
No. of cycles	168	20	80	15
No. of cycles transferred	153	20	70	15
Cancellation rate (%)	8.9	–	12.5	–
No. of previous failed cycles	3.8 ± 0.2	3.0 ± 0.0	3.0 ± 0.2	3.0 ± 0.0
Age (years)	33.7 ± 0.3	33.2 ± 2.8	39.1 ± 0.6	38.6 ± 5.2
Etiology of infertility (%)				
tubal factor	12.6	10	–	–
male factor	60.2	65	–	–
endometriosis	8.9	10	–	–
unknown cause	5.9	–	–	–
polycystic ovaries	7.9	10	–	–
low response	4.5	5	50	46.6
IVF failure	–	–	21.2	26.7
ovarian failure	–	–	28.8	26.7

Table 3 Reproductive outcomes in ovum donation patients with implantation failure who had embryos co-cultured with autologous endometrial epithelial cells (AEEC) and blastocyst transfer compared to routine day-2 transfer. Where applicable, values are mean ± SD

	AEEC blastocyst transfer	*Day-2 transfer*
Fertilization rate/patient (%)	80.9	77.9
Total no. of embryos	544	67
No. of day-2 embryos	6.8 ± 0.2	6.3 ± 0.4
Blastocysts on day 6 (%)	61.2	–
No. of blastocysts obtained	332	–
No. of blastocysts/embryos transferred*	2.3 ± 0.1	4.5 ± 0.9
Pregnancy rate (%)*	54.3	13.3
Implantation rate (%)*	32.7	4.5
Pregnancies	38	2
multiple	8 (21%)	1 (50%)
miscarriage	8 (21%)	–
ectopic	0	–
ongoing	18	–
live births	12	3

*$p < 0.05$

owing to embryonic development failure (Table 4). Patients with implantation failure undergoing IVF and day-2 embryo transfer had similar implantation and pregnancy rates (10.7% and 35%, respectively)[25] (Table 4).

Table 4 Reproductive outcome in *in vitro* fertilization patients with implantation failure who had embryos co-cultured with autologous endometrial epithelial cells (AEEC) and who underwent blastocyst transfer compared to those who underwent routine day-2 transfer. Where applicable, values are mean ± SD

	AEEC blastocyst transfer	*Day-2 transfer*
Fertilization rate/patient (%)	90.1	78.2
Total no. of embryos	1240	93
No. of day-2 embryos	8.1 ± 0.3	9.3 ± 0.4
Blastocysts on day 6 (%)	49.2	–
No. of blastocysts obtained	607	–
No. of blastocysts/embryos transferred*	2.3 ± 0.1	4.6 ± 0.9
Pregnancy rate (%)*	20.2	35.0
Implantation rate (%)*	11.9	10.7
Pregnancies	30	7
multiple	7 (23.3%)	1 (14.3%)
miscarriage	6 (20%)	2 (28.6%)
ectopic	1 (3.3%)	1 (14.3%)
ongoing	8	–
live births	15	5

*$p < 0.05$

We have achieved a clear improvement in implantation rates in ovum donation patients with implantation failure: 32.7% (optimal uterine receptivity/blastocyst) vs. 4.5% (optimal uterine receptivity/day-2 embryos). These differences were not obvious when patients with induction of ovulation were considered: 11.9% (suboptimal uterine receptivity/blastocyst) vs. 10.7% (suboptimal uterine receptivity/day-2 embryos). Data are not conclusive, but these figures suggest that, in patients with optimal uterine receptivity, the improvement of the embryonic factor makes an important difference, whereas when uterine receptivity is suboptimal, the amelioration of the embryonic factor makes almost no contribution to the implantation process.

CONTRIBUTION OF EMBRYONIC AND ENDOMETRIAL FACTORS TO THE OCCURRENCE OF EARLY PREGNANCY LOSS

For normal implantation to occur, it is necessary to have a morphologically and chromosomally normal embryo. On the other hand, a normal endometrium is also crucial and the interaction between the endometrium and the blastocyst is of great relevance[21,22,26]. It could be said that, in addition to endocrine regulation, complex intrauterine cellular communication mechanisms exist between the embryo and the endometrium to foster implantation.

To evaluate the embryonic and endometrial factors in the incidence of early pregnancy losses in IVF and oocyte donation cycles, we used a standardized microparticle enzyme immunoassay (MEIA) to measure urinary β-hCG in 145 patients undergoing IVF and 92 patients undergoing oocyte donation, in a prospective study[27]. Pregnancy loss before missed menses, which would generally go undetected, is referred to as early pregnancy loss.

The reproductive outcome of IVF was as follows: positive implantation was recorded in 60.7% (88/145) of cycles of embryo transfer. However, only 20.7% (30/145) of cycles resulted in viable pregnancies, and the remaining 58 miscarried. Early pregnancy loss accounted for 72.4% of these miscarriages. In oocyte donation, positive implantation was recorded in 69.6% (64/92) of cycles of embryo transfer. A total of 32.6% (30/92) achieved viable pregnancies, whereas the remaining 34 pregnancies ended in miscarriage, and early pregnancy loss accounted for 70.6% of pregnancy losses. The incidence of early pregnancy loss in IVF was 47.7%; in oocyte donation 37.5% showed β-hCG rises prior to menses[27] (Table 5).

This study shows that there is a high implantation rate in ART cycles. Comparing our results with published data on natural cycles[1,3,28–30] from studies that employed assays as sensitive as the one used in our study, we can conclude that implantation is significantly higher in ART (61–69%) than in natural conception cycles (29.2%), whereas the percentage of viable pregnancies is higher in natural cycles (59%) than in ART (34–47%). These results support the concept that appropriate endocrine and paracrine environments affecting the endometrium are necessary for successful implantation.

What these results indicate is that we are lacking a key element, which is the understanding and improvement of uterine receptivity in IVF patients. A pitfall resulting from embryological studies is the opinion that implantation is the result of good embryonic quality only. Although this is true and necessary, it is not the whole truth, because the endometrial factor is the real limiting factor, as demonstrated in these studies.

Table 5 Comparison of the outcome of natural cycles, *in vitro* fertilization (IVF) and oocyte donation

	Natural cycles		*IVF*		*Oocyte donation*	
	n	%	*n*	%	*n*	%
No. of total positive implantations/no. of embryos implanted	593/2033	29.2*	88/145	60.7	64/92	69.6
No. of viable pregnancies/no. of positive implantations	350/593	59.0*	30/88	34.1	30/64	46.9
No. of early pregnancy losses/no. of positive implantations	181/593	30.5†	42/88	47.7	24/64	37.5
No. of clinical abortions/no. of positive implantations	62/593	10.5	13/88	14.8	6/64	9.4

Natural cycle values were collected from references 1, 3, 28–30
*$p < 0.0001$ (vs. IVF and oocyte donation); †$p = 0.02$ (vs. IVF)

REFERENCES

1. Miller JF, Williamson E, Glue J, *et al.* Fetal losses after implantation. *Lancet* 1980; 2:554–6
2. Hertig AT, Rock J, Adams EC, *et al.* Thirty-four fertilized human ova, good, bad and indifferent, recovered from 210 women of known fertility: a study of biologic wastage in early human pregnancy. *Paediatrics* 1959;23:202–11
3. Wilcox AJ, Weinberg CR, O'Connor JF, *et al.* Incidence of early losses of pregnancy. *N Engl J Med* 1988;319:189–94
4. Society for Assisted Reproductive Technology, The American Society for Reproductive Medicine. Assisted reproductive technology in the United States: 1996 results generated from the American Society for Reproductive Medicine/Society for Assisted Reproductive Technology Registry. *Fertil Steril* 1999;71:798–807
5. Paulson RJ, Sauer MV, Lobo RA. Embryo implantation after human *in vitro* fertilization: importance of endometrial receptivity. *Fertil Steril* 1990;53:870–4
6. Garcia JE, Acosta AA, Hsiu JG, *et al.* Advanced endometrial maturation after ovulation induction with human menopausal gonadotrophin/human chorionic gonadotrophin for *in vitro* fertilization. *Fertil Steril* 1984;41:31–7
7. Bladford AJ, Najmabadi S, Paulson RJ. Ultrastructural characteristics of the luteal phase endometrium in donors undergoing controlled ovarian hyperstimulation. *Fertil Steril* 1997;67:625–30
8. Simón C, Mercader A, Frances A, *et al.* Hormonal regulation of serum and endometrial IL-1α, IL-1β and IL-1ra: IL-1 endometrial microenvironment of the human embryo at the apposition phase under physiological and supraphysiological steroid level conditions. *J Reprod Immunol* 1996;31:165–84
9. Fossum GT, Davidson A, Paulson RJ. Ovarian hyperstimulation inhibits embryo implantation in the mouse. *J In Vitro Fertil Embryo Transfer* 1989;6:7–10
10. Smith MG. On the interruption of pregnancy in the rat by injection of ovarian follicular extract. *Johns Hopkins Hosp Bull* 1926;39:203–14
11. Pellicer A, Ruiz A, Castellví RM, *et al.* Is the retrieval of high numbers of oocytes desirable in patients treated with gonadotrophin-releasing hormone analogues (GnRHa) and gonadotrophins? *Hum Reprod* 1989;4:536–40
12. Tarín JJ, Pellicer A. Consequences of high ovarian response to gonadotrophins: a cytogenetic analysis of unfertilized human oocytes. *Fertil Steril* 1990;54:665–70
13. Simón C, Cano F, Valbuena D, *et al.* Clinical evidences for a detrimental effect on uterine receptivity of high serum estradiol levels in high and normal responder patients. *Hum Reprod* 1995;10:2432–7
14. Pellicer A, Valbuena D, Cano F, *et al.* Lower implantation rates in high responders: evidence for an altered endocrine milieu during the preimplantation period. *Fertil Steril* 1996;65:1190–5
15. Testart J, Belaisch-Allart J, Forman R, *et al.* Influence of different stimulation treatments on oocyte characteristics and *in vitro* fertilizing ability. *Hum Reprod* 1989;4: 192–7
16. Toner J, Brzyski R, Oehninger S, *et al.* Combined impact of the number of preovulatory oocytes and cryopreservation on IVF outcome. *Hum Reprod* 1991;6:284–9
17. Chenette PE, Sauer MV, Paulson RJ. Very high serum estradiol levels are not detrimental to clinical outcome of *in vitro* fertilization. *Fertil Steril* 1990;54:858–63
18. Simón C, Garcia Velasco JJ, Valbuena D, *et al.* Increasing uterine receptivity by decreasing estradiol levels during the preimplantation period in high responders with the use of a follicle-stimulating hormone step-down regimen. *Fertil Steril* 1998;70:234–9

19. Tarín JJ, Sampaio MC, Calatayud C, *et al*. Relativity of the concept 'high responder to gonadotrophins'. *Hum Reprod* 1992;7:19–22
20. Fauser BCJM, Donderwinkel P, Schoot DC. The step-down principle in gonadotrophin treatment and the role of GnRH analogues. In JLH Evers, ed. *Baillière's Clinical Obstetrics and Gynaecology. Ovulation Induction: the Difficult Patient*. London: Baillière Tindal, 1993
21. De los Santos MJ, Mercader A, Frances A, *et al*. Role of endometrial factors in regulating secretion of components of the immunoreactive human embryonic interleukin-1 system during embryonic development. *Biol Reprod* 1996;54:563–74
22. Simón C, Gimeno MJ, Mercader A, *et al*. Embryonic regulation of integrins $\beta 3$, $\alpha 4$ and $\alpha 1$ in human endometrial epithelial cells *in vitro*. *J Clin Endocrinol Metab* 1997;82:2607–16
23. Remohí J, Gartner B, Gallardo E, *et al*. Pregnancy and birth rates after oocyte donation. *Fertil Steril* 1997;67:717–23
24. Navot D, Bergh P, Williams M, *et al*. An insight into early reproductive processes through the *in vivo* model of ovum donation. *J Clin Endocrinol Metab* 1991;72: 408–14
25. Simón C, Mercader A, Garcia-Velasco J, *et al*. Coculture of human embryos with autologous human endometrial epithelial cells in patients with implantation failure. *J Clin Endocrinol Metab* 1999;84:2638–46
26. Simón C, Moreno C, Remohí J, *et al*. Molecular interactions between embryo and uterus in the adhesion phase of human implantation. *Hum Reprod* 1998;13:101–14
27. Simón C, Landeras J, Zuzuarregui J, *et al*. Early embryonic losses in ART. *Fertil Steril* 1999;72:1061–5
28. Zinaman MJ, Clegg ED, Brown CC, *et al*. Estimates of human fertility and pregnancy loss. *Fertil Steril* 1996;65:503–9
29. Edmonds DK, Lindsay KS, Miller JF, *et al*. Early embryonic mortality in women. *Fertil Steril* 1982;38:447–53
30. Hakim RB, Gray RH, Zacur H. Infertility and early pregnancy loss. *Am J Obstet Gynecol* 1995;172:1510–17

19

Preimplantation assessment of human embryos from women of advanced age and patients with recurrent miscarriage

A. Pellicer, C. Rubio, A. Ruiz, J. Navarro, J. Remohí and C. Simón

THE EFFECTS OF AGE ON THE REPRODUCTIVE ORGANS

There is an evident decline in fecundity with age, clearly observed in populations in which contraception has not been employed[1]. In such circumstances, fecundity decreases and infertility increases with age, suggesting that the hypothalamus–pituitary axis, the uterus and/or the ovary are responsible for this impairment of fertility.

The endocrine profile of older women has not been completely characterized. The most consistent finding has been a subtle rise in serum levels of follicle stimulating hormone (FSH), which is not usually accompanied by a rise in luteinizing hormone (LH). Whether this monotropic FSH rise represents a primary neuroendocrine change or a response to changes in feedback signals from the aging ovary remains controversial. Recent studies suggest that a primary neuroendocrine change is associated with reproductive aging, which in turn may be responsible for the rise in serum FSH and changes in the menstrual pattern[2].

The aging of the uterus is also a controversial subject. Ovum donation is a good *in vivo* model to study, because many variables influence the final outcome of pregnancy, and the manipulation of the artificial cycle and selection of donors may help to standardize conditions in order to test appropriate hypotheses. Using this model, we performed a prospective study in which oocytes from the same cohort of follicles were randomly distributed between women of < 40 and of > 40 years undergoing ovum donation[3]. Pregnancy and implantation rates were similar between the groups. However, the rate of miscarriage was significantly increased in the group of recipients of > 40 years as compared to younger patients. From this study it could be inferred that waning oocyte quality, rather than reduced uterine receptivity, is responsible for the age-related decline in female fertility potential in natural and assisted reproduction cycles. However, some changes also occur at the uterine level; these result in turn in a decreased incidence of term pregnancies. We also tested the possibility that these changes were related to a restriction in the blood supply to the uterus in older women as compared to younger individuals. We performed a series of prospective studies employing color Doppler ultrasound to evaluate the uterine vascularization in both circumstances, and no difference was found between younger and older patients[4].

The ovary may be the major site of senescence within the reproductive axis. Besides a decrease with age in the population of follicles that can be stimulated[5], and the health of the follicles that can be recruited with drugs[6], there are substantial changes in the quality of the enclosed oocytes that are to be fertilized. Studies performed on unfertilized human oocytes showed a significant increase in chromosome abnormalities in women of > 35 years of age[7].

Similarly, Battaglia and colleagues[8] studied the influence of maternal age on the meiotic apparatus. Using high-resolution confocal microscopy they observed that the meiotic spindle in older women was frequently abnormal, showing up to 79% of aneuploid conditions as compared to 17% in younger patients.

In addition, recent studies employing fluorescence *in situ* hybridization (FISH) in human preimplantation embryos have shown that aneuploidy was more frequent in women of > 40 years than in younger patients[9], suggesting that the quality of the oocyte and the resulting embryo in women of > 40 years may be one of the factors involved in the decline of fecundity with age.

Moreover, Janny and Menezo[10] performed embryo cultures up to the blastocyst stage and showed that embryos derived from women of advanced age arrested at the morula stage to a higher degree than those derived from younger patients, suggesting again that the quality of the oocyte plays a crucial role in embryo development. They also showed a negative linear correlation between blastocyst expansion and patient's age[10]. Thus, when fertility in older patients is considered, the quality of the oocyte and the resulting embryo should be considered a priority.

PREIMPLANTATION DIAGNOSIS AS A TOOL TO INCREASE PREGNANCY RATES

Considering that chromosomal aberrations may represent the major cause of failed implantation in the older patient, it is conceivable that preimplantation diagnosis may be employed as a diagnostic tool to discard chromosomally abnormal embryos, thus increasing the percentage of normal embryos replaced, and enhancing pregnancy rates. This technique consists of the biopsy of one or two blastomeres from an eight-cell embryo and the analysis of its chromosomal status, and enables the selection of the chromosomally normal embryos that will be transferred back to the mother.

This concept was first tested by Gianaroli and co-workers[11,12], who treated patients with poor prognosis in *in vitro* fertilization (IVF), employing preimplantation diagnosis (PID). They were able to study 196 embryos from 36 women, of whom some carried a poor prognosis because of age[12]. They found 63% abnormal embryos in the age group, which was comparable to the percentage in women with repeated IVF failures (57%) or mosaic karyotype (62%). Initial reports of the outcome of embryo replacement were very enthusiastic[11], but reanalysis of the data with increased numbers showed that the pregnancy rate was not higher than 15% when preimplantation diagnosis was employed.

These studies have introduced new concepts in our efforts to improve implantation in IVF. However, they have failed so far to be considered as a practical alternative in patients with poor prognosis. Moreover, the lack of appropriate controls prevents the drawing of valid conclusions about the effect of age on the oocytes of these patients.

PREIMPLANTATION DIAGNOSIS IN OLDER PATIENTS AND WOMEN WITH REPEATED PREGNANCY LOSSES OF UNKNOWN ETIOLOGY

Recurrent spontaneous abortion is a distressing condition affecting up to 1% of couples in their reproductive years[13]. Despite the existence of well-defined causes of recurrent spontaneous abortion, almost 50% of the cases remain classified as of unknown etiology after appropriate infertility work-up[14–16]. The biological mechanisms involved in repetitive pregnancy losses remain obscure[17], and treatments are empirical in many circumstances, with no real improvement being noted in the total live-birth rates[18].

It is known that chromosomal abnormalities are implicated in first-trimester spontaneous abortions. In live births, chromosomal abnormalities occur at an incidence of 0.6%[19]; a ten-fold increase (6%) is present in still-births[20] and a 100-fold increase (60%) in spontaneous abortions[21].

Cytogenetic evaluations of spontaneous abortions, made directly from fetal tissue, have revealed an overall incidence of chromosomal abnormalities of 50–70%[22–25]. Analysis by chorionic villus sampling showed an even higher percentage of chromosomal abnormalities (83%), probably due to the elimination of misdiagnosis due to maternal cell contamination[26].

Based on the above evidence, our hypothesis was that chromosome abnormalities, arising *de novo* from random errors produced during gametogenesis and embryonic development, may be important etiological factors in patients with unexplained recurrent spontaneous abortions. Accordingly, we conducted a prospective study to assess the incidence of chromosomal abnormalities in preimplantation embryos of couples suffering from recurrent spontaneous abortions who were undergoing preimplantation diagnosis. Since we are familiar with the chromosomes more frequently disrupted in spontaneous abortions, the aim of our study was to estimate the incidence of aneuploidy for chromosomes 13, 16, 18, 21, 22, X and Y in preimplantation human embryos obtained from patients with recurrent spontaneous abortions. This screening would cover approximately 70% of the chromosome abnormalities detected in spontaneous abortions. The approach enabled us to learn about the etiology of this form of reproductive failure and to discuss whether IVF plus preimplantation diagnosis would be an appropriate treatment in such cases[27–29].

For preimplantation diagnosis, patients underwent an assisted reproduction cycle, and intracytoplasmic sperm injection (ICSI). Fertilization was assessed 17–20 h following microinjection and embryos were examined every 24 h. Embryo biopsies were performed early on the 3rd day after insemination at the eight-cell stage, allowing the removal of one or two blastomeres without detriment to the development of the embryo. After the biopsy, the embryos were cultured until the blastocyst stage, before being transferred back to the mother.

Blastomeres were analyzed initially by triple FISH using X, Y and 18 chromosome-specific probes. After signal elimination[29], nuclei were sequentially labelled using dual FISH with locus-specific probes for chromosomes 13 and 21 and then, in a third hybridization round, dual FISH with a centromeric probe for chromosome 16 and a locus bcr probe for chromosome 22. The percentages of abnormal embryos in each group were estimated as the number of affected embryos divided by the number of embryos analyzed, regardless of the probe employed.

In our earlier studies[27,28], a high incidence of abnormal embryos was found in couples suffering recurrent spontaneous abortions (16/33 and 29/50), but a control group was not included. These preliminary results were confirmed in a study conducted on nine couples with 3.9 ± 0.6 (range 3–6) previous spontaneous miscarriages in whom the possibility of studying chromosomal abnormalities in their embryos was offered[29]. We present the data collected so far in an ongoing study that involves three different groups of patients undergoing preimplantation diagnosis. The first group comprised women with recurrent spontaneous abortions ($n = 17$) who were < 36 years of age (mean 33.3 ± 0.5, range 30–35). A second group was made up of 18 women of the same age (mean 33.8 ± 0.6, range 30–36) who underwent preimplantation diagnosis because of a risk of transferring sex-linked diseases, primarily hemophilia and Duchenne's disease, who were considered reproductively normal for the purposes of this study. Another group of 12 patients was formed with the same characteristics of the former, except that the women were > 36 years old (mean 38.7 ± 1.8, range 37–41). This last (control) group was included because age has been identified as a major cause of embryonic abnormalities in IVF cycles[30].

A total of 135 embryos were biopsied in the study group, 119 of which were analyzed and 26 transferred in 17 IVF cycles. Four clinical pregnancies were achieved, resulting in an early miscarriage (46,XY) and the birth of three healthy babies. In the control group, 124 embryos were biopsied, and 104 finally analyzed. Forty embryos were replaced in 16 IVF cycles, resulting again in four clinical pregnancies, from which an early miscarriage and three normal pregnancies resulted. In the group of older patients, 74 embryos were biopsied and 66 analyzed by FISH. Twenty embryos were transferred in eight cycles; however, no pregnancies resulted.

The percentage of abnormal embryos was significantly ($p = 0.0001$) increased in patients with recurrent spontaneous abortions (68.1%) as compared to young controls (26.0%). The rate of chromosomal abnormalities in the control group was similar to that previously described when mosaics were excluded from a study group[30]. In our study, however, mosaicism was not studied because only one or two blastomeres were analyzed in most of the cases, since the embryos were used for replacement and not for research purposes. Numerical abnormalities for other chromosomes and other structural anomalies could also have escaped our screening. However, mosaicisms seem not to be frequent in the karyotypes of fetuses from women with recurrent spontaneous abortions[30]. Therefore, although this type of embryo screening is not totally comprehensive, we feel that it is sufficient to define causes of recurrent spontaneous abortion in some couples, and to select normal embryos for replacement.

Also, age was a parameter that significantly ($p = 0.0045$) increased the proportion of abnormal embryos (51.5%) as compared to embryos collected from young control patients. However, from the older patients and those with recurrent abortions, there was no difference in the percentage of normal and abnormal embryos identified by FISH (Table 1).

A detailed analysis of the chromosomal abnormalities in the three groups (Table 2) revealed a significant ($p = 0.027$) increase in the incidence of abnormalities in chromosomes 13, 16, 21 and 22 in the patients with recurrent

Table 1 Descriptive analysis of the patients and embryos entering the study

	Women with recurrent miscarriage (≤ 36 years)	*Control women* (≤ 36 years)	*Older women* (> 36 years)
No. of cycles	17	18	12
No. of biopsied embryos	135	124	74
No. of embryos analyzed	119	104	66
No. of embryos transferred	26	40	20
No. of abnormal embryos	81 (68.1%)^{a}	27 (26.0%)^{b}	34 (51.5%)^{c}
No. of normal embryos	38 (31.9%)	77 (74.0%)	32 (48.5%)
No. of transfers	12	16	8
No. of pregnancies	4 (33.3%)	4 (25.0%)	0
No. of miscarriages	1 (25.0%)	2 (50.0%)	0
Implantation rate	5/26 (19.2%)	5/40 (12.5%)	0

$^{ab}p < 0.0001$; $^{ac}p = 0.0282$; $^{bc}p = 0.0048$

Table 2 Descriptive analysis of the chromosomal abnormalities found in the embryos analyzed

	Women with recurrent miscarriage	*Control women*	*Older women*
No. of sex chromosome abnormalities/no. of embryos analyzed for this chromosome	13/104 (12.5%)	8/104 (7.7%)	7/58 (12.1%)
monosomy	8	4	5
trisomy	5	3	1
tetrasomy	0	1	1
No. of chromosome 13 abnormalities/no. of embryos analyzed for this chromosome	22/102 (21.6%)[a]	2/51 (3.9%)[b]	11/49 (22.4%)[c]
nullisomy 13	2	0	0
monosomy 13	14	2	7
trisomy 13	4	0	4
tetrasomy 13	2	0	0
No. of chromosome 16 abnormalities/no. of embryos analyzed for this chromosome	26/103 (25.2%)[d]	3/42 (7.1%)[e]	4/49 (8.2%)[f]
nullisomy 16	2	0	0
monosomy 16	18	2	2
trisomy 16	6	1	2
tetrasomy 16	0	0	0
No. of chromosome 18 abnormalities/no. of embryos analyzed for this chromosome	11/84 (13.1%)	5/104 (4.8%)	8/57 (14.0%)
nullisomy	2	0	0
monosomy 18	7	3	5
trisomy 18	2	1	3
tetrasomy 18	0	1	0
No. of chromosome 21 abnormalities/no. of embryos analyzed for this chromosome	29/116 (25.0%)[g]	5/54 (9.3%)[h]	13/50 (26.0%)[i]
nullisomy 21	1	0	0
monosomy 21	20	4	10
trisomy 21	7	1	3
tetrasomy 21	1	0	0
No. of chromosome 22 abnormalities/no. of embryos analyzed for this chromosome	21/99 (21.2%)[j]	2/44 (4.5%)[k]	6/36 (16.7%)[l]
nullisomy 22	1	0	0
monosomy 22	17	2	5
trisomy 22	1	0	1
tetrasomy 22	2	0	0

Table 2 *Continued*

Table 2 *Continued*

No. of haploid embryos/total no. of embryos analyzed	7/119 (5.9%)	2/104 (1.9%)	0
No. of triploid embryos/total no. of embryos analyzed	0	2/104 (1.9%)	2/66 (3.0%)
No. of tetraploid embryos/total no. of embryos analyzed	1/119 (0.8%)	4/104 (3.8%)	0

$^{ab}p = 0.0041$; $^{bc}p = 0.0071$; ^{ac}NS; $^{de}p = 0.0124$; ^{ef}NS; $^{df}p = 0.0157$; $^{gh}p = 0.0224$; $^{hi}p = 0.0366$; ^{gi}NS; $^{jk}p = 0.0128$; ^{kl}NS; ^{jl}NS

abortions and older patients as compared to controls. Interestingly, anomalies affecting chromosome 16 were found only in embryos of patients with recurrent spontaneous abortions. In embryos from these patients, autosomal monosomies were more frequent than trisomies. However, in the control group and older patients the incidence of autosomal monosomies and that of trisomies was comparable.

These findings support the hypothesis that in IVF the chromosomal status of embryos from couples with recurrent abortions is poorer than from patients not suffering recurrent abortions. This abnormality may explain some, but not all, cases of unexplained recurrent spontaneous abortion. In addition, the findings support the concept that age is associated with an increased incidence of abnormal embryos.

We are also analyzing the hypothesis that monosomic embryos may be eliminated during the implantation process, since we found a different ratio of monosomies versus trisomies in the groups established. In this sense, autosomal monosomies may impair embryo implantation ability, whereas a chromosomal excess (trisomies) may not affect implantation. In keeping with this concept, the role of chromosome 13 in recurrent spontaneous abortion should be further investigated because abnormalities in this chromosome were almost characteristic of this particular group of patients.

IS THERE AN INDICATION FOR ROUTINE PREIMPLANTATION DIAGNOSIS IN OLDER PATIENTS AND WOMEN WITH REPEATED MISCARRIAGE?

The data presented here confirm that aneuploidy for autosomes 13, 16, 18, 21, 22 and the sex chromosomes X and Y is higher in embryos obtained after IVF from patients with unexplained recurrent abortions than in normal controls. Age is also a factor influencing the chromosomal status of the embryo, as has been previously shown, employing the same technique of genetic analysis[9]. Furthermore, in our study the rate of aneuploidy for chromosome 16 was significantly increased in habitual aborters as compared to both controls and older patients. These findings corroborate the hypothesis that the chromosomal status of embryos from recurrent aborters is poorer than from other patients undergoing IVF, as we have previously reported[27–29]. Therefore, this could be a possible cause of unexplained recurrent abortion. However, it must also be emphasized that at least one patient miscarried despite the transfer of normal embryos (Table 1). Thus, numerical chromosome abnormalities cannot be regarded as the only possible explanation for reproductive failure in all couples with unknown causes of miscarriage. Nevertheless, we believe that these data clearly support the concept that preimplantation diagnosis should be indicated in couples with recurrent spontaneous abortions of unknown etiology as a treatment alternative.

The problem is more controversial concerning age. Gianaroli and colleagues[11,12] suggested the use of preimplantation diagnosis in couples with poor prognosis in IVF. Their data, however, showed a 15% pregnancy rate, which is far from being a positive result in assisted reproduction today. Our own data also show no pregnancies in any of the 12 patients analyzed in the older group (Table 1). These poor results clearly question the use of preimplantation diagnosis as a tool to increase implantation by selecting normal embryos in this population.

Moreover, the data obtained following routine IVF suggest that a selection against the implantation of abnormal embryos may be active in nature. Figures 1 and 2 have been retrospectively created from our IVF files of the past 5 years. The general process of ovarian stimulation and IVF techniques employed in our laboratories have been described elsewhere[29,31]. In Figure 1 we represent those patients who had a fixed number of embryos available for transfer. The characteristic of these data is that we were unable to select one or more embryos for transfer (usually the 'best looking' embryos), because patients had a restricted number of embryos available. Patients have been classified in several groups according to age, and the figure also takes into account the number of embryos replaced. As can be observed, women of < 36 years maintained a constant rate of embryonic implantation regardless of the number of embryos replaced. The same was true of the other two age groups, although there was a clear decrease in implantation rates as age advanced.

Figure 1 also shows miscarriage rates in the three groups of patients. Again, women of < 36 years had a constant rate of miscarriage despite the number of embryos transferred. The same was true for women aged 37–40 years. However, for patients aged 41–43, the percentage of miscarriages clearly increased as the number of embryos replaced was increased. This figure suggests that spontaneous abortion in these women was probably due to the quality of the embryos. In the groups of < 36 and 37–40 years, the proportion of abnormal embryos replaced must not have been too high and therefore the figure shows a constant percentage of miscarriage, women aged 37–40 having more abnormal embryos thus having more miscarriages. However, the figure also suggests that in the group of women of > 40 years the proportion of abnormal embryos must have been extremely high and, as a consequence, the more embryos transferred, the higher the abortion rates.

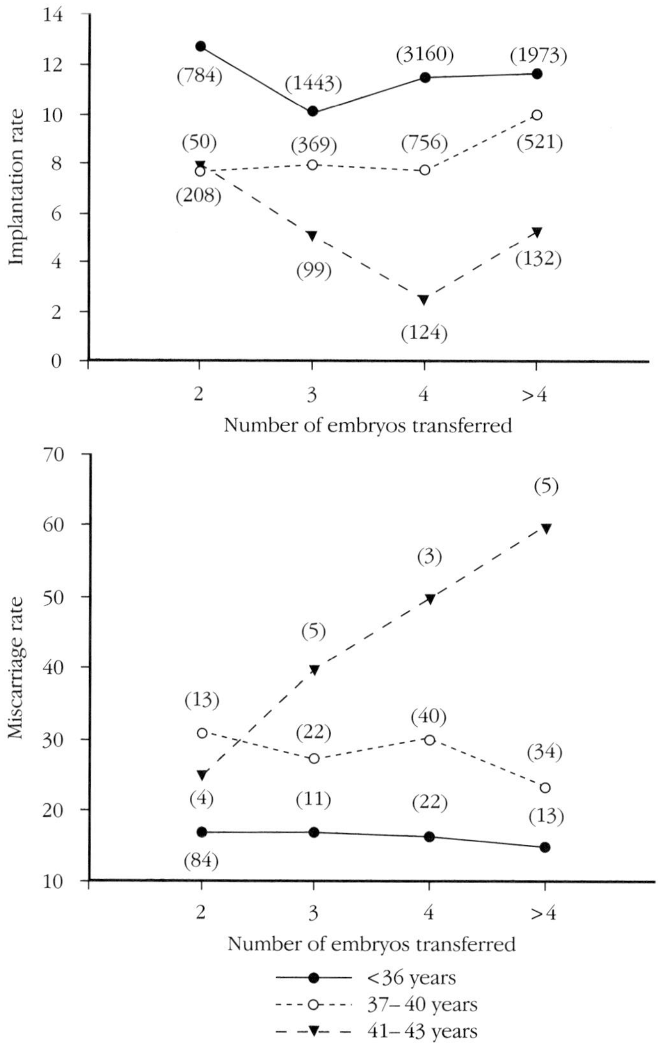

Figure 1 Implantation and miscarriage rates in IVF patients (classified by age) according to the number of embryos replaced in cases in which the selection of embryos for transfer was not possible (all embryos available were replaced). Numbers in parentheses represent embryos transferred in the upper panel and pregnancies in the lower panel

Figure 2 includes a different population of IVF patients. In this particular case, we have includes those cases in which the number of embryos available for transfer allowed us to select the 'best looking', while the remaining were cryopreserved. There is a clear difference from the patients in Figure 1. As a rule in our IVF laboratory, the faster cleaving embryos with fewer

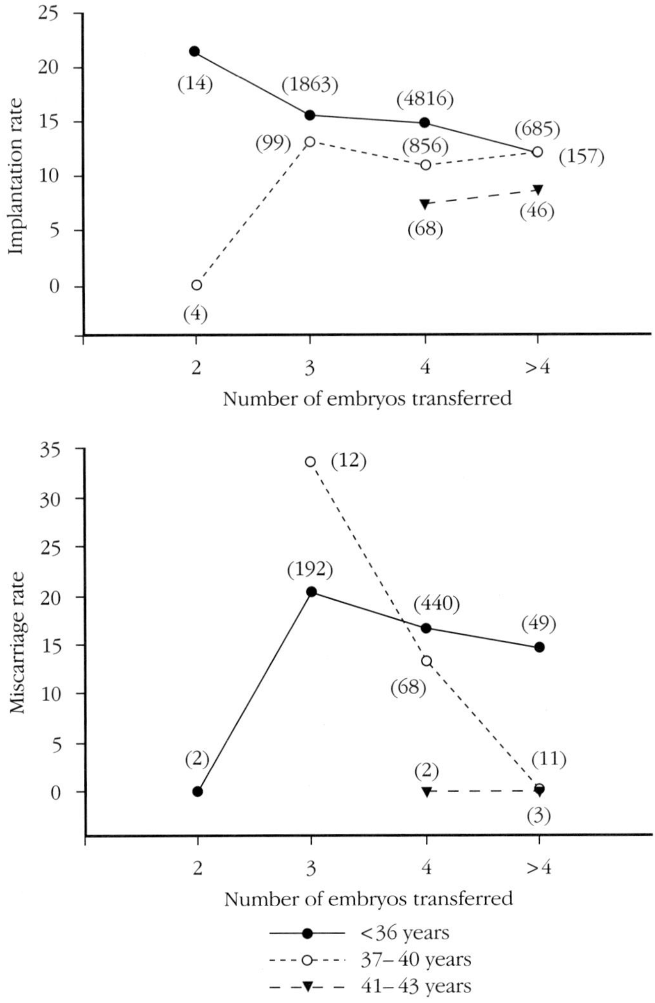

Figure 2 Implantation and miscarriage rates in IVF patients (classified by age) according to the number of embryos replaced in cases in which embryos were selected from a pool for replacement. Numbers in parentheses represent embryos transferred in the upper panel and pregnancies in the lower panel

fragments are usually selected for transfer, when possible. As a result, implantation rates in the upper panel in Figure 2 are higher than in Figure 1 in the three age groups. What is interesting is the bottom panel, in which miscarriage rates are represented. As can be observed, the selection of the embryos corrected the miscarriage rates in the two groups of advanced age, suggesting that nature may be playing a role in embryo selection *in vivo*, allowing the development of only normal embryos.

This hypothesis is very difficult to confirm but in practice we face two different situations in older patients. First, we have some women with a good response to gonadotropins in whom the number of embryos available for biopsy or selected transfer is high. In this case, biopsy may not be necessary, because if we choose the 'best looking' embryos for transfer, we may override the problem introduced by age. This has been shown in our data and was previously published by Widra and co-workers[32], who showed that the policy to increase delivery rates in IVF in older patients was to increase the number of embryos replaced.

The second, albeit more frequent, situation, is the older patient with a poor response to gonadotropins. In this case, the prognosis is poor regardless of the procedure employed. If we transfer the embryos, implantation is decreased and miscarriage increased, as our figures show. If we perform preimplantation diagnosis, the chances of having no embryos available for transfer are high, taking into consideration the low numbers, the probability of damage to the embryos during the diagnosis procedure and the final percentage of abnormal embryos. This was the case in our population, and was the experience of Gianaroli and colleagues[12].

CONCLUSIONS

The data presented show that chromosomal abnormalities are frequent in patients with a poor prognosis for having a normal delivery. In this case, we have carefully studied the embryos derived from women with recurrent spontaneous abortions and older patients employing preimplantation diagnosis, and compared them to embryos from young patients also undergoing IVF plus preimplantation diagnosis, mainly because of the possibility of inherited diseases. We have shown a significantly higher proportion of abnormalities in sex chromosomes and autosomes 13, 16, 21 and 22 in the first two groups of patients as compared to controls. Of particular interest is the fact that aneuploidy for chromosome 16 was only present in the group with recurrent spontaneous abortions. The data suggest that this may be a cause for recurrent miscarriage of unknown etiology, and therefore it is worth introducing preimplantation diagnosis as a treatment alternative in these cases.

We have also analyzed our experience with implantation and miscarriage in conventional IVF according to the number of embryos replaced and the age of the patient. We observed that implantation decreased with age, regardless of the possibility for selecting the 'best looking' embryos for transfer. However, when the embryos were not selected, miscarriage increased with age and also the rate of pregnancy loss correlated positively with the number of embryos replaced. In cases in which embryo selection was feasible, this dramatic increase in miscarriage was corrected, suggesting that nature has its own natural mechanism of selection. This fact, plus the lower rate of success of preimplantation diagnosis in cases of older patients, does not support the use of preimplantation diagnosis as a diagnostic tool to detect normal embryos for transfer in older women, as pregnancy rates are only theoretically increased.

REFERENCES

1. Menken J, Trussell J, Larsen U. Age and infertility. *Science* 1986;233:1389–94
2. Klein NA, Battaglia DE, Fujimoto VY, *et al*. Reproductive ageing: accelerated ovarian follicular development associated with a monotropic follicle-stimulating hormone rise in normal older women. *J Clin Endocrinol Metab* 1996;81:1038–45
3. Cano F, Simón C, Remohí J, Pellicer A. Effect of ageing on the female reproductive system: evidence for a role of uterine senescence in the decline in female fecundity. *Fertil Steril* 1995;64:584–9
4. Guanes PP, Remohí J, Gallardo E, *et al*. Age does not affect uterine resistance to vascular flow in patients undergoing oocyte donation. *Fertil Steril* 1996;66:265–70
5. Pellicer A, Marí M, De los Santos MJ, *et al*. Effects of ageing on the human ovary: the secretion of immunoreactive α-inhibin and progesterone. *Fertil Steril* 1994;61:663–8
6. Gougeon A, Ecochard R, Thalabard JC. Age-related changes of the population of human ovarian follicles: increase in the disappearance rate of non-growing and early-growing follicles in ageing women. *Biol Reprod* 1994;50:653–63
7. Plachot M, Veiga A, Montagut J, *et al*. Are clinical and biological IVF parameters correlated with chromosomal disorders in early life: a multicentric study. *Hum Reprod* 1988;3:627–35
8. Battaglia DE, Goodwin P, Klein NA, *et al*. Influence of maternal age on meiotic spindle assembly in oocytes from naturally cycling women. Hum Reprod 1996;11:2217–22
9. Munné S, Alikani M, Tomkin G, *et al*. Embryo morphology, developmental rates, and maternal age are correlated with chromosomal abnormalities. *Fertil Steril* 1995;64:382–91
10. Janny L, Menezo YJR. Maternal age effect on early human embryonic development and blastocyst formation. *Mol Reprod Dev* 1996;45:31–7
11. Gianaroli L, Magli MC, Ferraretti AP, *et al*. Preimplantation genetic diagnosis increases the implantation rate in human *in vitro* fertilization by avoiding the transfer of chromosomally abnormal embryos. *Fertil Steril* 1997;68:1128–31
12. Gianaroli L, Magli MC, Munné S, *et al*. Does preimplantation genetic diagnosis assist patients with a poor prognosis to achieve pregnancy? *Hum Reprod* 1997;12:1762–7
13. Stirrat GM. Recurrent miscarriage I: definition and epidemiology, causes and management. *Lancet* 1990;336:673–5
14. Tho P, Byrd JR, McDonough PG. Etiologies and subsequent reproductive performance of 100 couples with recurrent abortion. *Fertil Steril* 1979;32:389–95
15. Coulam C. Unexplained recurrent pregnancy loss. *Clin Obstet Gynecol* 1986;29: 999–1004
16. Clifford K, Rai R, Watson H, Regan L. An informative protocol for the investigation of recurrent miscarriage: preliminary experience of 500 consecutive cases. *Hum Reprod* 1994;9:1328–32
17. Tulppala M, Palosuo T, Ramsay T, *et al*. A prospective study of 63 couples with a story of recurrent spontaneous abortion: contributing factors and outcome of subsequent pregnancies. *Hum Reprod* 1993;8:764–70

18. Plouffe L, White EW, Tho SP, *et al*. Etiological factors of recurrent abortion and subsequent reproductive performance of couples: have we made any progress in the past 10 years? *Am J Obstet Gynecol* 1992;167:313–21
19. Nielsen J. Chromosome examination of newborn children. Purpose and ethical aspects. *Humangenetik* 1975;26:215–22
20. Machín GA, Crolla JA. Chromosome constitution of 500 infants dying during the perinatal period. *Humangenetik* 1974;23:183–8
21. Boué JG, Boué A. Chromosomal anomalies in early spontaneous abortion. Their consequences on early embryogenesis and *in vitro* growth of embryonic cells. *Curr Top Pathol* 1976;62:193–208
22. Boué J, Boué A, Lazar P. Retrospective and prospective epidemiological studies of 1500 karyotyped spontaneous human abortions. *Teratology* 1975;12:11
23. Hassold TJ, Matsuyama A, Newlands IM, *et al*. A cytogenetic study of abortions in Hawaii. *Ann Hum Genet* 1978;41:443–54
24. Plachot M. Chromosome analysis of spontaneous abortions after IVF. A European survey. *Hum Reprod* 1989;4:425–9
25. Eiben B, Bartels I, Bahr-Porch S, *et al*. Cytogenetic analysis of 750 spontaneous abortions with the direct preparation method of chorionic villi and its implications for studying genetic causes of pregnancy wastage. *Am J Hum Genet* 1990;47:656–63
26. Strom CM, Ginsberg N, Applebaum M, *et al*. Analysis of first-trimester spontaneous abortions by chorionic villus sampling and karyotype. *J Assist Reprod Genet* 1992;9: 458–61
27. Simón C, Rubio C, Vidal F, *et al*. Increased chromosome abnormalities in human preimplantation embryos after *in-vitro* fertilization in patients with recurrent miscarriage. *Reprod Fertil Dev* 1998;10:87–92
28. Vidal F, Giménez C, Rubio C, *et al*. FISH preimplantation diagnosis of chromosome aneuploidy in recurrent pregnancy wastage. *J Assist Reprod Genet* 1998;15:309–12
29. Pellicer A, Rubio C, Vidal F, *et al*. *In vitro* fertilization plus preimplantation genetic diagnosis in patients with recurrent miscarriage: an analysis of chromosome abnormalities in human preimplantation embryos. *Fertil Steril* 1999;71:1033–9
30. Daniely M, Aviram-Goldring A, Barkai G, *et al*. Detection of chromosomal aberrations in fetuses arising from recurrent spontaneous abortion by comparative genomic hybridization. *Hum Reprod* 1998;13:805–9
31. Pellicer A, Ruiz A, Castellví RM, *et al*. Is the retrieval of high numbers of oocytes desirable in patients treated with gonadotrophin-releasing hormone analogues (GnRHa) and gonadotrophins? *Hum Reprod* 1989;4:536–40
32. Widra E, Gindoff P, Smotrich D, *et al*. Achieving multiple-order embryo transfer identifies women over 40 years of age with improved *in vitro* fertilization outcome. *Fertil Steril* 1996;65:103–8

Index